# Concise Surgery

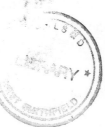

# Concise Surgery

## An Illustrated Guide

Edited by

### Kevin Lafferty MS, FRCS

Consultant Surgeon, Basildon and Thurrock General Hospitals NHS Trust,
Basildon, Essex, United Kingdom

### John Rennie MS, FRCS

Consultant Surgeon and Senior Lecturer,
King's College Medical and Dental School, London, United Kingdom

**ARNOLD**

A member of the Hodder Headline Group
LONDON • SYDNEY • AUCKLAND
Co-published in the USA by Oxford University Press, Inc., New York

First published in Great Britain 1998
Arnold, a member of the Hodder Headline group,
338 Euston Road, London NW1 3BH
**http://www.arnoldpublishers.com**

Co-published in the United States of America by
Oxford University Press, Inc.,
198 Madison Avenue, New York, NY10016
Oxford is a registered trademark of Oxford University Press

Whilst the advice and information in this book is believed to be true and
accurate at the date of going to press, neither the author[s] nor the publisher
can accept any legal responsibility or liability for any errors or omissions
that may be made. In particular (but without limiting the generality of the
preceding disclaimer) every effort has been made to check drug dosages;
however, it is still possible that errors have been missed. Furthermore,
dosage schedules are constantly being revised and new side-effects
recognized. For these reasons the reader is strongly urged to consult the
drug companies' printed instructions before administering any of the drugs
recommended in this book.

Publisher: Fiona Goodgame
Project Editor: Catherine Barnes
Production Editor:  Julie Delf
Production Controller:  Helen Whitehorn

12/7/99
M

British Library Cataloguing in Publication Data
A catalogue record for this book is available from the British Library

Library of Congress Cataloging-in-Publication Data
A catalog record for this book is available from the Library of Congress

ISBN 0 340 70611 2

1 2 3 4 5 6 7 8 9 10

Typeset in 10pt Sabon by Phoenix Photosetting, Chatham, Kent
Printed and bound by The Bath Press, Bath, Avon

# DEDICATION

To the memory of Leonard Cotton

# CONTENTS

# CONTRIBUTORS

**Brian Andrews  MS, FRCS**
Senior Surgical Registrar, King's Healthcare NHS Trust, King's College Hospital, London, United Kingdom

**Paul Baskerville  MA, DM, FRCS**
Consultant Vascular Surgeon & Clinical Director of Surgery, Vascular Surgical Unit, King's Healthcare NHS Trust, King's College Hospital, London, United Kingdom

**Irving S Benjamin  BSc, MD, FRCS(Glas), FRCS(Eng)**
Professor and Head of Surgery, Academic Department of Surgery, King's College Medical and Dental School, London, United Kingdom

**Matthew Button  MB BS**
Surgical Senior House Officer, Basildon and Thurrock General Hospitals NHS Trust, Basildon Hospital, Basildon, Essex, United Kingdom

**Michael D Catterall  FRCP, FRCP(Ed)**
Consultant Dermatologist, Basildon and Thurrock General Hospitals NHS Trust, Basildon Hospital, Basildon, Essex, United Kingdom

**C Richard G Cohen  MD, FRCS**
Resident Surgical Officer, St Mark's Hospital, Harrow, Middlesex, United Kingdom

**Dominic G Corry  MSc, FRCS**
Surgical Registrar, Southend Hospital, Southend, Essex, United Kingdom

**Mark Davenport  ChM, FRCS(Paeds), FRCS(Eng), FRCPS(Glas)**
Consultant Paediatric Surgeon, King's Healthcare NHS Trust, King's College Hospital, London, United Kingdom

**Jatin B Desai  FRCS(RCPSG), FRCS, C.Th(Edin), FRCS(Eng)**
Consultant Cardiothoracic Surgeon, King's College Medical and Dental School, London, United Kingdom

**David Gertner  BSc, MRCP**
Consultant Physician and Gastroenterologist, Basildon and Thurrock General Hospitals NHS Trust, Basildon Hospital, Basildon, Essex, United Kingdom

**Nigel D Heaton  MB BS, FRCS**
Consultant Liver Transplant Surgeon, King's Healthcare NHS Trust, King's College Hospital, London, United Kingdom

**Richard Jeffery  MB BS, FRCS**
Honorary Consultant Surgeon and Undergraduate Teaching Director, Basildon and Thurrock General Hospitals NHS Trust, Basildon Hospital, Basildon, Essex, United Kingdom

**Kevin Lafferty MS, FRCS**
Consultant Surgeon, Basildon and Thurrock General Hospitals NHS Trust, Basildon Hospital, Basildon, Essex, United Kingdom

**Andrew J M Leather MB BS, MS, FRCS**
Consultant General/Colorectal Surgeon, King's Healthcare NHS Trust, King's College Hospital, London, United Kingdom

**Ian P Linehan MS, FRCS**
Consultant General/Colorectal Surgeon, Basildon and Thurrock General Hospitals NHS Trust, Basildon Hospital, Basildon, Essex, United Kingdom

**D Mulvin**
Consultant in Urology, King's Healthcare NHS Trust , King's College Hospital, London, United Kingdom

**H G Naylor MB BS, FRCS**
Consultant Surgeon and Medical Director, Basildon and Thurrock General Hospitals NHS Trust, Basildon Hospital, Basildon, Essex, United Kingdom

**David R Osborne MS, FRCS**
Consultant Urologist, Basildon and Thurrock General Hospitals NHS Trust, Basildon Hospital, Basildon, Essex, United Kingdom

**Savvas Papagrigoriadis MD**
Lecturer in Surgery, Academic Department of Surgery, King's College Medical and Dental School, London, United Kingdom

**John Rennie MS, FRCS**
Consultant Surgeon and Senior Lecturer, King's College Medical and Dental School, London, United Kingdom

**Bernard F Ribeiro MB BS, FRCS**
Consultant General Surgeon with an interest in Gastroenterology, Basildon and Thurrock General Hospitals NHS Trust, Basildon Hospital, Basildon, Essex, United Kingdom

**Lindsey T A Rylah MBA, MB BS, FRCA**
Honorary Senior Lecturer at St Bartholomew's Hospital and the Royal London Hospital, London and Consultant Anaesthetist, Basildon and Thurrock General Hospitals NHS Trust, Basildon Hospital, Basildon, Essex, United Kingdom

**Roger J Sage MB BS, MRCP, FRCPath**
Consultant Medical Microbiologist, Basildon and Thurrock General Hospitals NHS Trust, Basildon Hospital, Basildon, Essex, United Kingdom

**Ann Scase MB BS, FRCA**
Specialist Registrar in Anaesthetics, The Royal London Hospital Trust, Whitechapel, London, United Kingdom

**Chris Taylor MB BS, MRCP**
Consultant Physician in GU/HIV Medicine, King's Healthcare NHS Trust, King's College Hospital, London, United Kingdom

**Simon Thomson  MB BS, FRCA**
Consultant in Anaesthesia and Pain Management, Basildon and Thurrock General Hospitals NHS Trust, Basildon Hospital, Basildon, Essex, United Kingdom

**Shay F Tinloi  MB BS(Lond), MRCP(UK), FRCA**
Consultant Anaesthetist, Basildon and Thurrock General Hospitals NHS Trust, Basildon Hospital, Basildon, Essex, United Kingdom

**Eric J Watts  DM, FRCP, FRCPath**
Consultant Haematologist, Basildon and Thurrock General Hospitals NHS Trust, Basildon Hospital, Basildon, Essex, United Kingdom

**Peter J Weller  FRCS(Edin), FDSRCPS(Glas)**
Consultant Maxillofacial Surgeon, Basildon and Thurrock General Hospitals NHS Trust, Basildon Hospital, Basildon, Essex, and Southend NHS Trust, Southend, Essex, United Kingdom

**Alan J Wilson  MSc, MD, FRCS**
Consultant Surgeon, Whittington Hospital, London, United Kingdom

# PREFACE

*Concise Surgery* is derived from *A Short Textbook of Surgery* which was the brainchild of Selwyn Taylor and Leonard Cotton and first appeared in 1967. The sixth edition was published after considerable revision in 1986 as *A New Short Textbook of Surgery*. It is a testament to the quality of the original authorship that the book was still in print over 25 years after inception.

In recent years, however, the undergraduate medical curriculum has changed and broadened to the point where tomes of beautifully written text (no matter how '*short*') would appear to be too time con-suming for hard-pressed students to assimilate. Computers, CD-ROMs, the Internet and a move to holistic teaching and learning methods make books seem rather outdated and 'ordinary'. Nevertheless, students continue to carry small books in their white coat pocket so perhaps this medium is not yet dead.

*Concise Surgery* was produced by collaboration between a district general hospital (Basildon) and a teaching hospital (King's College). This has hopefully resulted in a successful amalgam of everyday clin-ical experience and academic expertise. It aims to present basic general surgery in an acceptable and easily memorable form to the first year clinical student. The writing style is clipped and annotated in a manner which might mimic one's own handwritten notes. Wherever possible, illustrations, lists and line drawings are incorporated to eliminate large quantities of print. Most chapters are about 5000 words or less and so should not be too daunting. Any repetition of important topics or points in the text is entirely intentional.

Grateful thanks and appreciation are owed to the contributors, their staff, the photography depart-ments and students at Basildon and King's; and to Fiona Goodgame, Catherine Barnes and the Production team at Arnold.

KEVIN LAFFERTY
JOHN RENNIE

# chapter 1

# SURGERY:
# the basics

The speciality of surgery, in common with other branches of medicine, requires a working knowledge of pathology coupled with the clinical skills to apply this knowledge and treat patients. No doctor has ever failed to help a patient because he or she could not remember the minutiae of a particular topic; good basic medicine is the priority. The same applies to undergraduate examinations – it is basic knowledge, not minutiae, that is tested!

## CLINICAL SKILLS

All diagnoses are reached by:

1  Taking a history
2  Doing a clinical examination
3  Ordering special investigations.

> The order is very important because it is methodical, ensures that nothing is forgotten, and is what the Examiner wants to hear.

When taking a **history** it helps to have in mind a classification of disease such as:

● **Congenital**
Congenital – abnormality present from birth but not necessarily genetic
Inherited – genetic abnormality.

● **Acquired**
Trauma
Infection or inflammation
Neoplastic – benign or malignant: malignancy is primary or secondary

Collagen diseases
Autoimmune
Nutritional

Blood, blood vessels, the heart and circulation
Endocrine
Degenerative
Drugs.

Some diseases defy classification and are termed **idiopathic**, e.g. some psychiatric disorders.

The mnemonic TIN CAN BEDD is used commonly as an aid to memory.

The **clinical examination** must be orderly:

1 Observation
2 Palpation
3 Percussion
4 Auscultation.

Or alternatively, **Look, Feel, Tap, Listen.**

When reporting 'lumps and bumps' remember the rule of 'S's:

- **Site** – 'In the subcutaneous tissue overlying the left scapula...'
- **Size** – 'is a 5 × 5 cm...'
- **Surface** – 'smooth...'
- **Shape** – 'rounded lump...'
- **Special signs** – 'which is slightly fluctuant and is not attached to the skin. It is a lipoma.'
- **Nodes** – 'the left axilla is clear.'

It is especially important to **examine the loco-regional lymph nodes** – if they are not checked the examination is incomplete.

With **special investigations** keep it simple to start, e.g. test the urine for sugar or blood before ordering complex radiology.

## PATHOLOGY

Having reached a diagnosis using the clinical skills outlined above, it is necessary to understand and be able to discuss the pathology of the condition. This section highlights some basic elements of pathology which arise commonly in surgical practice and examinations.

### ACUTE INFLAMMATION – The response of living tissues to injury

There are five **local** effects caused by increased blood flow, migration of white cells and exudate formation (Figure 1.1):

1 Heat (calor)
2 Redness (rubor)
3 Pain (dolor)
4 Swelling (tumour)
5 Loss of function.

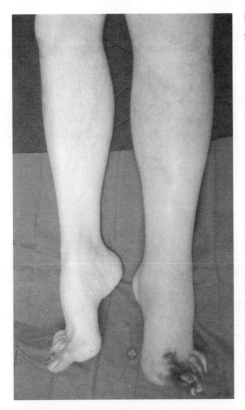

**Figure 1.1** Inflammation — cellulitis left leg secondary to gangrenous toes

Many surgical conditions need an understanding of acute inflammation and its results in order to appreciate the natural course of the disease and the possible complications – appendicitis and cholecystitis are good examples.

**Systemic** effects include fever, raised white count, high ESR, anaemia, lymphatic hyperplasia, pyaemia, septicaemia and toxicity.

The **outcome of acute inflammation** varies depending on severity and host response:

- Complete resolution – no residual effects
- Resolution with fibrosis – scarring
- Suppuration – abscess formation
- Gangrene – death of tissue in bulk
- Death – due to spreading infection or toxicity to vital organs, e.g. lungs, kidney, liver.

## WOUND HEALING

There are two recognized processes:

- Primary intention – no loss of tissue (surgical incisions) and rapid epithelial cover. There is minimal scarring.
- Secondary intention – loss of tissue with separated edges. Granulation tissue appears first, followed by slow epithelial cover. There is much scarring.

Wound healing is delayed by sepsis, dead tissue, foreign material, dirt and poor blood supply.

## HAEMORRHAGE

Haemorrhage may be **arterial** (pulsatile, bright red), **venous** (dark steady stream) or **capillary** (gentle ooze). It may be **revealed** (external), or **concealed** (into a body cavity). Haemorrhage is classified as:

- Primary – occurs at the time of injury or surgery
- Reactionary – occurs within 24 hours after primary haemorrhage and is caused by the rise in blood pressure following the hypotension produced by the original injury or anaesthesia, e.g. post-thyroidectomy bleeding
- Secondary – occurs usually about 7–10 days after injury and is caused by infection, e.g. post-haemorrhoidectomy.

## DISEASE CHARACTERIZATION

An individual disease or illness has certain characteristics which enable its identification. Once identified, a proven treatment can then be applied – **this is the essence of medical practice**. It follows that a system of characterizing disease is useful:

1 Incidence
2 Age
3 Sex
4 Geographical distribution
5 Predisposing factors
6 Macroscopic appearance
7 Microscopic appearance
8 Clinical features
9 Treatment
10 Prognosis.

Such a list is employed widely to recall the basic facts relating to any disease. Its use imparts confidence when speaking or writing in examinations and numerous amusing mnemonics are available. Employ it to determine knowledge of a particular condition.

## MALIGNANCY AND MALIGNANT SPREAD

Cancer is either primary or secondary to spread from elsewhere.

Cancer spreads in four ways:

1 Direct – directly into surrounding tissues
2 Blood – via the bloodstream
3 Lymph – via the lymphatics
4 Trans-coelomic – seeding throughout the pleura or peritoneum.

Many organs are only rarely affected with **primary** malignancy but are common sites for **secondary spread**, e.g. bone. This fact forms the basis of many a 'trick' examination question – for example, 'What is the most common malignant bone tumour?' is almost guaranteed to produce feeble mutterings about osteosarcoma, whereas the correct answer is 'secondary spread'.

## DEFINITIONS

Certain pathological conditions have precise definitions which are often quoted or asked for. Common ones are listed below.

| | |
|---|---|
| **Abscess** | collection of pus in a cavity lined by granulation tissue |
| **Adenocarcinoma** | malignant tumour of glandular epithelium |
| **Adenoma** | benign tumour of glandular epithelium |
| **Anaemia** | haemoglobin below normal for age and sex |
| **Aneurysm** | localized abnormal dilatation of an artery |
| **Carcinoma** | malignant tumour of epithelium |
| **Cyst** | abnormal cavity with well-defined lining |
| **Diverticulum** | a pouch arising from the wall of a viscus consisting of all layers (true diverticulum) or simply the mucosa (false diverticulum) |
| **Embolism** | transit within the bloodstream and impaction in some part of the vascular system of abnormal undissolved material |
| **Empyema** | collection of pus within a viscus or closed cavity, e.g. pleura, gall bladder |
| **Fistula** | abnormal communication or track between two epithelial surfaces |
| **Gangrene** | death of tissue in bulk. Can be dry (ischaemia) or wet (added putrefaction) |
| **Goitre** | enlargement of part or whole of the thyroid gland |
| **Hamartoma** | tumour containing a mixture of adult tissues normally present in the organ of origin |
| **Hernia** | abnormal protrusion of an organ through a defect in the wall of the cavity in which it lies |
| **Infarction** | an area of ischaemic necrosis caused by blockage to the blood supply |
| **Necrosis** | cell death |
| **Sarcoma** | malignant tumour of mesodermal connective tissue or its derivatives |
| **Sinus** | abnormal blind track in tissues that communicates with an epithelial surface |
| **Teratoma** | tumour containing tissue derived from all three germinal embryonic layers occurring at a site where these tissues are not normally found |
| **Thrombosis** | formation of a solid mass (thrombus) from the constituents of blood within the bloodstream during life |
| **Tumour** | an abnormal mass of tissue, the growth of which exceeds and is unco-ordinated with that of normal tissues, and which persists in the same excessive manner after cessation of the stimulus that evoked the change; a tumour can be benign or malignant |
| **Ulcer** | a localized loss of continuity of an epithelial surface (e.g. skin, intestine) |

# SURGICAL PRACTICE

Having reached a diagnosis using clinical skills and knowledge of pathology, it is necessary to consider whether surgery is indicated; are the risks and complications acceptable; and does the patient consent to undergo the procedure?

## INDICATIONS FOR SURGERY

All operations are potentially dangerous and may have unwanted side-effects or complications. Surgery, therefore, is indicated only when the potential risks are outweighed by the potential benefits. Indications for surgical treatment can be divided into:

- **Absolute** – situations or conditions in which surgery is the only available treatment option, e.g. life-threatening trauma or haemorrhage
- **Relative** – situations or conditions in which surgery (despite complications) has the potential to improve the quality of life, or reduce the risk of death, to a greater extent than other available treatment. The major part of surgery falls into this category.

Surgery is also used extensively for **diagnosis** (e.g. biopsy, laparoscopy) before instituting suitable treatment; and also as an **adjunct to medical therapy where this has failed or complications have arisen:**

**Q.** What are the indications for surgery in ulcerative colitis/Crohn's/peptic ulcer etc.?

**A.** Failure of medical treatment and/or complications.

## FITNESS FOR SURGERY

A patient must be physically capable of withstanding the trauma of any proposed surgical intervention and associated anaesthetic. In this context, pre-existing medical illness is an important consideration and individuals are routinely classified according to the American Society of Anesthesiology (ASA) criteria (Table 1.1).

Clearly, it is essential to review the ASA status of an individual patient and consider the magnitude of the proposed operation before deciding upon the suitability of surgical treatment, e.g. day surgery patients are usually ASA class 1 or 2.

## CLASSIFICATION OF OPERATION

From the patient's perspective, any operation is highly significant. However, operations are generally classified by surgeons and anaesthetists according to a **scale of magnitude** which relates broadly to the risks involved and the degree of physiological disturbance:

- Minor – e.g. skin lesions
- Intermediate – e.g. hernia repair

**Table 1.1** ASA classification

| Class | Condition of patient |
| --- | --- |
| Class 1 | Otherwise fit patient |
| Class 2 | Mild to moderate systemic disturbance, e.g. controlled diabetes; mild asthma; controlled hypertension |
| Class 3 | Severe systemic disturbance, e.g. limitation of activity from ischaemic heart disease; chronic airway limitation (CAL) |
| Class 4 | Severe, already life-threatening, systemic disorder, e.g. recent myocardial infarction; severe CAL |
| Class 5 | Moribund patient unlikely to survive |

- Major – e.g. cholecystectomy
- Complex major – e.g. colectomy and anastomosis
- Complex major plus – e.g. heart surgery.

Operations can also be classified by their degree of **urgency**:
- Emergency – immediate operation; resuscitation simultaneous with surgery; usually within 1 hour, e.g. leaking abdominal aortic aneurysm; severe trauma
- Urgent – delayed operation; as soon as possible after resuscitation; usually within 24 hours, e.g. peritonitis
- Scheduled – operation at time to suit both patient and surgeon, e.g. routine surgery.

Although the preceding stratification of patients and procedures seems perfunctory, such jargon is in everyday use and must be understood:

'I have a 50-year-old **ASA 3** male with peritonitis who needs an **urgent major** laparotomy.'

## COMPLICATIONS OF SURGERY

These can be classified as:
- Early – within 24 hours
- Intermediate – up to 3 weeks post-operative
- Late – any time thereafter, perhaps years.

Complications can be:
- Local – to do with the operation site itself
- General – affecting other systems of the body, e.g. cardiorespiratory.

This classification (see Table 1.2) can be used for any form of surgery, e.g. appendicectomy.

**Table 1.2** Complications of appendicectomy

|  | Local | General |
| --- | --- | --- |
| Early | Bleeding | Anaesthetic; cardiac<br>Urinary retention |
| Intermediate | Wound infection | Chest infection; DVT; PE |
| Late | Incisional hernia | Adhesions<br>Ugly scar<br>Faecal fistula |

Wound infection remains the most common post-operative complication of all operations (5–10%).

## INFORMED CONSENT

Patients must give their consent before submission to any form of medical or surgical treatment. Such consent may be implied, verbal or written, and in the past was given in the context of a paternalistic doctor/patient relationship, i.e. 'doctor knows best'. Informed consent has its origins in the 1950s and seeks to involve the patient with the complexities of choice of treatment and outcomes so that he/she can make an informed decision to proceed or not, i.e. 'self-determination'.

The doctrine of informed consent is a large and complex philosophical subject involving ethical and legal considerations which differ according to country and culture. Some important points are annotated.

### Ethical considerations
- Respect for the individual; autonomy; self-determination.
- Therapeutic privilege of the doctor to withhold information thought to be detrimental.
- Limited capacity of patient to comprehend.
- Engendering within the patient a positive attitude to illness or death.

### Legal considerations
- Patient has the legal right to give or withhold consent.
- Quality of consent, i.e. how much information needs to be given, and in what depth?
- Degree of disclosure of risks.
- Breach of medical duty to withhold information.

There are five basic prerequisites to be met before informed consent is considered valid:

1 Information – given at a suitable level and depth
2 Understanding – by the patient of the information

3 Willingness – to undergo the procedure
4 Competence – to give consent
5 Written or verbal authorization.

In surgical practice a patient should always be advised of the reasons for recommending a procedure and the risks involved. If this is not done, the patient may claim damages for subsequent complications or side-effects which, had they known of them, would have caused them to refuse surgery in the first place.

The vast majority of surgical complications fall into the categories of **bleeding, infection and thromboembolic disease** and it is good practice to include these in any preoperative consent. Other complications specific to the procedure should then be discussed and recorded. Although there is no absolute requirement for informed consent to be written, the signed **consent form** is standard practice and is often linked to an information sheet or booklet outlining the operation and its consequences.

## SCREENING FOR DISEASE

The screening of apparently healthy individuals for occult disease is well established in general medicine, obstetrics, gynaecology and neonatology. Screening for 'surgical' disease is a relatively recent concept. The criteria for effectively screening a population for a particular disease are:
- The disease must be common.
- It must pose a significant health problem.
- Its natural history and biological behaviour must be known.
- Effective treatment must be available.
- The screening test must have a high sensitivity and specificity (minimal false positive/negative rate).
- It must be cheap and easy to implement.
- The screening programme must be cost-effective.

A national mammographic breast cancer screening programme is already implemented. Other schemes for detection of colorectal cancer (faecal occult blood), aortic aneurysm (ultrasound scanning) and prostate cancer (PSA) have been suggested.

# chapter 2

# SHOCK:
# blood loss and replacement;
# abnormal clotting and bleeding

## SHOCK

Shock is a clinical syndrome caused by circulatory failure leading to tissue damage; if not recognized and corrected, it may rapidly lead to multi-organ failure and death.

The main features are **reduced systolic blood pressure** and **tissue hypoxia**. Other features will depend on the cause. The usual classification is:

1 **Hypovolaemic shock** – results from loss of fluid from the circulation, either directly (e.g. haemorrhage) or indirectly following fluid loss elsewhere (e.g. loss of plasma in burns; loss of water and electrolytes in diarrhoea; or internal, e.g. fluid shift into an inflammatory exudate in the peritoneum such as in pancreatitis).

2 **Cardiogenic shock** – occurs when venous return to the heart is adequate but cardiac output is reduced, i.e. the heart fails as a pump. Causes are myocardial infarction, acute massive pulmonary embolus, pericardial tamponade, severe dysrhythmias and, rarely, tension pneumothorax.

3 **Septic shock** – usually the result of a septicaemia with endotoxin-producing Gram-negative bacteria. The toxins cause vasodilatation of arterioles and capillaries and increase capillary permeability, i.e. make the capillaries more leaky, leading to loss of plasma from the vascular bed to the extravascular and interstitial spaces.

4 **Anaphylactic shock** – a severe and rare form of allergy, leading to release of inflammatory mediators causing vasodilatation and increased capillary permeability.

5 **Neurogenic shock** – a term for the acute circulatory collapse frequently associated with loss of consciousness that may occur following stimuli such as a sudden fright or severe pain. In mild forms this is referred to as a vasovagal attack or simple faint. It does not of itself cause the full syndrome of shock resulting in tissue damage, but it may complicate shock occurring from other causes. It is mediated by the autonomic nervous system and results in severe bradycardia and vasodilatation.

## CLINICAL FEATURES OF SHOCK

These will be determined partly by the cause but in general will result from **hypotension and reduced tissue perfusion** – this leads to organ failure and sets up a vicious circle with **hypoxia and acidosis**. Activation of complement and inflammatory mediators may occur along with increasing catecholamine release, causing vasoconstriction and further reducing tissue perfusion. The hypoxia reduces myocardial contractility, further exacerbating the problem (Figure 2.1).

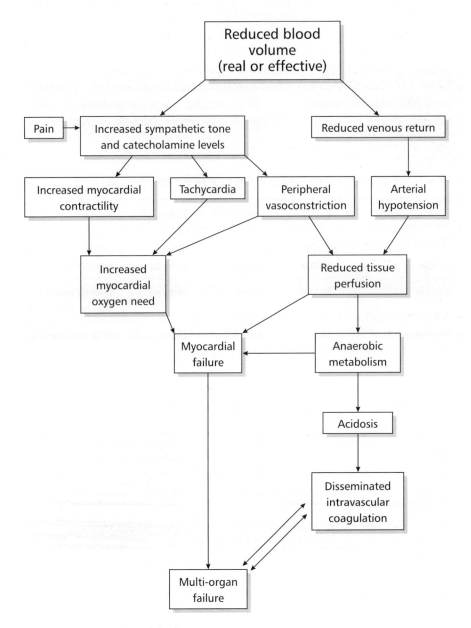

**Figure 2.1** Pathophysiology of shock

The circulatory response to hypotension is to conserve perfusion of the vital organs – the heart and brain – at the expense of other tissues. There is a progressive vasoconstriction of the skin, then splanchnic vessels, then renal vessels. If prolonged, renal cortical necrosis (acute tubular necrosis) occurs, causing acute renal failure.

### Hypovolaemic shock

In previously fit healthy young adults the systolic blood pressure (BP) may be maintained by peripheral vasoconstriction, despite appreciable blood loss (up to 2 litres). The diastolic BP may be temporarily increased because of the tachycardia. Such intense vasoconstriction cannot be maintained and hypotension eventually develops. Elderly patients or those with coronary artery disease may develop symptoms after losing 500 ml of blood; otherwise symptoms of weakness, tachypnoea and thirst tend to occur after loss of 1 litre. In severe hypovolaemia – blood loss greater than 2 litres or 40% – in addition to hypotension, typical features include skin pallor, tachycardia, confusion, tachypnoea, thirst, oliguria resulting from hypovolaemia and catecholamine effects. The physical signs depend on the amount of blood loss (Table 2.1).

**Table 2.1** Features of acute blood loss based on average adult blood volume of 5 litres

| Blood loss volume (ml) | 0–800 | 800–1500 | 1500–2000 | >2000 |
|---|---|---|---|---|
| Blood pressure | | | | |
| Systolic | Normal | Normal | Reduced | Severely reduced |
| Diastolic | Normal | Normal | Reduced | Severely reduced (may be unrecordable) |
| Pulse (beats/min) | Slight tachycardia | 100–200 | 120 (thready) | >120 (very thready) |
| Capillary refill | Normal | Slow >2 s | Slow >2 s | Undetectable |
| Respiratory rate | Normal | Normal | >20/min | >20/min |
| Urinary flow rate (ml/h) | >30 | 20–30 | 10–20 | 0–10 |
| Mental state | Alert | Anxious or aggressive | Anxious, aggressive or drowsy | Drowsy, confused or unconscious |

### Cardiogenic shock

This may give all the features of hypovolaemic shock with other features of heart failure, e.g. pulmonary oedema, severe dyspnoea, central cyanosis, sometimes pink frothy sputum, inspiratory crackles at the lung bases and a distinctive chest x-ray (bat's wing) appearance. If right heart failure is present there will be an elevated jugular venous pulse, often with hepatomegaly and peripheral oedema.

## Septic shock

The patient is usually febrile and may have had rigors. In contrast to hypovolaemia, the skin may be warm ('hot shock') because of the vasodilating effect of endotoxins. The other features will be similar to hypovolaemia.

## Anaphylactic shock

There will be recent exposure to an allergen such as a drug, seafood or a bee sting. There may be urticaria from histamine release and stridor from laryngeal oedema. Wheeze and facial oedema may also be present. There will also be severe hypotension due to vasodilatation which may lead to loss of consciousness.

## Neurogenic shock

The cause is usually obvious; the distinctive feature is bradycardia from vagal inhibition of the heart. Loss of sympathetic tone in the veins of the legs and splanchnic circulation lead to loss of consciousness with cold, clammy white skin.

## DIFFERENTIAL DIAGNOSIS

The clinical situation normally indicates the likely diagnosis – external haemorrhage or fluid loss will be obvious and a typical history of myocardial infarction may precede cardiogenic shock. Sudden pleuritic chest pain would suggest a pulmonary embolus. Anaphylactic and neurogenic shock occur instantly or within minutes of the stimulus.

If the cause is not apparent, a full clinical examination, paying particular regard to signs of heart failure or hidden internal bleeding, is necessary. **If doubt remains, the central venous pressure** must be measured. In hypovolaemia (or reduced effective blood volume) it will be low. In cardiogenic shock it will be high.

## TREATMENT OF SHOCK

Treatment is required immediately and the initial management decision is whether to give fluid resuscitation, which is life saving in hypovolaemia but may be fatal in cardiogenic shock.

## Hypovolaemic shock

Treatment consists of oxygen in high concentration by mask or nasal catheter and restoration of blood volume by intravenous fluids. **The fluid that has been lost must be replaced**, e.g. plasma for burns, crystalloid solution for diarrhoea and blood for haemorrhage. As time is required to prepare blood for transfusion, initial fluid replacement usually begins with normal saline. Up to 1 litre can be given as crystalloid run in as fast as possible. This will increase the intravascular compartment immediately but fluid will begin to move into the interstitial space. Next give a colloid solution such as albumin 4.5% or a gelatine solution which will stay within the vascular compartment for several hours. If more than 1.5 litres has been lost, then blood transfusion should be given and continued until normal blood volume is restored. **Fluid replacement can be accurately titrated using the central venous pressure.**

### Septic shock

Such patients usually need mechanical ventilation and treatment on an intensive care unit. The mainstay of therapy is appropriate antibiotics and attention to the source of sepsis. The blood pressure is maintained with saline and/or colloid, and inotropes if indicated.

### Cardiogenic shock

Treatment depends on the cause – for myocardial infarction, infusions of inotropes such as dopamine and dobutamine are given and occasionally other catecholamines. Dysrhythmias are treated as necessary. Pericardial tamponade and pneumothorax are treated by drainage and pulmonary embolus by anticoagulation with heparin or by thrombolysis.

### Anaphylactic shock

Give intravenous chlorpheniramine (antihistamine) and hydrocortisone immediately and repeat as necessary. Subcutaneous adrenaline may be necessary, followed by high-dose steroids if these measures are ineffective. Intravenous adrenaline can be given *in extremis* but may cause ventricular fibrillation.

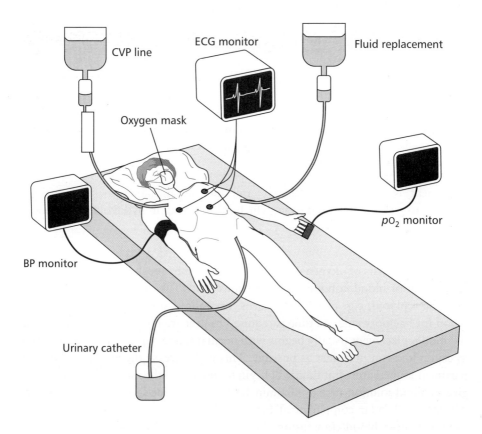

**Figure 2.2** Monitoring the shocked patient. BP, blood pressure; CVP, central venous pressure; ECG, electrocardiograph; $pO_2$, oxygen pressure

**Neurogenic shock**

In minor cases, it is only necessary to increase venous return to the heart by elevating the legs. In more severe cases, treatment is determined by the underlying cause. Potent analgesics may be required to relieve pain.

## GENERAL MEASURES

Once initial treatment is underway, intensive monitoring (Figure 2.2) is required, particularly pulse, blood pressure and oxygen saturation. Fluid replacement is most accurately judged by the central venous pressure. In severe cases, it is necessary to monitor renal output which requires bladder catheterization – adequate renal perfusion results in a urine output of >0.5 ml/kg/h. Oxygen by mask is always given and saturation of the blood can be measured by a pulse oximeter on an ear lobe or finger clip. **Saturation should be maintained above 90%; if it falls, intubation and mechanical ventilation may be required.** A haemoglobin of at least 8.0 g/dl is required and above 10.0 g/dl is preferred. Platelet count should be measured and a coagulation screen should be checked for evidence of disseminated intravascular coagulation (DIC). Arterial blood gas analysis may be required to monitor pulmonary function and acid–base balance.

## HAEMORRHAGE

Bleeding or haemorrhage can be the result of **local** or **general** causes or a combination of both. Local causes include lesions such as ulcers or tumours and injuries. General causes are normally deficiencies in blood clotting proteins. When bleeding is local, it may be **revealed** as from a lesion on the skin or a haematemesis, or **concealed** such as into the thigh in a fractured femur or into the peritoneum. It may be:

- Primary – occurring at the time of injury
- Reactionary – within 24 hours following a rise in blood pressure after cessation of the primary haemorrhage
- Secondary – usually 7–10 days after the initial event due to infection or ischaemia.

## TYPES

- Arterial – pulsatile and bright red from the proximal end of the vessel
- Venous – steady stream of dark blood from both ends of the vessel, easily controlled by local pressure
- Capillary – steady oozing, e.g. following dental extraction or abrasion.

## EFFECTS OF HAEMORRHAGE

**Acute severe haemorrhage**

Severe haemorrhage is defined as sufficient to reduce the blood pressure. After the initial vasoconstriction, fluid moves from the interstitial compartment into the bloodstream over 48 hours, causing a slow drop in haemoglobin – **the Hb is normal immediately after acute haemorrhage**. Once haemodilution has occurred **after an acute bleed the anaemia is normocytic and normochromic**; it is only after the iron stores are exhausted that the typical iron deficiency changes occur.

### Chronic haemorrhage

There are usually intermittent small bleeds rather than a steady continuous bleed which leads to depletion of the body's iron stores; when they are exhausted, further bleeding leads to iron deficiency anaemia. The blood count and film show the typical microcytic and hypochromic picture (Figure 2.3). In severe anaemia, fainting and blackouts may occur. Other symptoms include angina, exertional dyspnoea, claudication, ankle swelling and, rarely, a low fever. The clinical history may reveal bleeding, e.g. menorrhagia, haematemesis or melaena.

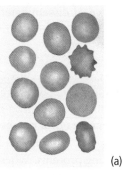
(a)

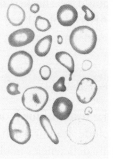
(b)

**Figure 2.3** (a) Normal and (b) iron-deficient blood film

## ESTIMATION OF BLOOD LOSS

The severity of acute blood loss is indicated by clinical assessment (Table 2.1). The pulse rate is the most sensitive guide and, although the blood pressure may be unchanged in the early stages in a recumbent patient, postural hypotension may be found in blood loss of around 1 litre.

For chronic haemorrhage the degree of anaemia is proportional to the blood loss. At operation, blood loss can be measured by weighing swabs and from measurement of blood aspirated from the operative field by the sucker. When large volumes of blood have been lost, central venous pressure monitoring is essential.

**Common causes of Fe deficiency**
- Peptic ulcers – gastric, duodenal
- Menorrhagia
- Carcinomas – colon, stomach, oesophagus
- Ulcerative colitis
- Gastritis (including drug-induced)
- Coeliac disease

**Possible causes**
- Hiatus hernia
- Diverticular disease
- Piles

## TREATMENT OF HAEMORRHAGE

### Local measures

These depend on circumstances and include suturing bleeding vessels, where they can be identified, and coagulation by diathermy. Pressure on a bleeding surface alone may stop the venous or capillary bleeding, e.g. a dressing and compression bandage over a cut on a limb or pack in a tooth socket. Epistaxis may require packing of the nasal cavity.

First aid measures for venous and capillary bleeding include lying the patient down and applying pressure. Cold packs may help by inducing vasospasm – the first aid acronym is ICE (I, immobilization; C, compression; E, elevation).

Fractured limbs should be immobilized to prevent further bleeding. At operation, hot packs may help promote coagulation by speeding the chemical processes of coagulation but the benefit may be outweighed by capillary and arteriolar vasodilatation. Vasoconstrictor substances can stop oozing from wounds, e.g. very dilute adrenaline solution applied directly. Gelatine foam and alginate can speed coagulation when applied to oozing wounds by providing a surface which activates coagulation factors.

Two specific vasoconstrictors can be given intravenously for local effects on relevant organs. Vasopressin may stop bleeding from oesophageal varices caused by portal hypertension through constriction of the splanchnic vessels but it can also increase the systemic blood pressure to a dangerous level and may cause a myocardial infarction in susceptible patients. Ergometrine contracts the uterus and can be given for post-partum and gynaecological bleeding.

### General measures

These consist of resuscitation with intravenous (i.v.) fluids and blood immediately it is available. Pain relief is given where necessary but if morphine is required, it should be given intravenously as peripheral vasoconstriction prevents absorption following intramuscular injection. When bleeding is due to haematological causes, specific blood component therapy is required.

## BLOOD TRANSFUSION

Blood transfusion is required when blood loss has been greater than 1.5–2 litres or when blood will be required for surgery. In normal circumstances, a patient's ABO blood group and rhesus type is identified and blood is cross-matched against the patient's serum or plasma. Blood of the same or compatible group is selected and cells from the donor unit are mixed with the patient's serum or plasma and examined for evidence of red cell agglutination or lysis. When taking samples and giving blood, identification of the patient and ensuring accurate documentation are vitally important; **86% of transfusion mishaps are the result of misidentification at the bedside.**

With modern techniques, a full cross-match (Figure 2.4) is usually complete within 1 hour and hospitals will have their own arrangements for issuing blood when required before this time – this is sometimes known as an **urgent** or **emergency** cross-match and will identify any antibody likely to lead to a major incompatibility. However, a shortened cross-match may not detect a weak antibody which could cause a delayed transfusion reaction. In rare, extremely urgent cases, uncross-matched blood, either of the patient's own group or, if it is not known, 'O Neg', may be given. In these cases, a sample for cross-match should be taken before the blood is given.

'O' rhesus negative blood should be used sparingly as only one in six donors are rhesus negative. If rhesus positive blood is given to a rhesus negative patient, then antibodies may be formed. If further rhesus positive blood is given, a transfusion reaction will result. If a woman with anti-rhesus antibodies carries a rhesus positive fetus, then rhesus haemolytic disease may affect the fetus, causing hydrops fetalis, kernicterus or death. **Therefore, rhesus positive blood should never be given to a rhesus negative woman of child-bearing age.**

Blood is collected from donors into an anticoagulant with additives such as saline, adenine, glucose and mannitol to preserve the red cells. In most cases, the plasma is separated and frozen instantly to be used later as fresh frozen plasma (FFP). Red cells are issued as concentrated or packed cells, one unit in a sterile plastic bag contains red cells from 450 ml of whole blood.

Whole blood is not normally used for transfusion because many components deteriorate on storage. Coagulation factors V and VIII have a half-life of between 6 and 12 hours only. When coagulation factors are necessary to correct bleeding, fresh frozen plasma is given. Refrigeration also slows the loss of potassium ions from the cell which can lead to hyperkalaemia with transfusions. Once removed from the body, blood platelets do not tolerate refrigeration and if platelets are required for transfusion, they are separated from the blood before it is refrigerated.

Although it is in theory attractive to use whole fresh blood for major haemorrhage, it is no longer feasible to supply it because of the potential for transmitting

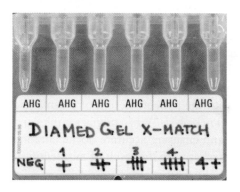

**Figure 2.4** Cross-match. From left (negative) no reaction between patient serum and donor cells through to right (4+) complete lysis of donor cells by patient's serum

infections. **Blood donors are questioned before donation regarding the risks of transmitting infections and blood is routinely screened for syphilis, HIV and hepatitis B and C.**

## COMPLICATIONS OF BLOOD TRANSFUSIONS

Serious complications are rare, provided procedures are followed properly. The most serious complication – a haemolytic transfusion reaction – occurs when the donor cells are lysed by antibodies in the patient's plasma. Usually, this occurs when A or B blood is given to an O patient. The symptoms include chest pain and breathlessness mimicking a myocardial infarction and loin pain may occur as red cell agglutinates are trapped in the renal glomeruli. The urine may be pink from haemoglobinuria. The same features can be caused by transfusion of infected blood.

> **Features of a severe haemolytic transfusion reaction**
> - Crushing chest pain
> - Shortness of breath
> - Loin pain
> - Anuria or pink urine

1 **Haemolytic transfusion reaction** is a medical emergency requiring oxygen, i.v. fluids and high-dose steroids. The unit of blood being transfused and a fresh sample taken from a distant site should be returned to the lab for re-cross-matching and a direct antiglobulin (Coombs') test to confirm the diagnosis. Disseminated intravascular coagulation may occur and generalized capillary bleeding at operation may be the first sign when an incompatible transfusion is given to an anaesthetized patient.
2 The most common complication of transfusions is a febrile, **non-haemolytic transfusion reaction**. This is normally due to antibodies against the patient's platelets, white cell or protein antigens and it is not possible to prevent these by cross-matching. Symptomatic measures such as paracetamol and cooling the patient may help but antihistamines and hydrocortisone may be necessary. This problem is particularly common in multiply transfused patients.
3 If the patient has a weak antibody which was not detected on cross-matching, a **delayed transfusion reaction** may occur. This results in immune destruction of the transfused red cells giving jaundice with a positive Coombs' test.

## ABNORMAL BLEEDING

The causes of abnormal bleeding include:
- Inherited deficiencies of coagulation factors
- Thrombocytopenia
- Acquired coagulation disorders
- Abnormalities of the vessel wall
- Drugs.

## INHERITED COAGULATION DEFICIENCIES

The commonest of these are:
- Haemophilia A – factor VIII coagulant protein deficiency
- Haemophilia B – factor IX deficiency
- von Willebrand's disease – a deficiency in the amount or composition of the high molecular weight von Willebrand factor multimers, which act as a carrier molecule for factor VIII.

Other factor deficiencies are rare. Severe deficiency presents as bleeding in early childhood and patients will be registered with their local Haemophilia Centre; however, milder abnormalities may only be diagnosed later. Treatment is replacement of the missing factor except for milder cases of haemophilia A and von Willebrand's disease where the low levels of factor VIII can be boosted by an infusion of desmopressin (DDAVP).

## THROMBOCYTOPENIA

Thrombocytopenia may cause bleeding, especially when the platelet count is less than $40 \times 10^9/l$. The cause is either increased destruction or decreased production, e.g. autoimmune, haematological disease (leukaemia, aplastic anaemia), drugs (cytotoxics). If autoimmune, steroids are the standard treatment but splenectomy is indicated in certain severe or recurrent cases.

## ACQUIRED COAGULATION DISORDERS

Apart from factor VIII, all coagulation factors are synthesized in the liver and therefore **liver disease may reduce their levels**. Factors II, VII, IX and X also require vitamin K for their synthesis. As vitamin K absorption may be reduced in obstructive jaundice, vitamin K injections may restore normal levels. Otherwise, as with hepatocellular problems, treatment is with fresh frozen plasma (FFP).

**Disseminated intravascular coagulation** (DIC) may complicate many serious illnesses. There is a generalized activation of coagulation causing fibrin strands and microthrombi to form – they are usually lysed in the circulation but may lodge in the renal or pulmonary circulation, causing further organ dysfunction. Coagulation factors and platelets are consumed in the process, leading to prolonged clotting times and thrombocytopenia. Elevated levels of fibrinogen degradation products (FDPs) and cross-linked fibrin degradation products (XDPs) help to confirm the diagnosis but they may also be elevated after thrombosis or an operation.

## ABNORMALITIES OF VESSEL WALL

Vessel wall abnormalities include rare connective tissue diseases, immune vasculitis and scurvy. In the case of Henoch–Schonlein (H–S) purpura, a purpuric rash due to allergic vasculitis may occur at the same time as abdominal pain due to vasculitis affecting the bowel wall; it usually resolves spontaneously.

## DRUGS

Anticoagulant drugs such as heparin and warfarin may cause bleeding, especially when the appropriate clotting times (APTT for heparin, INR for warfarin) are over the therapeutic range. Continuous monitoring of anticoagulant therapy is essential.

Anti-inflammatory drugs such as aspirin may cause bleeding by reducing platelet function and through gastric irritation.

## ABNORMAL CLOTTING

The causes of thrombosis are still best classified exactly as they were by Virchow in the nineteenth century – abnormalities in the vessel wall; the state of flow; and alterations in the blood. Stasis and alterations in the blood are more important in venous thrombosis and changes in the vessel wall, e.g. atheroma, are more important in arterial thrombosis.

### THROMBOPHILIA

Natural anticoagulant proteins (**protein S, protein C, and antithrombin III**) inactivate activated clotting factors, particularly factors V and VIII. Inherited deficiency of natural anticoagulant proteins is found in around 20% of cases of spontaneous venous thrombosis in patients under 40 years of age. These are sometimes known as the thrombophilias and may be responsible for cases of premature thrombosis – especially when it occurs in an unusual site such as the mesenteric vessels.

An inherited **abnormal factor V (factor V Leiden)** has also been discovered – the mutated form does not bind to protein C and therefore cannot be inactivated. At present it appears to be involved in 25% of cases of unprovoked thrombosis in young patients.

The long-term treatment of these patients depends on the frequency and severity of thrombosis – some patients require lifelong treatment with warfarin – less seriously affected patients only require prophylaxis to cover high risk situations, e.g. surgery and childbirth. Subcutaneous heparin is effective for most cases requiring prophylaxis but for more severe cases who would normally be taking warfarin, long-term i.v. heparin is necessary if the patient is nil by mouth.

## CRIB BOX – SHOCK: BLOOD LOSS AND REPLACEMENT; ABNORMAL CLOTTING AND BLEEDING

**A definition of shock** – a clinical syndrome resulting from reduced effective circulating blood volume; characterized by low blood pressure and decreased tissue perfusion leading to tissue hypoxia, acidosis and death. Types are:

- Hypovolaemic
- Cardiogenic
- Septic
- Anaphylactic
- Neurogenic

### Haemorrhage

- **Local** – injury; ulcer; tumour
- **General** – clotting disorder

- **Revealed** – superficial injury, etc., blood is seen
- **Concealed** – hidden in body cavity, gut or fracture

- **Primary** – at time of injury or surgery
- **Reactionary** – within 24 hours following restoration of blood pressure
- **Secondary** – within 7–10 days; sepsis, inflammation, ischaemia

### Blood transfusion

- Three complications – haemolytic transfusion reaction; non-haemolytic transfusion reaction; delayed transfusion reaction

### Abnormal bleeding

- Inherited coagulation deficiency – haemophilia A, B; von Willebrand's
- Thrombocytopenia – autoimmune; haematological disease; toxic drugs
- Acquired coagulation disorder – liver disease; DIC
- Vessel wall abnormalities – collagen disorders; vasculitis; scurvy; H–S purpura
- Drugs – anticoagulants; asprin; NSAIDS

### Abnormal clotting

- Virchow's triad – vessel wall; blood; blood flow
- Thrombophilia – deficient protein S, C, antithrombin III; factor V Leiden

# chapter 3

# FLUID BALANCE AND NUTRITION

An understanding of fluid and nutritional requirements in health and disease is of vital importance in the management of the patient on the surgical ward. An adequate plasma volume, water and electrolyte distribution provides the correct environment for cell function, while nutrition provides the substrates and the source of energy to keep the body healthy.

## FLUID BALANCE

### FLUID DISTRIBUTION

In the normal healthy male adult, about 60% of the body weight is water. This water is distributed through two main compartments:
- Intracellular (ICF) – this lies inside the cells of the body
- Extracellular (ECF) – this lies outside the cells.

The ECF is itself subdivided further:
- Intravascular (plasma)
- Interstitial.

A diagrammatic representation in a hypothetical 70 kg man is shown in Figure 3.1.

An adult female has relatively more fat than the adult male and thus has slightly less body water (55% body weight) whilst a baby has relatively more water (75% in a newborn).

Some water is present in the abdominal cavity, lumen of the gastrointestinal tract and pleural cavity. This normally represents only a small amount. However, in some disease states (such as pancreatitis, ileus) a significant proportion of the body water may be sequestrated in these spaces and therefore lead to marked loss from the other compartments – particularly the ECF.

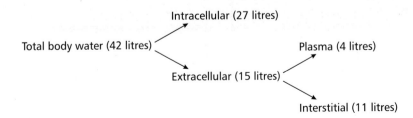

**Figure 3.1** Fluid compartments in 70 kg man

## FLUID COMPOSITION

In health, the volumes and composition of the compartments are kept remarkably constant although there is vast interchange of water and electrolytes between the intravascular compartment and the interstitial compartment (across the capillary membrane) and between the interstitial compartment and the ICF (across the cell membrane). The distribution of the main cations and albumin in the various compartments is summarized in Figure 3.2.

The total volumes are kept constant by a fine balance between intake of fluid and excretion. The relative volumes and composition are kept constant by the forces acting across the boundaries of the fluid compartments. It is the interchange across these boundaries that facilitates the transfer of oxygen and nutrients from the bloodstream to the cells and the transfer of the products of metabolism (e.g. $H^+$, $CO_2$, and urea) from the cells to the bloodstream and eventual excretion by the lungs and kidneys.

An understanding of the forces that cause the water and electrolyte shifts between the compartments is essential to enable the correct fluid management of a patient.

### Interchange across the capillary membrane

The capillary membrane is a selectively permeable membrane. It allows free passage of small molecules (water and electrolytes) and thus allows quick equilibration according to concentration and electrical gradients. However, it is almost

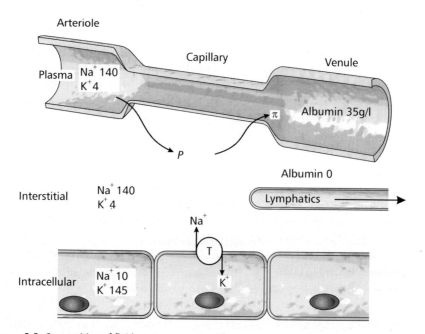

**Figure 3.2** Composition of fluid compartments and forces across cell membranes: $P$, hydrostatic pressure; $\pi$, colloid osmotic pressure; T, active transport pump

impermeable to large molecules such as albumin (molecular weight 69 000) and other proteins.

In the blood, hydrostatic pressure ($P$) forces water and electrolytes out of the capillary and this is opposed by the colloid osmotic pressure ($\pi$) (Figure 3.2). The colloid osmotic pressure is due to the large molecules which cannot diffuse out of the capillary. In a normal person, albumin is responsible for approximately 80% of the colloid osmotic pressure.

At the arterial end of the capillary, hydrostatic pressure is greater than colloid osmotic pressure, so that there is a movement of water, electrolytes and other small molecules out into the interstitial space.

At the venous end there is a net inward force because the colloid osmotic pressure is greater than the hydrostatic pressure. This draws water, electrolytes and small molecules back into the capillary.

The net result is a transfer of a small amount of fluid into the interstitial space but this is absorbed by the lymphatics so that the relative volumes of the two compartments remain constant.

In disease, however, this may not be so – as in **cardiac failure** when the net hydrostatic pressure is raised, or in **conditions where the capillary membrane becomes permeable to albumin**, or in hypoalbuminaemia.

### Interchange across the cell membrane

The cell membrane is also a selectively permeable membrane. It is freely permeable to water but not to sodium or potassium ions. An active transport pump (T, Figure 3.2) exists which pumps sodium ions into the interstitial compartment and potassium ions into the cell.

Water moves between ECF and ICF according to the osmotic gradient generated by the difference between the ECF and the ICF osmolality. A decrease in the concentration of electrolytes in the ECF will therefore lead to a shift of water from ECF to ICF. Conversely, an increase in concentration of electrolytes in the ECF will shift water from ICF to ECF. As sodium is the main ECF cation, it is largely responsible for ECF osmolality and thus the ECF volume.

### Significance

- A colloid such as albumin or gelatin given intravenously will stay in the intravascular compartment for hours until the colloid is metabolized or excreted. This type of solution is ideal for restoring the circulating intravascular volume.
- An electrolyte solution (e.g. normal saline) which has a similar osmolality to plasma will distribute itself readily through the ECF. This solution can be used in cases where there has been significant loss from the ECF, such as in bowel obstruction or vomiting.
- A non-electrolyte solution, such as 5% dextrose, once the dextrose is metabolized, is essentially water, and will distribute itself throughout the body water. This solution is useful if there have been losses from the ICF as well as the ECF, e.g. as in dehydration.

## NORMAL FLUID BALANCE

### Water balance

The average water balance for a 70 kg man is as shown in Table 3.1.

If the oral intake of fluid is excessive, the kidneys will increase the urinary excretion so that the balance is maintained.

If the intake has been too little, the kidneys retain water, and urinary excretion is reduced. At the same time the thirst mechanism is stimulated to increase oral fluid intake – so that the fluid balance is again maintained.

If the losses are such that even maximal reabsorption by the kidneys cannot maintain the balance, and the person is deprived of fluid (as is possible in hospitals), he will become progressively more fluid depleted. Organ perfusion will be impaired, and there is also a very real danger of acute renal failure developing.

**Table 3.1** Water balance in 70 kg man

| Daily intake | | Daily output | |
|---|---|---|---|
| Drink | 1500 ml | Lungs | 400 ml |
| Food | 750 ml | Sweating | 600 ml |
| Metabolic | 250 ml | Faeces | 100 ml |
| | | Urine | 1400 ml |
| Total | 2500 ml | | 2500 ml |

An adequate urine output (>0.5 ml/kg/h) is an indication of an adequate fluid intake.

### Electrolyte balance

The daily electrolyte balance is also finely regulated, and the healthy person can cope with a wide range of sodium and potassium intake.

The average daily requirement of sodium is about 100 mmol/day and potassium about 80 mmol/day.

The kidneys are especially efficient at conserving sodium, particularly in times of surgery and trauma (stress response to trauma). However, a low intake of sodium in the face of continued losses may lead to a contraction in the ECF compartment with resultant poor organ perfusion. A consistently high sodium intake, on the other hand, may lead to an expansion of the ECF volume (if the kidneys cannot cope) and this may precipitate heart failure.

Potassium is essentially an intracellular ion, so the body has to be markedly depleted in potassium before the plasma becomes hypokalaemic. As it is a sudden change in plasma potassium that is clinically important, in the initial stages of fluid and electrolyte therapy it is not necessary to administer potassium supplements. If, however, plasma potassium concentration starts to fall or if there are large potassium losses, potassium supplements are indicated.

## FLUID PREPARATIONS AVAILABLE

The approximate compositions of some commonly used fluids are given in Table 3.2. Only the concentrations of the important ions are shown. The colloid molecular weight, where appropriate, is also given.

**Table 3.2** Approximate composition of important ions in commonly used fluids

|  | Electrolyte content (mmol/litre) | Molecular weight |
| --- | --- | --- |
| **COLLOIDS** | | |
| Albumin 4.5% | $Na^+$ – 150 | 69 000 |
| Dextran 70 | $Na^+$ – 150 | 70 000 |
| Gelatin | $Na^+$ – 150 | 35 000 |
| Starch | $Na^+$ – 150 | 200 000–400 000 |
| **CRYSTALLOIDS** | | |
| 0.9% NaCl | $Na^+$ – 150; $Cl^-$ – 150 | |
| Ringer's lactate | $Na^+$ – 130; $K^+$ – 5; Lactate – 30 | |
| 0.18% NaCl/4% dextrose | $Na^+$ – 30; $Cl^-$ – 30 | |
| 5% Dextrose | Nil | |

### Colloids

These fluids are used for restoring circulating volume (either whilst awaiting availability of blood for transfusion or if there has been plasma loss). They have to be administered with care, particularly in the patient with cardiac disease, as they rapidly increase the circulating volume.

**Albumin** Albumin is, theoretically, the colloid of choice, as it is the naturally occurring colloid. Albumin is the main agent responsible for colloid osmotic pressure. It also has a wide number of functions in the body. However, in practice, it has significant disadvantages:

- Expense
- Significant advantage over other colloids not clinically proven.

**Dextrans** The dextrans are high molecular weight dextrose polymers. They are little used nowadays in view of their potential for allergic reactions and interference with the clotting mechanism.

**Gelatins** These solutions are produced by the hydrolysis of bovine collagen, the different preparations available differing in their average particle size and therefore their half-life in the intravascular space. They are less allergenic than dextrans and have a long shelf-life. Haemaccel and Gelofusine are very commonly used plasma expanders.

**Starch solutions** These solutions contain molecules of high molecular weight, several times that of albumin. The starch molecules are similar to glycogen and are metabolized by endogenous amylase, and the small fragments are readily excreted by the kidneys.

They have a prolonged half-life in the circulation (some up to 24 hours) and, because of the very low incidence of allergic reactions, are, arguably, better plasma expanders than the gelatins. They are, however, more expensive.

### Crystalloid solutions
These fluids are used to restore extracellular and intracellular fluid volume.

**0.9% NaCl** – 0.9% NaCl ('normal saline') is a commonly used solution to restore ECF volume. It has a higher concentration of sodium (150 mmol/l) than plasma so care has to be taken not to overload the patient with sodium. As previously explained, this may lead to an expansion of the ECF with its potential risk of inducing a fluid overload.

**Ringer's lactate** – Ringer's lactate (Hartmann's solution) has no advantage over 0.9% NaCl. Moreover, it contains lactate ions. This is potentially dangerous in any patient who is at risk of developing lactic acidosis (such as diabetic patients or any patient with poor tissue perfusion). In view of this, indications for using Hartmann's solution rather than 0.9% NaCl are minimal.

**0.18% NaCl/4%** – dextrose 0.18% NaCl and 4% dextrose ('dextrose saline') distributes itself in all compartments and is useful in situations where there is depletion of all the fluid compartments. It has a low sodium content (30 mmol/l). The clinician has to ensure that the total sodium intake is adequate if this solution is prescribed on its own – as in the post-bowel surgery patient, where the sodium loss may be high.

**5% Dextrose** – This solution is used not because it provides calories, but in situations where there is fluid loss from both the ECF and the ICF (e.g. excessive sweating and hyperventilation). It is often used in combination with 0.9% NaCl in a fluid regimen that provides both enough sodium and water.

## PRESCRIBING FLUID REGIMENS

Prescribing a fluid regimen is a clinical task that must be undertaken with the utmost care, particularly in the very sick patient or the patient who has had major surgery:
- Too little fluid and the patient risks developing dehydration and acute renal failure
- Too much and the patient becomes overloaded
- The wrong type of fluid, and the fluid ends up in the wrong compartment.

The factors that must be considered are:
- The pre-existing fluid status of the patient
- The normal requirements of the patient
- The nature of continuing excessive losses
- The pre-existing medical condition of the patient.

## Pre-existing fluid status

The surgical patient often presents with signs of dehydration due to a number of factors (e.g. inadequate intake, excessive sweating, vomiting, diarrhoea, intestinal obstruction). Such patients require fluid resuscitation. It is important to exclude and treat bleeding as the cause of the fluid loss with the appropriate blood and blood product therapy (see Chapter 2). An estimate of the amount and type of deficit can be made from the history, examination, investigation and occasionally invasive monitoring.

Features of dehydration are:
- Thirst
- Obtunded mental state
- Dry tongue
- Loss of skin turgor
- Low central venous pressure (jugular venous pressure, JVP)
- Poor urine output (<0.5 ml/kg/h)
- Raised haematocrit and urea.

Such a patient needs vigorous fluid resuscitation (**at least 10 ml/kg**) in addition to maintenance therapy. The type of fluid is dependent on the assessment of the nature of the loss. If this is primarily from the ECF (e.g. vomiting, ileus, diarrhoea, peritonitis) the replacement fluid should be normal saline. If there are also losses from the ICF (e.g. reduced intake, excessive sweating) solutions such as 5% dextrose are needed in addition.

If the patient presents with gross dehydration in shock (cold and clammy, hypotension and fast thready pulse) and particularly if there has been intravascular albumin loss due to inflammation (e.g. acute pancreatitis), the solution of choice is, initially, a colloid in order to rapidly restore the intravascular volume. Once the shock state has been treated, attention can then be turned to replacing the fluid losses from the other compartments.

In any patient where the fluid resuscitation does not produce the expected clinical improvement and a return of an adequate urine output, central venous pressure (CVP) measurement using a CVP line should be considered (Figure 3.3).

Using a centrally placed venous line, the pressure in a central (close to the right atrium) vein can be measured. As this pressure reflects the filling pressure of the right atrium, the adequacy of the venous return and hence the volume status of the patient can be inferred. A normal CVP is 5–10 cmH$_2$O as measured from the level of the heart, with the patient supine (Figure 3.4).

### Normal maintenance

This has been discussed previously. For an adult, a fluid volume of 2500 ml/day containing about 100 mmol of sodium should be sufficient to meet most normal needs. Examples of a daily regimen that provides the above are:

- 1000 ml of normal saline and 1500 ml of 5% dextrose (2500 ml and 150 mmol Na)
- 2500 ml of 0.18% NaCl and 4% dextrose (2500 ml and 75 mmol Na).

For the paediatric patient, the fluid given is usually 0.18% NaCl and 4% dextrose. The maintenance calculations are as given in Table 3.3, the maximum volume prescribed being as in an adult.

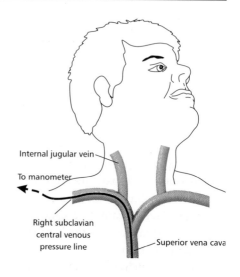

**Figure 3.3** CVP line placement

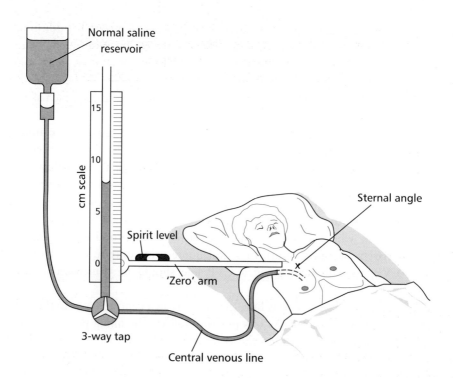

**Figure 3.4** CVP measurement

**Table 3.3** Paediatric maintenance fluid

| Weight (kg) | ml/kg/h |
|---|---|
| 0–10 | 4 |
| 10–20 | 2 |
| > 20 | 1 |

Example: a 25 kg child needs
$4 \times 10 + 2 \times 10 + 1 \times 5 = 65$ ml/h of fluid

## Continuing losses

The surgical patient often loses extra fluid and electrolytes depending on: nature of surgical condition, trauma of operation, vomiting, intestinal ileus, excessive sweating. So the prescribed regimen may have to be modified to take into account the above.

- A typical daily regimen is 1000 ml normal saline and 2000 ml 5% dextrose – this provides 3000 ml of water and 150 mmol of sodium per day. Potassium supplements are indicated if there are clinically suspected large losses or if hypokalaemia develops. An initial daily supplement of 80 mmol potassium can be added to the regimen.
- The actual fluid and electrolyte requirement has to be modified according to the extent of the estimated losses, the clinical response and the results of laboratory monitoring of haematocrit and electrolytes. CVP measurement may be required.
- Continuing blood loss should be treated by blood, blood product or colloid replacement according to the estimated loss.

## Pre-existing medical conditions

The previously medically fit patient can cope with a fairly wide range of prescribed intravenous fluid volume and electrolytes – by virtue of a compliant circulation, healthy cardiac muscle and efficient kidneys. The patient with significant pre-existing medical conditions has, however, to be treated with the utmost caution. Any excess or deficiency of water or electrolytes may lead to a worsening of the underlying condition.

**Cardiac disease** The patient cannot cope with too much sodium or fluid as the increase in circulating volume can induce cardiac failure. Care should be exercised with the volume and amount of sodium prescribed.

**Liver disease** The patient with severe liver disease has a poor glycogen store, is intolerant of sodium (despite a low plasma sodium value), and may become encephalopathic if dehydrated. 5% Dextrose is usually the appropriate fluid. Sufficient sodium is often present in the drugs the patient is already taking.

**Chronic renal disease** The patient with chronic renal disease tends to be acidotic and to retain potassium. Such a patient can be overloaded very easily with water but, on the other hand, hypovolaemia can very quickly cause a further deterioration of renal function.

## MONITORING OF FLUID THERAPY

In the majority of patients on intravenous fluid therapy, careful clinical observations together with simple laboratory tests are sufficient to establish the effectiveness of the prescribed therapy.

The features the clinician should monitor regularly are:
- Signs of dehydration
- Signs of possible fluid overload, e.g. raised JVP, crepitations at lung bases
- Fluid balance – input and output balance – allowing for insensible and other (e.g. ileus) losses
- An adequate urine output (>0.5 ml/kg/h)
- Normal daily electrolyte estimation.

It is only in the severely ill or unstable patient that more invasive monitoring (e.g. CVP monitoring, cardiac filling pressure and cardiac output estimations) is required.

# NUTRITION

## EFFECTS OF STARVATION

The stress response to trauma and surgery consists of a neuroendocrine response leading to increased production of pituitary hormones, insulin, and increased sympathetic activity. This results in increased catabolic activity:
- Hyperglycaemia
- Increase in whole body protein turnover
- Fat breakdown.

The surgical patient is not only at risk because of a reduced food intake, but also because of the extra demand caused by the stress response. If the supply of carbohydrates, protein and fat is not maintained, the patient can rapidly develop the features of starvation, notably:
- Depletion of glycogen stores
- Muscle weakness
- Respiratory complications
- Tendency to infections.

Patients who are prone to develop these complications are those who have pre-existing malnutrition, and those who are very sick (e.g. the septic patient). It is important, therefore, to identify the at-risk group so that the appropriate nutritional treatment is instituted as early as possible.

## NUTRITIONAL ASSESSMENT

Many sophisticated methods have been described to identify the malnourished patient. On the surgical ward, simple clinical indicators are usually sufficient:

- Inadequate intake, excessive loss or demand (as in septic patient)
- Body weight: >10% unintentional weight loss
- Muscle wasting and weakness
- Albumin <35 g/l.

The severity of the malnutrition is indicated by the severity of the above features.

## NUTRITIONAL CONTENT

Nutritional planning and the method by which the feed is administered is usually done in conjunction with the hospital nutrition team. Regardless of the method of administration, the contents of the food should include:

- A source of energy
- A source of nitrogen
- Water and electrolytes
- Vitamins and trace elements.

### Energy

The energy requirements for a normal person are of the order of 1500–2000 kcal/day. If the patient is in a rapid phase of fat and protein breakdown (so-called hypercatabolic phase), as in the very sick, up to 4000 kcal/day may be required (Table 3.4). This energy is supplied as a combination of carbohydrates (e.g. glucose) and fats (including the essential fatty acids).

### Nitrogen

The normal person requires about 9 g of nitrogen per day, and if the patient is hypercatabolic, the requirements may be as much as 25 g nitrogen per day. It is important to note that each gram of nitrogen needs at least 120 kcal of energy for assimilation in the body. This nitrogen may be provided as protein or peptides in enteral feeding or as amino acids in parenteral feeding.

### Water and electrolytes

The provision of water and electrolytes has to be in accordance with the principles of fluid and electrolyte balance as described in the earlier part of this chapter.

**Table 3.4** Energy and nitrogen requirements in the malnourished

|  | Normal | Mildly catabolic | Hypercatabolic |
|---|---|---|---|
| Energy (kcal/day) | 2000 | 3000 | 4000 |
| Nitrogen (g/day) | 9 | 14 | 25 |
| 1 g Nitrogen = 6.25 g protein | | | |

In a patient who is parenterally fed, the volume of fluid (including drugs) that the patient is already receiving often limits the amount of feed the patient can receive.

### Vitamins and trace elements

These have to be included in small amounts as they are vital for the various enzymatic reactions in the cells of the body. Examples of trace elements are manganese, zinc, cobalt.

## METHODS OF ADMINISTRATION

### Enteral feeding

Whenever possible, enteral feeding should be used rather than parenteral feeding – because of the potential complications of parenteral feeding. Enteral feeding depends on the functional integrity of the lower part of the intestinal tract. Examples of methods of enteral feeding are:

- By mouth
- By nasogastric tube
- By nasojejunal tube
- By feeding jejunostomy tube.

The type and consistency of the food is determined by the clinical state of the patient and the method chosen. The patient should be considered for enteral feeding as early as is practicable.

Some malnourished patients, such as those who have an oesophageal stricture or similar problem, may need a feeding jejunostomy for pre- and post-operative nutrition.

### Parenteral feeding

This is intravenous feeding using a specially designed cannula. This method is used only if enteral feeding is not possible, e.g.:

- Inflammatory bowel disease
- Loss of small bowel
- Non-functioning bowel, e.g. long-standing ileus
- Severe cachexia
- Hypercatabolic states.

Parenteral feeding should be started if the patient cannot be fed by the enteral route, and is likely to become grossly malnourished by the time the enteral route becomes available.

Traditional **total parenteral nutrition** (**TPN**) has to be given via a centrally placed feeding line because of the high concentration of dextrose in the feed and the high osmolality of the solution which causes severe thrombophlebitis if given into a peripheral vein. TPN via the central route is extremely dangerous in view of the large number of potential complications:

- Related to insertion of central line
- Infection

- Hyperglycaemia
- Electrolyte disturbances
- Fluid overload.

Newer methods use a feed which contains less dextrose and relatively more lipids to provide the same number of calories. This solution can be infused into a peripheral vein via a special intravenous feeding catheter. So far the results are very promising and may lead to traditional TPN via the central route being used in only very few patients.

### Monitoring

The patient who is enterally or, especially, parenterally fed has to be monitored carefully. The patient needs:

- A fluid balance chart
- Regular blood sugar estimations
- Daily urea and electrolytes.

If the patient is hypercatabolic and is on TPN, a daily estimate of the nitrogen balance is helpful to determine whether the feed given is sufficient. Nitrogen is lost mainly as urea in the urine, and hence an estimation of the urea loss in a 24-hour urine collection can be used to determine the nitrogen loss. A correction has to be made for other small urinary nitrogen loss and any change in blood urea.

---

**CRIB BOX – FLUID BALANCE AND NUTRITION**

**Fluid replacement**

The prescribed fluid should take account of:

- Pre-existing fluid status
- Normal maintenance requirement
- Continuing losses
- Pre-existing medical condition

Learn the daily fluid and electrolyte requirements AND a prescribing regimen

**Nutrition**

Patients should be adequately fed to reduce morbidity

- Feeding should be started as early as possible
- Enteral feeding is the method of choice
- Parenteral feeding should be considered if enteral feeding is not possible

Learn the daily nutritional requirements

# chapter 4

# PAIN MANAGEMENT

There are obvious ethical and humanitarian reasons for treating pain, be it acute or chronic. However, studies have shown that the majority of patients complain of either moderate (53%) or severe (41%) pain after surgery.

**Post-operative pain impairs mobilization and breathing, prolongs in-patient stay, and increases the incidence of deep vein thrombosis and chest infection.** Poorly managed chronic pain results in financial crisis for the individual and is a major drain on social security and health agencies. In the United Kingdom, chronic back pain alone causes annually an estimated 60 million days lost to industry at a cost of £3.8 billion. Unremitting pain is sadly a common feature of terminal disease.

## WHAT IS PAIN?

Pain is defined as 'an unpleasant sensory and emotional experience associated with actual or potential tissue damage, or described in terms of such damage'.

The perception of pain relates to three factors (Figure 4.1):

1 Physical
2 Psychological
3 Behavioural.

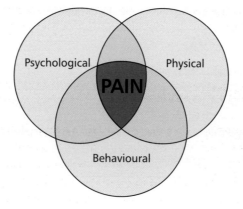

Figure 4.1

These three factors vary in importance between patients and circumstances; for example, in pain following a planned inguinal herniorrhaphy the most important factor is physical, but in pain resulting from cancer, psychological factors may have a greater role. In patients with chronic back pain, behavioural and psychological factors may be the most important. These factors together produce the concept of 'total pain'.

## THE NEUROPHYSIOLOGICAL BASIS OF PAIN

There is no single pathway responsible for the perception of pain because the nervous system is not a 'hard-wired' system of circuits; changes that occur in chronic pain show that it is a plastic system. Release of peptides in the spinal cord in response to injury can result in long-term changes in the way in which information is processed. The receptive field of individual nociceptors in the dorsal horn may expand after repeated stimulation ('wind-up'). Central sensitization of the nervous system explains how pain can continue even after the precipitating injury has healed (e.g. phantom limb pain). Damaged nerve membranes may behave abnormally, developing continuous activity resulting in an increasing receptive field and loss of normal inhibitory mechanisms.

Perception of pain is modulated at every level of the nervous system, either enhancing or inhibiting the final sensation. In the dorsal horns transmission to higher centres is modulated by a **gating system**, depending on the relative activities of C fibres and A-beta fibres which can act to close the 'gate' and inhibit pain transmission. Impulses that reach the dorsal horn are modulated by descending inhibition and facilitation from the higher centres, which can also influence the gating mechanism. Further extensive modulation then occurs in the brain, with the frontal cortex playing a major role in the final integrated motor response.

This integrated system results in **perceived pain being a function of the whole nervous system**, including complex emotional and behavioural responses.

As pain is not one simple pathway with one-way traffic, it is hardly surprising that simple single treatments often fail and that a multimodal treatment schedule is often required.

## MEASUREMENT OF PAIN

Since pain is a subjective experience, its measurement is fraught with difficulties. The most frequently used method of pain intensity scoring is the 10 cm visual analogue scale (VAS) (Figure 4.2). The patient is asked to mark a point on the line which best defines his/her pain. Many patients find linear visualization of their pain a difficult concept and although results are not always reliable, a VAS is simple and quick.

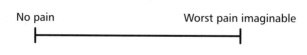

**Figure 4.2** Visual analogue scale (VAS)

Another simple method of measurement is the verbal rating scale (Figure 4.3). It is often better to measure pain both at rest and after a standardized movement, for example coughing.

Pain measurement in paediatric practice depends upon the child's development. In pre-verbalizing children an observational physiological and behavioural assessment is used (e.g. the Children's Hospital of Eastern Ontario Pain Scale, CHEOPS). A graduated pain scale which uses a series of faces ranging from smiling to crying (Figure 4.4) is used commonly to give some measure of suffering and children as young as 5 years have been taught to use visual analogue scales.

No pain        Mild pain        Moderate pain        Severe pain        Incapacitating pain

**Figure 4.3** Verbal rating scale

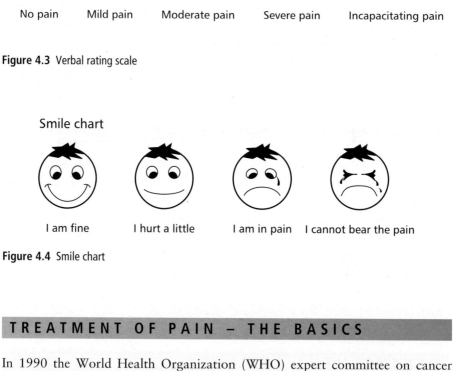

**Figure 4.4** Smile chart

## TREATMENT OF PAIN – THE BASICS

In 1990 the World Health Organization (WHO) expert committee on cancer developed a ladder (Figure 4.5) to guide the management of pain. Initial treatment begins at step 1 with non-opioids such as paracetamol and aspirin. If this is ineffective, move to step 2 with mild opiates such as codeine or dihydrocodeine. These are used with or without non-steroidal anti-inflammatory drugs (NSAIDs) and other co-analgesic medications. If the patient remains in pain, then move to step 3 with strong opioids such as morphine. This approach to pain management leads to rapid pain control in the majority of patients. The ladder can be

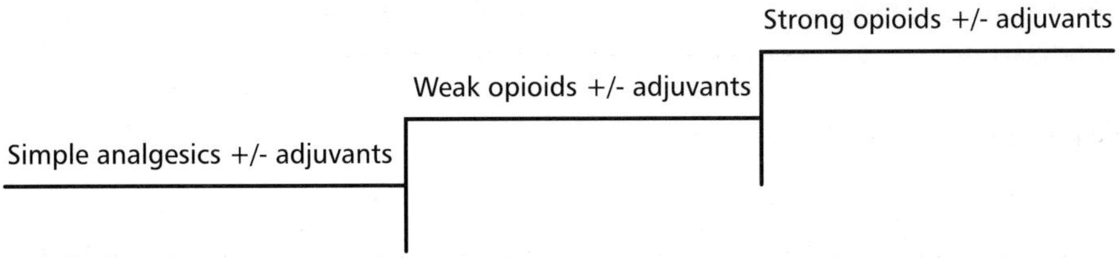

Strong opioids +/- adjuvants

Weak opioids +/- adjuvants

Simple analgesics +/- adjuvants

**Figure 4.5** WHO ladder

commenced on any step and movement can be up the ladder as described or down as the patient recovers, but there is no benefit to be derived from changing drugs on the same step apart from a change in side-effect profile.

> The aim of treatment is to relieve pain and improve function. Management of any pain involves three basic concepts:
>
> 1 Prescribe regular medication – not on an as-required basis
> 2 Give a large enough dose – tailored to the individual patient
> 3 Correct use of the WHO ladder.

## THE ACUTE PAIN SERVICE

Many hospitals run an Acute Pain Service using the skills of a consultant anaesthetist, a clinical nurse specialist, a pharmacist and trainees. The aims of an Acute Pain Service are:
- To set local guidelines for the management of acute pain
- To educate staff in pain management techniques
- Trouble-shooting for difficult pain problems
- Audit.

## ACUTE PAIN MANAGEMENT

The simplest way to manage acute pain is to use a **limited pharmacopoeia**; in this way a few selected drugs and their side-effects become well known. A regularly updated **pain assessment chart** is vital; it should include a measure of pain intensity, drugs given and observations of sedation, respiratory rate and vital signs. Drugs should be given regularly and in large enough quantities to render the patient pain free, taking into account factors such as age, site of incision, weight and medical condition.

'**Balanced analgesia**', that is, the combination of **an opioid** with or without **a non-steroidal anti-inflammatory** drug, with or without **a local anaesthetic** block, is becoming a popular technique resulting in improved pain control and increased mobilization.

## OPIOIDS

Morphine is generally regarded as the gold standard of pain control. It is reliable, in common usage both in and out of the operating theatre and doses can be easily adjusted to suit the individual patient. It can be given by many different routes:

- **Intravenous bolus** – this is useful to establish pain relief in theatre, recovery and casualty prior to commencing regular analgesia. It should be diluted and given slowly to obtain maximum analgesia with minimum side-effects.
- **Intravenous infusion** – this requires careful monitoring of the patient. The rate of infusion is controlled by nursing staff in relation to subjective pain scores. It is best used in intensive care or a high dependency units.
- **Patient controlled analgesia (PCA)** (Figure 4.6) – this is a device that allows the patient to self-administer a small bolus of opioid intravenously and adjust the level of analgesia to suit his/her needs, e.g. the patient can increase his/her analgesia prior to physiotherapy or movement. Patients still require close observation although overdosage and significant respiratory depression are rare. Overdosage is prevented by the requirement for conscious activation by the patient, a 'lockout' interval between doses, and nursing observations. There is a high level of patient satisfaction with this mode of delivery.
- **Intramuscular** – this is often painful and depends on nursing availability for regular dosing. It is unreliably absorbed in the shocked or hypothermic. It can be given hourly until pain relief is achieved and then should be given on a 4-hourly basis.
- **Intraspinal** – opioid receptors are present in both the brain and the spinal cord. Application of opioids directly via the intrathecal route or by dural transfer via the epidural route can provide profound analgesia. There are complications such as urinary retention and itching, which can limit the widespread use of this technique. Intraspinal opiate analgesia should only be used if there is an acute pain service.

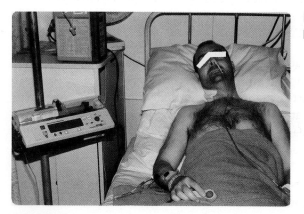

**Figure 4.6** PCA device (demand button in patient's right hand)

## NON-STEROIDAL ANTI-INFLAMMATORY DRUGS (NSAIDS)

These can be used either as an adjuvant to opioids or occasionally instead of them. These, too, should be given regularly. They act by inhibiting prostaglandin synthesis which accounts for their wide range of side-effects. There is a theoretical increased risk of bleeding due to their effect on platelet function, although this rarely has a clinical effect.

Care must be taken in those with renal insufficiency or dependent on diuretics as there is an increased incidence of acute renal failure or salt and water retention in this group. Asthmatics may be sensitive to NSAIDs (5–10%) and in those with asthma and nasal polyps 7–20% can be extremely sensitive. These drugs should be avoided in patients with known sensitivity or nasal polyps.

There is a low incidence of gastrointestinal irritation in patients given NSAIDs in the short term for acute pain.

NSAIDs can also be given by a variety of routes:
- **Oral** – good bioavailability, only useful in those able to take at least sips of water.
- **Rectal** – may have variable absorption, often a useful route in those nil by mouth.
- **Intramuscular** – injections can be painful.
- **Intravenous** – can be as effective as morphine, especially in musculoskeletal pain.

## LOCAL ANAESTHETICS

A variety of local anaesthetic techniques can be used to provide analgesia post-operatively for most surgical procedures:
- **Simple techniques** – infiltrating the wound or performing peripheral nerve blocks with long-acting local anaesthetic at the time of surgery will provide useful analgesia well into the post-operative period, e.g. ilio-inguinal nerve block in hernia repair.
- **Plexus blocks** – these can be performed as a single shot technique or the period of analgesia can be extended by using a continuous infusion via a catheter, e.g. brachial plexus infusion via an axillary catheter following hand surgery.
- **Regional anaesthesia** – catheters placed in the epidural space are commonly used to provide analgesia, e.g. after thoracic, pelvic or abdominal surgery or during labour. Low doses of dilute local anaesthetics can be combined with opioids or alpha-2 blockers to provide profound analgesia by using a continuous infusion technique.

## ACUTE PAIN IN SPECIAL CIRCUMSTANCES

### DAY SURGERY

Effective day surgery demands high quality surgery, anaesthesia and nursing. Patient advice concerning post-operative morbidity, such as pain and swelling, is essential. Before discharge patients should have their pain controlled. Most day case anaesthetics will include combinations of local anaesthetic infiltration or nerve blocks, NSAIDs and opioids (i.e. 'balanced analgesia').

## PAEDIATRICS

Children, like adults, can be treated with simple analgesics, mild opiates and morphine. Doses must be given on a mg/kg basis and adjusted with reference to regular pain assessment. The use of needles should be avoided and drugs are often given via a subcutaneous cannula which can be inserted in theatre or using local anaesthetic cream. There is also a place for the use of epidural analgesia, nerve blocks, infiltration with local anaesthetics and in older children PCAs have been used successfully.

## ELDERLY

For complex social, cultural and environmental reasons, the elderly often under-report pain. Multiple pathology is common, thus dosage of opioids and NSAIDs must be adjusted appropriately. Opioids are given in dilute, gradually increasing quantities until the patient is pain free, when the regular dose can be calculated.

## TRAUMA

Analgesia should be given after resuscitation and neurological assessment. Pain relief reduces sympathetic stimulation improving cardiac, endocrine and metabolic functions. Opioids are generally the most effective and in view of potential hypovolaemia, should be given in dilute slowly increasing quantities until pain relief is achieved.

## RENAL DYSFUNCTION

Opioids are excreted via the kidneys and therefore dosage intervals may need to be lengthened as blood levels will remain high for longer. NSAIDs should be avoided as renal function may deteriorate further with their use.

## HEPATIC DYSFUNCTION

Smaller doses of morphine are used as it is metabolized in the liver before excretion.

## DRUG ABUSERS

The acute post-operative period is not the time to attempt detoxification. Drug abusers have behavioural, physical and psychological factors which make pain control more difficult. Opioid abusers will require the morphine equivalent of their usual maintenance dose as well as the 4-hourly amount required for pain control. Continuous local anaesthetic techniques and NSAIDs can be helpful.

## SHORT PAINFUL PROCEDURES

The aim is to obtain pain relief for the length of the procedure only. Methods by which this can be achieved are for example:

- Entonox – a 50:50 mixture of nitrous oxide and oxygen
- Haematoma blocks – infiltration with local anaesthetic of the haematoma associated with a fracture
- Intravenous regional analgesia – the distal veins of a limb are emptied of blood, a tourniquet applied and the vessels filled with local anaesthetic (**Bier's block**).

## NON-MALIGNANT CHRONIC PAIN MANAGEMENT

Chronic pain has been defined as **pain which persists past the time when healing is expected to be complete.**

The pathophysiological factors causing chronic pain are multidimensional and the concept of 'total pain' involving physical, psychological and behavioural factors is very important in both diagnosis and management. The complex nature of such pain means that multiple treatment modalities may be required simultaneously. A combination of drugs, neural blockade, stimulation-induced analgesia, physiotherapy and psychological strategies may be used. In some it is not possible to obtain complete pain relief and the goal of treatment shifts emphasis to increasing function and quality of life. The management of chronic non-malignant pain is complex. Stimulation-induced analgesia has a useful place and will be briefly highlighted.

### STIMULATION-INDUCED ANALGESIA

Sensory pathways can be electrically or mechanically stimulated resulting in modulation of pain perception:

- **Acupuncture** – a mechanical or electrical stimulation of peripheral points results in stimulation of sensory pathways that can produce analgesia.
- **Trancutaneous electrical nerve stimulators (TENS)** – a small electrical current is passed across the skin between electrodes placed on either side of the painful area. They are usually kept on for several hours at a time and give the sensation of strong but pleasant tingling.
- **Spinal cord stimulators** – an electrode is placed in the epidural space to modulate descending and ascending impulses by stimulating the dorsal columns. The electrodes are connected via an extension cable tunnelled through the subcutaneous fat to a pulse generator usually implanted in the abdominal wall. The patient develops paraesthesia over the area stimulated. Spinal cord stimulation is being used to help manage neuropathic pain such as that seen in peripheral neuropathy and failed back surgery. Spinal cord stimulation also relieves the pain of ischaemia in inoperable peripheral vascular disease and angina pectoris.

## MANAGEMENT OF PAIN IN CANCER

Over the last 30 years the management of symptoms in cancer has developed into the speciality of palliative medicine. The **Palliative Medicine Service** in most hospitals is a consultant-led service involving specialist palliative care nurses, the pain management service, community services and psychological support services.

The assessment of pain in cancer once again involves visual analogue scales and questionnaires, as well as taking into account the psychological and social effects that the pain and diagnosis of cancer have on the patient and their family. The concept of 'total pain' is nowhere more relevant than under these circumstances.

The WHO ladder for the management of pain was originally conceived for use in the palliative setting. The rules of pain management are simple – medication should be given orally if at all possible; it should always be given regularly, adhering to the WHO ladder.

**Pain management**

- By mouth
- By the clock
- By the ladder

### DRUG TREATMENT

- Management of severe pain in cancer begins with full assessment including a pain chart.
- If pain is severe, morphine is prescribed and given as regular oral doses 4-hourly, with further morphine available for breakthrough pain.
- Every 24 hours consideration is given to increasing the morphine dose by 33–50%, until analgesia is adequate.
- When the pain is controlled the amount of morphine required to maintain analgesia over 24 hours can be calculated and converted to a slow release formulation of morphine given regularly once or twice a day, depending on the preparation. Under these circumstances symptom control is paramount and concerns of addiction are irrelevant and unfounded.
- Bone pain may require treatment with NSAIDs and in appropriate cases the use of adjuvant analgesics such as antidepressants or anticonvulsants may be necessary.
- Patients unable to take oral medication, for example in obstruction or dysphagia, may be given drugs parenterally by the subcutaneous or intravenous route.
- Intramuscular administration should almost never be required in the terminally ill patient.

There are some patients whose pain is difficult to control even after following the above guidelines and they are managed best by insertion of an intraspinal catheter. The system for drug delivery will depend on the patient concerned and local resources. The equipotent doses of morphine given by different routes are thought to have the following approximate ratios:

ORAL (30 mg) : PARENTERAL (10 mg) : EPIDURAL (1 mg) : INTRATHECAL (0.1 mg)

Most patients suffering from pain during cancer illness will achieve adequate control using the WHO guidelines. There are patients who continue to have severe pain despite utilizing these guidelines. There are many interacting reasons for this and the patient will require the services of an integrated palliative care and pain management team.

## INTERVENTIONAL PAIN MANAGEMENT TECHNIQUES

The choice of interventional pain management technique will depend upon the pain diagnosis, patient condition, prognosis and informed consent of the patient and their carers.

- **Neurolytic plexus blocks** – such as destruction of the coeliac plexus with alcohol can deliver excellent pain relief in up to 90% of people with visceral pain arising from foregut cancer, e.g. pancreatic cancer, hepatic secondaries and gastric cancer.
- **Subarachnoid neurolysis** – can provide relief in the last few weeks of life, for example in malignant pelvic recurrence.
- **Cervical cordotomy** – can provide pain relief for a few months in unilateral limb pain, such as tumours invading the lumbar or brachial plexus.
- **Continuous intraspinal opioid delivery systems** – using external tunnelled catheters, implanted patient activated reservoirs or implantable fixed or variable rate reservoirs and pumps are now becoming established as the fourth rung of the WHO ladder.

---

**CRIB BOX – PAIN MANAGEMENT**

**Pain is an 'unpleasant sensory and emotional experience associated with actual or potential tissue damage, or described in terms of such damage'**

**Chronic pain** – persists past the time when healing is expected to be complete

**Three factors** – physical; psychological; behavioural

**Pain pathways** are complex and modulated at all levels of the nervous system

**Good pain control requires appropriate pain measurement records**, e.g. VAS

**Use the WHO ladder**

**Manage pain** by mouth; by the clock; by the ladder

**Stimulation induced analgesia** – acupuncture; TENS; spinal cord stimulator

**Interventional techniques** – neurolysis; cordotomy; intraspinal opioids

# chapter 5

# INFECTIONS AND SURGERY

At any one time, **20–25%** of hospitalized patients will be suffering from a bacterial infection, making it the single most common pathogenic process encountered. Half are **community-acquired infections (CAIs)**, requiring hospitalization for treatment.

The remainder are **hospital-acquired infections (HAIs)**, being a complication of initial underlying pathology, and are **iatrogenic**. The consequences of HAI are considerable, including increased morbidity, mortality and economic cost for patient and institution.

Prevention of HAIs (as opposed to treatment) is not only preferable but clearly possible. Frequently prevention focuses on antibiotic prophylaxis, ignoring many other important factors, such as aseptic technique, clean environment and surgical technique.

> In the United Kingdom, **antibiotics account for approximately one-quarter of pharmaceutical expenditure**. Antibiotics tend to be viewed as a panacea for the treatment and prevention of bacterial disease, whereas in reality they are only one element in a strategy. Rational use of antibiotics is imperative, not only to achieve the best outcome for an individual, but to prevent the emergence of bacterial resistance in the general population.
>
> **Many hospitals are experiencing serious difficulties with multiple antibiotic-resistant microbes generated by the irrational use of antibiotics.**

Although much attention is paid to bacterial infections in hospitalized patients, consideration needs to be given to other microbes and in particular to viruses. HIV and hepatitis B have obvious risk implications for both patients and health care workers.

## HOST/MICROBE/ENVIRONMENT

Manifestations of infection are the result of complex interactions between microbe and host (Figure 5.1). Almost infinite variability exists, as both components are biological and therefore ultimately dependent on genetics. In the normal host there is a benign and sometimes symbiotic relationship with billions of bacteria, yet in the immunocompromised, normally innocuous organisms can produce serious disease.

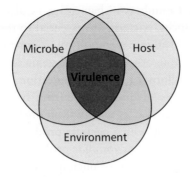

**Figure 5.1** Host/microbe/environment interactions

Thus the concept of non-pathogenic organisms or commensals is outdated; it is more practical to consider the relative virulence of any microbe with reference to the ability of the host to resist infection.

Superimposed upon this already complex situation are the effects of the environment on both man and microbe. Whilst a variety of micro-organisms, including viruses, bacteria and protozoa, can cause significant disease in man, it is bacterial disease that currently produces the most significant problem in hospital medicine. Unfortunately hospitals *par excellence* bring together all the worst risk factors found in man, microbe and environment. It is difficult to determine the relative influence of each of these three factors. Nevertheless, some generalizations can be made about each factor.

## BACTERIA

Unicellular bacteria-like organisms have been in existence for at least three billion years. A brief, if somewhat simplistic, look at some of their basic properties can graphically illustrate their potential and our relative impotence.

- **Size and numbers** – it is an understatement to say that bacteria are small. Vast numbers colonize humans. Counts are especially high in the oropharynx, female genital tract and the lower gut.
- **Doubling time** – many bacteria of medical importance will, under ideal circumstances, double every 20 minutes. Simple arithmetic demonstrates that in a little over 7 hours there will be over one million progeny of an original bacterium.
- **Survivability** – over the aeons of existence, bacteria have adapted to survive in a wide variety of circumstances. The genetic potential and hence adaptability of bacteria is enormous. Of great medical importance is the ability of bacteria to deactivate antibacterial agents produced by other primitive life forms, e.g. the production of antibiotics by fungi.
- **Genetics** – bacteria are also capable of exchanging genetic information in the form of transposons and plasmids. The exchange is much more common than at first thought and certainly occurs across 'genus barriers'.

Man is colonized by vast numbers of bacteria; so-called commensals or normal flora. In some circumstances, bacteria are essential to the well-being of the host, helping, as in the gut, with vitamin metabolism. Commensals also serve some protective function in preventing other more pathogenic organisms multiplying.

**Suppression of normal flora leads to superinfection**, e.g. *Candida*.

There are large numbers of disease-producing bacteria. The pathogenicity, often referred to as virulence, varies widely from organism to organism. Broadly there are three mechanisms by which bacteria produce disease:

- **Invasiveness** – *Streptococcus pneumoniae* probably provides the best example of pure invasiveness. In meningitis or pneumonia, there is little evidence of toxicity other than that generated by the invasion of organisms alone.
- **Toxin production** – botulism provides the paradigm of disease produced by toxin production. All the signs and symptoms are a manifestation of toxin production by *Clostridium botulinum*. Botulism is rare but many other organisms cause significant disease by the production of exotoxins: tetanus, diphtheria and some staphylococcal diseases are examples.
- **Hypersensitivity** – hypersensitivity reactions require prior exposure to a pathogen. As far as infectious disease is concerned, the most important is type IV hypersensitivity. Tuberculosis is the most widely used example.

A single mechanism may be responsible but more frequently there is a mixture, e.g. *Staphylococcus aureus* can be invasive, producing boils and carbuncles, but may also express a variety of exotoxins (toxic epidermal necrolysis, toxic shock syndrome). The ability to exploit these mechanisms is an expression of the micro-organisms' virulence.

In some circumstances virulence factors can be identified or hypothesized – molecular genetics and cell biology are undoubtedly increasing understanding. Factors that have been documented to enhance pathogenicity include:

- Adherence to epithelial cells with the aid of pili, e.g. *Neisseria gonorrhoeae*
- Avoidance of phagocytosis with the development of capsules
- The use of enzymes to destroy tissue and aid invasion, e.g. haemolytic streptococci and clostridia
- The expression of endotoxins – most Gram-negative rods; the lipopolysaccharide in the cell wall being a potent human toxin
- Exotoxins – potent toxins include those produced by *Staphylococcus aureus* (toxic shock syndrome toxin); and *Pseudomonas* (exotoxin A).

## HOST DEFENCES

Many of the manifestations of infection result from host defence mechanisms – the immune response.

It is important to recognize that the immune system is **integrated** and that damage to any one component will lead to reduced ability to combat infection. The pattern of infection in immune compromised individuals is likely to vary, depending upon the part of the immune system most affected. The greater the of immune compromise, the greater the diversity of organisms likely to produce disease – e.g. in the severely neutropenic patient, many so-called commensal organisms are likely to become pathogenic: the most commonly seen bacteraemia in neutropenic patients is *Staphylococcus epidermidis*.

**The immune system consists of three integrated components:**
- Mechanical barriers to infection, such as the skin, mucous membranes and cilia in the respiratory tract. There are other non-specific mechanisms, such as gastric acid. Serum proteins, called interferons, also act in a non-specific way to combat infectious agents.
- The humoral mediated immune system consists largely of circulating and fixed phagocytes, such as neutrophils and monocytes. **The hallmark of the humoral immune system is inflammation.** It is relatively non-specific and may occur in response to factors other than infection, e.g. trauma and chemical damage.
- The cell mediated immune system requires a so-called immunological memory and can only be employed on a subsequent exposure to an infecting agent when specific antibodies will be produced to neutralize the infecting agent.

---

**The three integrated components of the immune system**

- Mechanical barriers to infection
- Humoral mediated immune system
- Cell mediated immune system

---

In most surgical circumstances, it is the mechanical and humorally mediated immune responses that are of primary importance. Cell mediated immune response plays a relatively minor part, being directed more at intracellular organisms.

Once a bacterium breaches the primary defences, the immune response is initially that of the classical inflammatory response. The purpose is to attempt to localize the infection. *Staphylococcus aureus* boils are a typical example.

Failure to localize the invading microbe leads to cellulitis and lymphangitis of regional lymph nodes, a common manifestation of *Streptococcus pyogenes* infection. Further dissemination leads to septicaemia, the classical manifestations of which are fever, rigors and septic shock, with multiple organ failure ensuing, e.g. *Neisseria meningitidis* septicaemia.

---

The immune response is an integrated, complex mechanism and the failure of any one part impacts upon the rest. Surgery, underlying pathology, or both, cause an immune defect.

---

## ENVIRONMENT

The hospital environment compounds the risks of infection:
- At any one time, the number of infected patients in an acute hospital is likely to be in excess of 20%; approximately half the infections will be hospital-acquired.

- Somewhere in the region of 25–40% of patients will be receiving antimicrobial therapy, undoubtedly significantly increasing the levels of antimicrobial resistance.
- Many infected patients shed large numbers of pathogenic organisms. Health care workers become transiently colonized and frequently transmit organisms from patient to patient.

Other factors may play a role in the development of HAIs, but are much less easy to define and quantify: the level and quality of **domestic activity**; the **patient mix** and throughput of a ward; the **microbiological quality of food**. Concern has been expressed at the difficulty of **decontaminating complex medical equipment**.

## PREVENTION OF HAI

### GENERAL STRATEGY

**Prevention is better than cure.** Nowhere is this more relevant than in infectious disease.

Antibiotics play a minor role in treatment and prevention, but in the current culture are too often viewed as the most significant factor. Semelweiss and Lister (an obstetrician and a surgeon) pioneered the concept of bacterial decontamination of surgeon and patient using simple antibacterial agents such as hypochlorite and carbolic. Their work led to the concept of the modern theatre where asepsis is the key.

**Skin preparation and environment play a crucial role in preventing surgical infection.** Many of the techniques have tended to become devalued, with reliance placed heavily on antimicrobial agents. Rather like the immune system, an integrated approach is necessary.

The most important issue relating to HAI is that of good hygienic practice, e.g.:
- Hand washing
- Sterile/aseptic technique
- Environmental control in operating theatre
- Surveillance/audit – infection rates in wounds can drop by up to one-third after surgeons are informed on a regular basis of their sepsis rates.

Such simple procedures stem from the pre-antibiotic era, but still remain appropriate.

### ANTIBIOTIC PROPHYLAXIS

Antibacterial prophylaxis (Table 5.1) is of undoubted benefit in surgery, provided it is used rationally. Some simple rules need to be applied:
- Antibiotics should be given when contamination of a wound is expected or when operations on a contaminated site may lead to bacteraemia. The majority of 'clean' operations do not warrant prophylaxis. The exception is when

**Table 5.1** Antibiotic prophylaxis

| Site of operation | Antibiotic | Comments |
| --- | --- | --- |
| Urinary tract | Single dose gentamicin 2 mg/kg | Anti-pseudomonal agents essential |
| Gall bladder | Azlocillin 5 g at induction | Anti-anaerobic agents not required |
| Orthopaedic implants and vascular grafts | 1st generation cephalosporins | Gram-positive skin flora main problem |
| Large bowel | Augmentin or cefuroxime + metronidazole | Prophylaxis reduces wound infection rates from 40% to 10% |
| Gynaecology | Augmentin or cefuroxime + metronidazole | Also consider *Chlamydia*, especially in TOP |

prosthetic material is to be implanted where the consequences of infection are grave.

- Prophylactic regimens should be directed against the most relevant pathogens. It is impossible to cover all organisms. Regimens that decrease the total number of pathogens are usually sufficient.
- Antibiotics are usually best given parenterally **at the time of induction of anaesthesia** to ensure effective tissue levels during surgery when there is a maximum risk of local contamination or dissemination.
- **There is no evidence that prolonged prophylaxis has any advantage over short courses** (24 hours). Indeed, prolonged administration tends to lead to the emergence of resistant organisms, superinfection and is also expensive. If surgery is prolonged, e.g. >2 hours, top up doses should be given during surgery.
- Prophylaxis against *Clostridium tetani* or *Clostridium welchii* is an exception, requiring a minimum of 5 days of antibiotics.
- Prophylaxis is inappropriate if there is established infection (e.g. where there is established peritonitis due to visceral perforation, or an infected prosthesis). Full courses of antibiotics will be required.

## TREATMENT OF HAI

### RISK EVALUATION

The management of infections in surgery is a matter of risk assessment; protocols play a part, but must not be adhered to in an unthinking manner. In many infections, supportive care is more critical than antibiotics. There are a minimum of five basic criteria to be assessed.

## Underlying pathology

Probably the most significant factor to evaluate before deciding upon an antibiotic regimen is the patient's underlying pathology. It will broadly reflect the patient's immune system. Those with rapidly fatal underlying pathology are the most likely to succumb to infection. Broad spectrum empirical therapy is necessary and probably has significant influence on outcome. With lesser pathology,

| Treatment of HAIs |
|---|
| Risk evaluation |
| • Underlying pathology |
| • HAI vs CAI |
| • Putative organism |
| • Site of sepsis |
| • Age of patient |

the outcome is far less dependent on finding the appropriate antimicrobial agent. Indeed, fit, healthy young people have a considerable ability to combat infection, and antibiotic therapy plays a comparatively minor part.

## HAIs vs CAIs

Most community-acquired organisms remain relatively sensitive to antibiotics. This at least in part reflects the levels of antibiotic usage in the community versus hospitals. Acute wards in hospitals are likely to have 25–40% of patients receiving antibiotics in contrast to less than 1% in the community. Benzylpenicillin still plays a major part in the treatment of CAI, with organisms such as *Streptococcus pyogenes*, pneumococci and *Neisseria* spp. remaining largely sensitive, at least in the UK. Monitoring and knowledge of local, national and international ecology is important.

## Putative organism

The organisms likely to be involved in an infectious process must be considered. In some circumstances, the likely pathogens can be confined to a very narrow list, e.g. CAI meningitis or pneumonia, with largely predictable antibiotic sensitivity. The range of organisms involved in HAI post-surgery sepsis are very much more diverse, but aerobic Gram-negative rods and anaerobes are much more likely to be involved and therefore empirical antibiotic therapy needs to be tailored. The greatest diversity is likely to occur in the intensive care environment, where the most compromised ill patients are managed, broad spectrum empirical therapy often being necessary.

## Site of sepsis

In any case of serious sepsis, it is important to attempt to identify the site of the source. Some sites are much more easily treated. Many antibiotics are excreted unchanged in the urine, thus making even serious complicated urinary tract infections relatively easily treated. By contrast, pneumonia and meningitis are relatively difficult, because penetration of antibiotic is variable and often poor. Antibiotic penetration of bone is particularly poor and it is necessary to give protracted courses. When prosthetic material is introduced, antibiotic therapy becomes particularly difficult.

## Age

The extremes of age influence antibiotic therapy. Metabolism and excretion of antibiotics, and poor immune response are just examples of the considerations necessary. Renal function is variable at both ends of the age spectrum. Care must therefore be exercised in both choice and dosage of antimicrobials.

## MANAGEMENT OF SPECIFIC INFECTIONS

### URINARY TRACT

Simple cystitis is a disease almost exclusively of women. When a well-documented urinary infection occurs in men, it requires further investigation. Obstruction, reflux and anatomical abnormality are the likely predisposing conditions. Gram-negative rods of gut origin, frequently referred to as 'coliforms', are the most frequent organisms involved (*Escherichia coli*, *Klebsiella*). *Proteus* spp. are particularly associated with calculi and *Pseudomonas* spp. with hospitalization and instrumentation. **Manipulation or instrumentation in patients with bacteriuria is likely to precipitate bacteraemia, and prophylactic antibiotics should be administered.** A single dose prior to the procedure is usually adequate. Aminoglycosides (gentamicin) are often useful, being active against most Gram-negative organisms, including *Pseudomonas*. With single dose therapy, nephrotoxicity is rarely, if ever, a problem.

Many catheterized patients develop bacteriuria but remain asymptomatic. Antibiotic therapy in most circumstances is unnecessary. It is only when signs or symptoms of ascending infection (i.e. fever, rigors, loin pain) develop that antibiotics are indicated. If treatment is used, it is essential that the indwelling catheter is changed during therapy, otherwise antibiotic resistance will inevitably develop. Aminoglycosides, some third generation cephalosporins and quinolones are all likely to be effective, but knowledge of local resistance problems is important.

### SKIN AND SOFT TISSUE INFECTION

#### Boils and carbuncles

Boils and carbuncles (Figure 5.2) are usually community-acquired. Gram-positive organisms predominate and are therefore likely to be relatively antibiotic sensitive. Simple staphylococcal boils and carbuncles may require surgical drainage, but unless there is a failure to localize, antibiotics are unlikely to contribute. Multiple recurrent boils are invariably due to chronic staphylococcal carriage and require topical decontamination – disinfectant antibacterial creams, such as mupirocin.

Rarely, there is failure to localize staphylococcal lesions, regional lymph nodes become involved and systemic antibiotics are necessary – flucloxacillin, fusidate and erythromycin are likely agents.

#### Cellulitis

Failure to localize infection and widespread cellulitis tend to be more frequently associated with haemolytic streptococci. *Streptococcus pyogenes* (Lancefield group A streptococci) is the most common.

Cellulitis is most frequently community-acquired and affects the peripheral limbs. The portal of entry of the streptococcus may be a minor graze or abrasion, or via damage resulting from underlying pathology as diverse as tinea pedis and diabetes mellitus. Local cellulitis may rapidly spread to local lymph channels, leading to **lymphangitis** and a characteristic red line. Spread to local lymph nodes must be considered serious and warrants urgent parenteral therapy. Local disease may progress to massive cellulitis, streptococcal gangrene and necrotizing fasciitis. Widespread dissemination may occur, resulting in septic shock. Not only will high doses of parenteral antibiotics be required, but surgical intervention in terms of fasciotomy and/or debridement may be required.

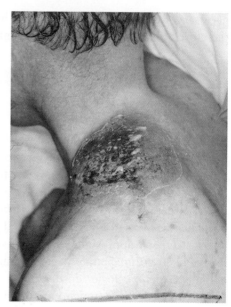

**Figure 5.2** Carbuncle on shoulder

*Staphylococcus aureus* and occasionally Gram-negative organisms may be involved in cellulitis. Usually the patient has significant underlying pathology. Diabetics in particular are prone to severe lower limb cellulitis, where broader spectrum antibiotics would be appropriate. Gentamicin or a quinolone in combination with benzylpenicillin provide reasonable empirical therapy.

Whatever the cause, the key to diagnosis must rest initially with suspicion. Empirical treatment needs to be started urgently, and whilst organisms other than streptococci may be involved, **high-dose penicillin is imperative**, unless the patient is highly allergic, in which case vancomycin is indicated.

### Infectious gangrene

The terminology surrounding infectious gangrene is complex and confusing. Descriptions relate to clinical, microbiological and anatomical manifestations, added to which are a number of eponyms. Some initial generalizations can nevertheless be made:

- Individually, all forms of infectious gangrene are rare, but morbidity and mortality are high, whatever the aetiology.
- Recognition of the problem is critical and treatment is invariably urgent.
- A variety of specialists, including physician, surgeon, intensivist and microbiologist, need a co-ordinated, integrated strategy for treatment.

Much is often made of the clinical differences between forms of infectious gangrene. Pain, fever, toxicity, crepitus and underlying pathology may help to distinguish forms of serious soft tissue infection (see Table 5.2). In practice, the systemic signs and symptoms are more likely to reflect the extent of disease and the patient's underlying condition rather than the aetiology. Useful distinguishing features may, however, occur:

**Table 5.2** Differential diagnosis of gangrenous infections of subcutaneous tissues and skin

| | Bacterial synergistic gangrene | Necrotizing fasciitis and cellulitis | Streptococcal gangrene | Gas gangrene |
|---|---|---|---|---|
| Predisposing conditions | Usually follows wound infection; draining sinus | Wound infection; perineal infections | Occasionally diabetes or myxoedema, but often none; after abdominal surgery | Local trauma to deep soft tissues |
| Pain | Severe | Variable | Severe | Severe |
| Toxicity | Minimal | Marked | Marked | Very marked |
| Fever | Minimal or absent | Moderate | High | Moderate or high |
| Crepitus | Absent | Frequent | Absent | Frequent |
| Aetiology | Microaerophilic streptococcus plus S. aureus (or Proteus) | Usually a mixture of aerobic and anaerobic organisms | Primarily group A streptococci | Cl. perfringens (occasionally other clostridia) |
| Progress | Slow | Rapid | Rapid | Rapid |

- The presence of crepitus around a lesion invariably indicates anaerobic organism involvement, as would evidence of gas formation on x-ray (Figure 5.3). Suspect clostridial myonecrosis or bacterial synergistic gangrene.
- A foul odour will indicate the involvement of anaerobes and/or microaerophilic organisms.
- Extensive cellulitis with bullae formation and superficial gangrene of the skin will suggest streptococcal disease.
- Many of the diseases involving mixed and/or anaerobic organisms are consequent upon contaminated surgery.

The aetiology of infectious gangrene directs the emphasis of treatment, e.g. streptococcal gangrene is primarily a medical emergency needing supportive surgery, whilst anaerobic infection requires urgent surgery with medical and microbiological support. All cases may require intensive care and plastic surgery.

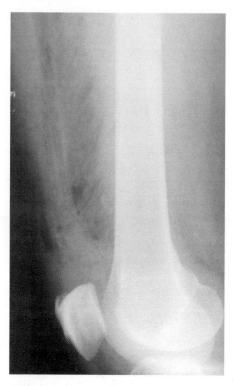

**Figure 5.3** Gas gangrene in muscles of the thigh – gas outlines the muscle structure

## BONE INFECTION

Primary infection of bone is uncommon today. Prior to *Haemophilus influenzae* vaccine, Haemophilus infection occurred in children under the age of 5 years. Now most bone infection is a consequence of trauma, orthopaedic surgery or occasionally a bacteraemic episode.

Orthopaedic surgically related infection is dominated by infection with Gram-positive skin flora, the most common being *Staphylococcus aureus*. Much more difficult to assess is that caused by coagulase-negative staphylococci such as *Staphylococcus epidermidis*. Particular difficulty emerges in the significance of microbiological isolates in low grade infection of prostheses. Often empirical and prolonged anti-staphylococcal therapy is necessary over weeks or months.

## GASTROINTESTINAL SURGERY

The microbiology of the gastrointestinal tract varies considerably. Antibiotic treatment and organisms of the various sites are shown in Table 5.3.

**Table 5.3** Antibiotic treatment

| Site | Organisms | Antibiotics | Comments |
|---|---|---|---|
| Urinary tract | Gram-negative rods 'Coliforms' | Gentamicin or quinolone | *Pseudomonas* a frequent cause; anaerobes rarely involved |
| Bone and soft tissue | *Staphylococcus aureus* β-Haemolytic streptococci | Flucloxacillin, fusidate Benzylpenicillin | Combination therapy often required |
| Intra-abdominal involving viscera | Gram-negative rods Faecal streps + anaerobes | Metronidazole + gentamicin or quinolone or 3rd generation cephalosporins | Frequently mixed infections |
| Respiratory tract Lower (post-op) | *Streptococcus pneumoniae* *Haemophilus influenzae* | Amoxycillin Quinolone + amoxycillin or 3rd generation cephalosporins | Choice will depend heavily on risk assessment |
| Lower (ITU) | Gram-negative rods | Imipenem | |
| Gynaecology | Gram-negative rods Anaerobes Group B streptococci *Chlamydia* | 3rd generation cephalosporins Quinolone + metronidazole Erythromycin | *Chlamydia* are probably the most common cause of pelvic inflammatory disease (PID) |

## Mouth and oropharynx

Normally α-haemolytic streptococci predominate. Lifestyle and disease lead to significant changes. The hygienically neglected mouth, with periodontal disease or gingivitis, may harbour vast numbers of anaerobes. Hospitalization and antibiotic therapy destroys the relatively sensitive oral streptococci and replaces them with intrinsically resistant Gram-negative rods. These organisms may remain as colonists, but have the potential to lead to significant infection, especially in the critical care environment.

## Stomach and duodenum

Relatively small numbers of bacteria colonize the hostile environment of the stomach and duodenum. Special mention needs to be made of *Helicobacter* spp. and their role in gastric ulcer and duodenal ulcer. The identification of the role of helicobacters has dramatically shifted the emphasis of treatment from surgery to conservative medical management. Emphasis is now on acid reduction and bacterial eradication using short (1–2 weeks) courses of proton pump inhibitors and antibiotics.

## Gall bladder and bile duct

Disease may be associated with acute infection in the form of acute cholecystitis or ascending cholangitis. Coliforms of gut origin are the likely pathogens. Anaerobes are infrequently involved unless there is abscess formation. The increasing use of endoscopic techniques has tended to lead to a greater diversity of organisms. Hospitalization, medical device and previous antibiotics must be taken into consideration when infection is clinically apparent.

## Colon

Bacterial counts in the large bowel may reach $10^{11}$–$10^{12}$/g of content. Clearly there is enormous potential for primary infection and for infection complicating surgery. The large bowel has colossal numbers of anaerobic bacteria. They outnumber the 'coliforms' by at least 10:1. Invariably operation or perforation at such sites potentially leads to significant numbers of bacteria contaminating the wound and potentially the bloodstream. Prior to antibiotic prophylaxis, serious wound infections following large bowel surgery were of the order of 40%. Prophylaxis has led to a reduction to the order of 10%. Most infectious are a synergistic combination of coliform and anaerobe. On occasions, this may lead to the serious problem of synergistic necrotizing infection.

The incidence of gastroenteritis has increased year on year for the last two decades. Campylobacters and salmonellas lead the causes of bacterial infection, often accompanied by systemic symptoms, fever, rigors, abdominal cramps and pain, and bloody diarrhoea. Confusion with appendicitis and other surgical pathologies is common. Detailed history, examination and microbiological investigation in the form of stool and blood culture are mandatory.

Superinfection in the oropharynx and large bowel with *Candida* and *Clostridium difficile* can occur following therapy for infection elsewhere. It is most commonly seen in the intensive care environment after prolonged use of broad spectrum antibiotics which suppress normal flora.

## CHEST SURGERY

Although infections in operative wounds do occur in cardiothoracic surgery, they are relatively uncommon and usually caused by skin flora, e.g. sternal osteomyelitis following cardiac surgery. Serious lower respiratory tract infections can complicate any surgery and are associated with pre-existing lung pathology and post-operative pain interfering with coughing. *Haemophilus influenzae* and *Streptococcus pneumoniae* are the likely community-acquired organisms involved, but as elsewhere the environment in which patients are cared for prior to surgery is important. Hospitalization and antibiotics will lead, for example, to coliforms and pseudomonas playing a more significant role.

## GYNAECOLOGY

The female genital tract is heavily colonized with coliforms and anaerobes. Group B streptococci are also found in a significant number of women. Antibiotic prophylaxis is undoubtedly indicated when operations are likely to involve entry into the vagina.

## VIRAL INFECTIONS

A wide variety of viruses may be transmitted via blood, but hepatitis B and HIV have been the dominant concerns in recent years. Hepatitis C is becoming increasingly important.

### HEPATITIS B VIRUS (HBV)

Carriage of hepatitis B surface antigen (HBsAg) is uncommon in the UK, but in parts of the world rates may be as high as 10–20%. Central Africa and SE Asia are high risk areas, where vertical transmission of the virus is common. It is important to look at markers other than HBsAg, as these provide an index of infectivity. Individuals that are hepatitis B e antigen (HBeAg) positive are highly infectious. HBeAg positive surgeons are restricted from invasive surgery in the UK. Vaccination of health care workers is common practice in Western countries and will give protection to approximately 95% of individuals.

### HEPATITIS C VIRUS (HCV)

Hepatitis C is transmitted in much the same way as hepatitis B, i.e. sexually, through drug abuse, etc. Much less is known of the epidemiology, although it appears to be more common than HBV. It is known that chronic carriage of HCV leads to chronic liver disease. No vaccine is available, so protection is by good practice.

## HUMAN IMMUNODEFICIENCY VIRUS (HIV)

Transmission, as with HBV and HCV, is by inoculation, but appears to require a larger inoculum. The great concern is the high morbidity and mortality associated with the infection. To date, only one case of transmission from health care worker to patient has been documented. The reverse process is much more common, almost certainly following repeated needle-stick injuries. The screening of patients for HIV carriage leads to many problems, not least of which are ethical. The protection of health care workers currently rests entirely with observance of safe practice and so-called 'universal precautions'.

### CRIB BOX – INFECTIONS AND SURGERY

- HAIs are preventable and iatrogenic
- Around 10% of hospitalized patients have HAIs
- Virulence is host/microbe/environment dependent
- Prevention of HAIs is mainly by reducing cross-infection with physical means, e.g. hand washing, aseptic/sterile technique
- Antibiotic **prophylaxis** differs from **antibiotic treatment**

# chapter 6

# HIV AND THE SURGEON

## ABDOMINAL PAIN IN THE HIV POSITIVE PATIENT

The majority of HIV positive patients will experience gastrointestinal symptoms during the course of their HIV disease, one of the commonest being abdominal pain. Up to 15% of patients admitted to hospital with a previous AIDS diagnosis will require surgical evaluation because of severe abdominal pain. The number, however, who require surgical intervention will be smaller.

In making a clinical diagnosis in an HIV positive patient with abdominal pain it is important to take into consideration the patient's degree of immunosuppression:

- Patients with a well-preserved immune system and who are asymptomatic in terms of their HIV infection are more likely to have a non-HIV related cause for their abdominal pain.
- Patients who have AIDS or are significantly immunosuppressed are likely to have tumour or opportunistic infection as the cause of their pain.

Common causes of an 'acute abdomen' in HIV positive patients are:

- Cytomegalovirus infection
- Lymphoma
- Kaposi's sarcoma
- Acute appendicitis
- Cholecystitis and biliary disease.

## CYTOMEGALOVIRUS INFECTION

- Disease due to cytomegalovirus (CMV) infection in HIV positive patients is due to the reactivation of latent infection.
- Up to 80% of HIV positive patients will have evidence of previous exposure to CMV.
- Invasive CMV disease occurs in patients with advanced immunosuppression, usually with a CD4 lymphocyte count $<50/mm^3$.
- The most common manifestation of CMV disease is **retinitis**.

CMV infection can affect the whole of the gastrointestinal tract from oesophagus to the rectum. It most commonly affects the colon.

### Pathology

CMV infects both epithelial and endothelial cells. In arterioles supplying the sub-mucosa of the bowel it results in vasculitis and subsequent thrombosis. Histopathological biopsy specimens show characteristic intranuclear and intracy-toplasmic inclusion bodies with a perinuclear halo.

### Presentation

Patients with CMV colitis present with **abdominal pain, bloody diarrhoea and fever**. The abdominal pain tends to be non-specific and diffuse.

### Diagnosis and treatment

Radiology is unhelpful. The diagnosis is made histologically from endoscopic biopsies showing typical inclusion bodies (Figure 6.1). The treatment of uncomplicated CMV colitis is medical with antiviral drugs (ganciclovir; fos-carnet).

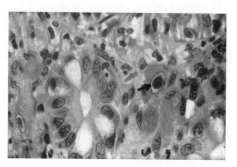

**Figure 6.1** CMV inclusion body (arrowed)

### Surgical complications of CMV colitis

- Perforation
- Haemorrhage
- Ischaemia
- Medically refractory toxic megacolon.

## LYMPHOMA

HIV positive patients have a 60–100 times increased risk of developing non-Hodgkin's lymphoma and 3% of patients present with lymphoma as their AIDS defining diagnosis. Gastrointestinal involvement is common (Figure 6.2).

### Pathology

Of the non-Hodgkin's lymphomas in HIV positive patients, 60–90% are high grade B-cell lymphomas, either small non-cleaved or immunoblastic types. Intermediate grade large cell tumours are also seen. Hodgkin's disease is also associated with HIV infection occurring predominantly in those infected via par-enteral drug use.

### Presentation

HIV related lymphomas typically present with extensive disease, often with extra-nodal involvement. B-cell symptoms are a feature in up to 80% of patients. Gastrointestinal involvement occurs in up to 45% of patients and has been reported throughout the gastrointestinal tract, particularly the ileum. Patients with gastrointestinal lymphoma may present with an abdominal mass or a surgi-cal complication.

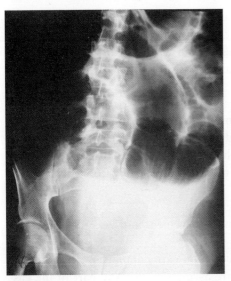

**Figure 6.2** Intestinal obstruction secondary to pelvic B-cell non-Hodgkin's lymphoma

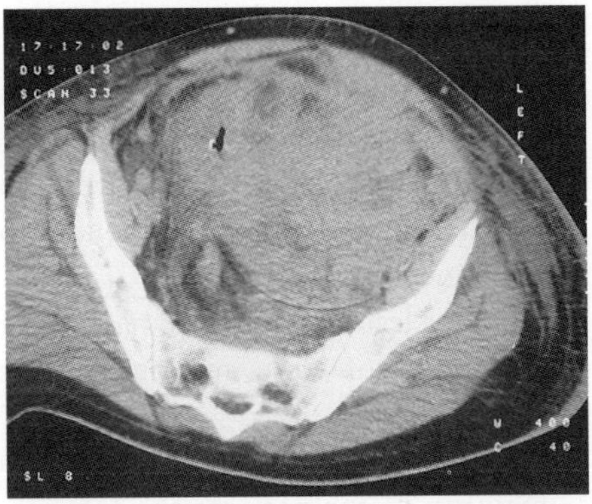

**Figure 6.3** B-cell non-Hodgkin's lymphoma. CT scan of pelvis. Same patient as in Figure 6.2

### Diagnosis and treatment

Wherever possible the diagnosis should be made non-surgically, by CT (Figure 6.3) or ultrasound guided biopsy. Complications may require surgical intervention and resection of involved bowel. Usually the disease is widespread with nodal involvement and patients usually require systemic cytotoxic chemotherapy.

### Surgical complications of lymphoma

- Obstruction
- Perforation
- Haemorrhage.

## KAPOSI'S SARCOMA

Kaposi's sarcoma (Figure 6.4) is **the most common HIV related tumour.** It is seen most frequently in homosexual men but also in black Africans and less commonly in patients who have acquired their HIV infection through injecting drug use or blood products.

### Pathology

Kaposi's sarcoma is thought to be an **endothelial neoplasm** of small vessels. Histologically, the tumour typically shows vascular proliferation with spin-

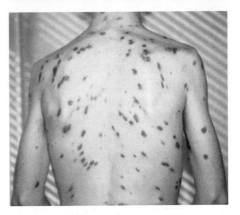

**Figure 6.4** Cutaneous Kaposi's sarcoma

dle shaped cells. There is usually evidence of extravasated red blood cells and haemosiderin which is a helpful diagnostic feature. Kaposi's sarcoma is associated with the recently described human herpes virus-8 which seems to act as a viral cofactor in both HIV related and 'classical' Kaposi's sarcoma.

### Presentation
- Kaposi's sarcoma usually appears as **multiple pink or violaceous skin lesions** which may be macular, papular or nodular in appearance.
- They can vary in size from several millimetres to confluent plaques of tumour over 10 cm in diameter and tend to be asymptomatic, apart from cosmetic disfigurement.
- Nodular lesions can cause pain and ulcerate.
- With HIV infection, mucous membrane involvement and visceral disease are common.
- The gastrointestinal tract is the most common extracutaneous site and in the majority of the patients the tumours are asymptomatic. Any part of the gastrointestinal tract may be involved but is most commonly seen in the **stomach and duodenum**.

### Diagnosis and treatment
Cutaneous lesions of Kaposi's sarcoma (Figure 6.4) usually present little diagnostic difficulty because of their typical appearance. The diagnosis, if in doubt, can be confirmed by punch biopsy. Gastrointestinal Kaposi's sarcoma is usually diagnosed on the basis of the endoscopic appearance of the tumours (Figure 6.5). Gastrointestinal tumours are usually up to 2 cm in diameter and as in the skin are violaceous in colour. They tend to arise in the submucosa and are therefore more difficult to biopsy endoscopically. Radiography is not as useful as endoscopy, but contrast studies may show raised nodular masses within the gut lumen. Surgical treatment is only warranted in the case of complications, principally obstruction or bleeding. Usually small tumours can be managed by primary resection.

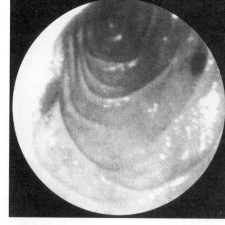

**Figure 6.5** Endoscopic appearance of oesophageal Kaposi's sarcoma

### Surgical complications of Kaposi's sarcoma
- Haemorrhage
- Obstruction.

## APPENDICITIS

- Acute appendicitis is at least as common in HIV infected individuals as in the non-infected population.
- Usually the cause is obstruction by a faecolith, although obstruction by non-Hodgkin's lymphoma and Kaposi's sarcoma can occur.
- The diagnosis may be delayed as signs of peritonitis may be less severe than in the immunocompetent.
- Appendicectomy in HIV positive patients is associated with similar mortality rates as for HIV negative patients and should be performed in the standard fashion.

## CHOLECYSTITIS AND BILIARY DISEASE

### ACALCULOUS CHOLECYSTITIS

- Acalculous cholecystitis may be associated with enteric infection in HIV positive patients.
- The usual presentation is with right hypochondrial pain, positive Murphy's sign and fever.
- Ultrasonic examination shows a thickened gall bladder and the absence of gall stones.
- Alkaline phosphatase is usually raised and radionucleotide scanning fails to visualize the gall bladder.
- Associated infection may respond to appropriate antimicrobial therapy; however, severe cases may require surgical intervention.
- Laparoscopic cholecystectomy is the treatment of choice.

**Enteric infections associated with acalculous cholecystitis**

- Salmonella
- Campylobacter
- CMV
- Cryptosporidiosis

### HIV-ASSOCIATED CHOLANGIOPATHY

- HIV-associated cholangiopathy is a condition usually related to opportunistic infection.
- **It consists of papillary stenosis with common bile duct dilatation or sclerosing cholangitis with focal strictures and dilatation of intra- and extrahepatic bile ducts.**
- Patients present with right upper quadrant pain and tenderness.
- Jaundice may occur but is uncommon. Alkaline phosphatase is raised in isolation in the majority of patients.

**Infections associated with HIV cholangiopathy**

- CMV
- Microsporidiosis
- Cryptosporidiosis
- *Mycobacterium avium intracellulare*

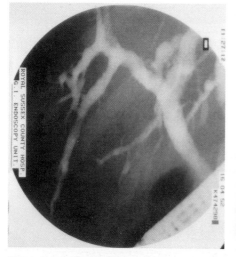

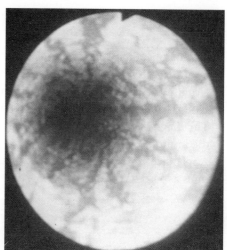

**Figure 6.6** ERCP appearance of HIV-associated cholangiopathy in a patient with CMV and cryptosporidiosis

**Figure 6.7** Endoscopic appearance of *Candida* oesophagitis

- Ultrasonography shows dilated intra- and extrahepatic bile ducts but may be normal.
- Endoscopic retrograde cholangiopancreatography (ERCP) (Figure 6.6) is required to the make the diagnosis. Biliary samples can be taken during the procedure to diagnose infection.
- Even with treatment of any underlying infection, symptomatic response is often disappointing although patients with papillary stenosis may improve following endoscopic sphincterotomy.

## DIFFERENTIAL DIAGNOSIS OF ABDOMINAL PAIN IN THE HIV INFECTED PATIENT

### EPIGASTRIC PAIN

- *Candida* oesophagitis (Figure 6.7)
- CMV oesophagitis/gastritis
- Peptic ulceration
- CMV duodenitis
- Pancreatitis.

### RIGHT UPPER QUADRANT PAIN

- Acalculous cholangitis
- AIDS-associated cholangitis
- Viral hepatitis.

## RIGHT ILIAC FOSSA PAIN

- Acute appendicitis.

## DIFFUSE ABDOMINAL PAIN WITH DIARRHOEA

- *Cryptosporidium*
- *Microsporidium*
- *Salmonella* species
- *Giardia lambia*
- *Campylobacter* species
- CMV
- *Mycobacterium avium* complex
- *Clostridium difficile.*

# ANORECTAL DISEASE IN HIV POSITIVE PATIENTS

Anorectal disease is common in HIV infected patients and is the most frequent reason for surgical referral. Anorectal disease is a result of anal intercourse and up to 15% will undergo anorectal surgery compared with 4% of non-homosexual HIV infected patients. The most frequent diagnoses in patients presenting with anorectal disease are:

- Anal and perianal warts (Figure 6.8)
- Anorectal ulceration
- Perianal sepsis
- Haemorrhoidal disease.

## ANOGENITAL WARTS

- Cutaneous warts **caused by human papilloma viruses (HPV)** are common in HIV infected individuals. They occur in the same areas as in non-infected individuals but tend to be greater in number and resistant to standard therapies.
- Anal and perianal warts unresponsive to topical therapy are the commonest indication for surgery in HIV infected patients, particularly in homosexual men. Anal HPV infection in the immunosuppressed can result in large cauliflower-like warts associated with anal discharge and perianal sogginess.

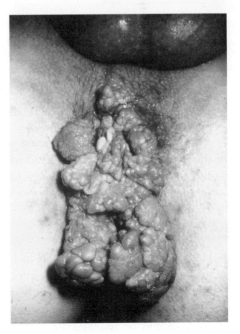

**Figure 6.8** Anal warts

- Treatment is by coagulation using electrocautery or scissor excision. Recurrence is common.
- **Squamous carcinoma of the anus** is seen more frequently in homosexual men and the immunosuppressed.
- HPV has been implicated in the pathogenesis of these conditions and therefore histological examination of warts in HIV positive patients should be routine.

## ANORECTAL ULCERATION

- The aetiology of the majority of cases of anorectal ulcers in HIV positive patients, particularly homosexual men, is infectious.
- **In all cases appropriate cultures and serological tests should be performed** before surgical referral.
- Ulceration due to herpes simplex virus infection (Figure 6.9) responds in the majority of cases to treatment with acyclovir; however, high doses may be required if the area of ulceration is extensive.
- In patients with anorectal ulcers resistant to medical therapy, surgical excision is recommended with histological examination for viral inclusion bodies of CMV and herpes simplex as well as evidence of malignancy.

> **Infectious causes of anorectal ulceration**
>
> - Herpes simplex
> - CMV
> - Syphilis
> - Chancroid
> - Lymphogranuloma venereum

## PERIANAL SEPSIS

- Perianal sepsis may be more common in HIV infected individuals although the evidence is conflicting. Perianal, low rectal and ischiorectal abscesses occur and can usually be managed by incision and drainage with good results.
- **Anorectal lymphoma is common** and this diagnosis must be considered when surgical treatment is considered for a suspected ischiorectal abscess.

## HAEMORRHOIDAL DISEASE

- Haemorrhoids are as common in HIV infected patients as in the non-infected population but are associated with receptive anal intercourse.
- They should be managed in a similar fashion to non-infectious patients.

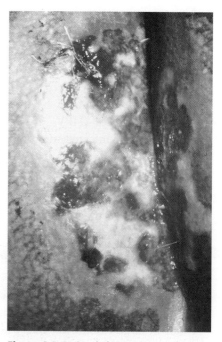

**Figure 6.9** Perianal ulceration caused by herpes simplex virus infection

# THE RISK OF OCCUPATIONAL HIV INFECTION IN HEALTH CARE WORKERS

The risk of HIV infection after percutaneous exposure to blood from HIV infected patients has been calculated as being between 0.1 and 0.36% – much lower than rates for patients infected with hepatitis B and C.

- **The major risk for acquiring HIV infection is from needle-stick injuries with hollow bore needles.**
- Needle-stick injuries from solid needles such as those used in suturing are associated with much lower rates of infection.
- Mucous membrane exposure is thought to have resulted in seroconversion in one health care worker – a nurse who sustained a mucous membrane and skin exposure with a large amount of HIV infected blood whilst unblocking an arterial line.
- There have been no reports of HIV seroconversion in health care workers as a result of aerosol exposure during orthopaedic surgery.

## PRECAUTIONS RECOMMENDED FOR OPERATING STAFF

All staff performing invasive procedures in all patients should adhere to the following:
- Be immunized against hepatitis B
- Cover all cuts and abrasions with waterproof dressings
- Do not pass sharps hand to hand
- Do not use hand needles
- Do not guide needles with fingers
- Do not re-sheath needles
- Dispose of all sharps safely into approved containers.

The following clothing should be worn when operating on high risk patients:
- Double gloves
- High efficiency masks
- Eye protection
- Boots
- Impervious gowns.

# PROPHYLAXIS AFTER OCCUPATIONAL EXPOSURE TO HIV

Although the mainstay of preventing occupationally acquired HIV infection is the safe handling of sharps, post-exposure prophylaxis (PEP) is recommended by the Ministry of Health in the United Kingdom and the US Public Health Service.

- Zidovudine given soon after percutaneous exposure reduces the risk of sero-conversion by up to 79%. Although most of the evidence for post-exposure prophylaxis is based on the use of zidovudine alone, more potent combinations of antiretroviral agents are now recommended.
- Health care workers exposed to high risk body fluids or tissues known to be, or strongly suspected to be, infected with HIV through percutaneous exposure, mucous membrane exposure or exposure through broken skin should be recommended to have a combination of:

  zidovudine 250 mg t.d.s. or b.d + lamivudine 150 mg b.d. + indinavir 800 mg t.d.s.

- Post-exposure prophylaxis should be taken as quickly as possible following exposure but may be considered up to 2 weeks after exposure.
- PEP should be taken for 4 weeks.

---

## CRIB BOX – HIV AND THE SURGEON

Abdominal pain is a frequent symptom in HIV positive patients

Common causes of an 'acute abdomen' are:

- Cytomegalovirus infection
- Kaposi's sarcoma
- Lymphoma
- Acute appendicitis
- Cholecystitis
- Biliary disease

Treatment is primarily medical and, apart from patients with acute appendicitis, surgery is only indicated in patients with complications, usually:

- Perforation
- Obstruction
- Ischaemia
- Haemorrhage
- Medically refractory toxic megacolon

15% of HIV infected homosexual men undergo surgery for anorectal disease; commonest indications are:

- Anorectal warts
- Anorectal ulceration
- Sepsis
- Haemorrhoids

The risk of seroconversion following percutaneous exposure to HIV blood is 0.1–0.36%

Needle-stick injuries with hollow bore needles are associated with the greatest risk

Post-exposure prophylaxis (PEP) is recommended in cases of percutaneous or mucous membrane exposure or exposure through broken skin to high risk body fluids. The recommended drug combination is:

- Zidovudine
- Lamivudine
- Indinavir

# chapter 7

# TRAUMA

The proper management of trauma can mean the difference between life and death, or full recovery and permanent disability.

Every doctor must have a basic knowledge of how to cope with a trauma victim, whether it be at the roadside or in the resuscitation room.

Deaths from major trauma occur in three phases:

1 **Immediate** (50%) – due to lethal injury
2 **Early** (30%) – within the first few hours due to intracranial bleeding and exsanguination from visceral injury or from multiple fractures
3 **Late** (20%) – after a period of weeks due to sepsis and multiple organ failure.

## MECHANISM OF TRAUMA

Trauma can be classified broadly into:

- Blunt, e.g. road traffic accidents (RTAs) (acceleration/deceleration injury); falls; assaults
- Penetrating, e.g. high and low velocity missiles; stab wounds.

> To have the best chance of survival and recovery, severely injured patients must be resuscitated within an hour – **'the golden hour'**.

There are three aspects to the management of the trauma victim:

1 Safety of the patient and attendant personnel
2 Primary survey and resuscitation (or 'A,B,C...')
3 Secondary survey and subsequent management.

## THE PREHOSPITAL PHASE

On arriving at the scene of an incident ensure that both you and the victim are safe. Note the **mechanism** and severity of the injury (e.g. was a seat belt worn; speed of vehicle; height of fall, etc.).

The initial treatment requires a **primary survey** of the victim, using the classic **'ABCs'** mnemonic:

- **A**irway and cervical spine control
- **B**reathing and ventilation
- **C**irculation and haemorrhage control
- **D**isability: neurological status
- **E**vacuation – exposure – environment

## AIRWAY AND CERVICAL SPINE CONTROL

- The **airway** must be inspected to ensure patency and any blockages removed.
- Maintain the airway in unconscious patients with a chin lift or jaw thrust.
- **Protect the cervical spine.** Neck movement should be avoided by the use of cervical splints, collar, or tape to the forehead to hold the patient's head in a neutral position. **A cervical spine injury must be assumed** in any major trauma.

## BREATHING AND VENTILATION

- The patency of the airway must be ensured.
- If the victim is not breathing, artificial respiration is commenced, with mouth-to-mouth breathing if masks and intubation facilities are not available. Oxygen, if available, should be given at the highest concentration possible.
- Certain injuries impair ventilation, including tension and open pneumothorax, flail chest and massive haemothorax.
- Fractured ribs and pulmonary contusion may compromise ventilation to a lesser degree.
- A sucking chest wound (**open pneumothorax**) should be covered and tension pneumothorax relieved by inserting a needle into the affected side.

## CIRCULATION AND HAEMORRHAGE CONTROL

- External blood loss is controlled by direct pressure, not tourniquets.
- Conscious level, colour, pulse rate and volume are a good guide to blood loss.
- An irregular pulse may signify heart or pericardial problems.

## DISABILITY AND NEUROLOGICAL STATUS

The neurological status is monitored and recorded, using the Glasgow coma scale if possible. Alternatively, the AVPU method is short and simple:
- **A**lert
- Responds to **V**ocal stimuli
- Responds to **P**ainful stimuli
- **U**nresponsive.

Grossly deformed fractured limbs should be straightened and splinted to avoid neurovascular complications.

## EVACUATION – EXPOSURE – ENVIRONMENT

- The patient should be evacuated to a trauma centre as soon as is practicable.
- The injury and status of the patient should be related to the centre.
- Measures should be taken to avoid hypothermia and continuing danger of injury to the patient.
- Appropriately trained staff may instigate fluid resuscitation and tracheal intubation before transfer.

Hospital 'trauma centres' are fully equipped and staffed to cope with all aspects of trauma, with specialist facilities such as neurosurgery and cardiothoracic surgery on site.

Helicopter transport expedites the transfer of patients from the accident scene to hospital.

## THE HOSPITAL PHASE

As soon as the patient arrives, the primary survey, using 'ABCs', is repeated and resuscitation commenced. Life-threatening conditions, the primary survey, and resuscitation are managed simultaneously.

### AIRWAY AND CERVICAL SPINE CONTROL

- Airway patency is maintained as necessary using an oro- or nasopharyngeal airway, oro- or nasoendotracheal intubation, or cricothyroidotomy.
- The cervical spine is protected throughout.
- **All patients require supplemental oxygen**, the delivery of which can be monitored with a pulse oximeter.

### BREATHING AND VENTILATION

- If breathing is impaired despite an adequate airway, intubation and **assisted ventilation** are instituted. Exposure and examination of the chest will reveal adequacy of chest excursions, air entry, pneumothorax, haemothorax, etc.
- A nasogastric tube will prevent aspiration of stomach contents into the chest.

### CIRCULATION

- The circulation must be assessed and intravenous access achieved with **at least two wide bore cannulae.** CVP monitoring may be indicated. Rapid fluid resuscitation with crystalloid is commenced – 2 or 3 litres may be required to effect a satisfactory haemodynamic response.
- Blood is taken for the following:
  Full blood count
  Urea and electrolytes, amylase
  Cross-matching
  Arterial blood gases.

- Shock is usually due to blood loss and cross-matched blood is given as soon as possible. *In extremis*, type-specific un-cross-matched blood, or O negative blood is used.
- ECG, ventilation, temperature, pulse and blood pressure monitoring is begun.
- A urethral catheter monitors urine output but should not be inserted if there is a possibility of urethral trauma (e.g. pelvic fracture).

## DISABILITY AND NEUROLOGICAL STATUS

- Neurological appraisal is continued throughout, bearing in mind that deterioration of haemodynamic state, oxygenation, ventilation, drugs, alcohol and intracranial bleeding will have effects.

## EXPOSURE – ENVIRONMENT

- All clothing is removed to facilitate thorough examination and the patient protected from hypothermia with warm blankets and a warm environment.
- Intravenous fluids should be warmed before use.

## SECONDARY SURVEY AND INVESTIGATIONS

The secondary survey consists of assessment of the adequacy of resuscitation (blood pressure, pulse, respiration and temperature). It begins only after the primary survey is completed. Falling blood pressure, tachycardia and other signs of shock indicate inadequate resuscitation or continued bleeding into a body cavity.

A **full history** is needed. If not available from the patient, family members and prehospital emergency service staff are consulted. The **mechanism, type** and possible **severity** of injury are clearly important. The mnemonic AMPLE is often used:

- Allergies
- Medication
- Past illnesses
- Last meal
- Events relating to the injury.

A **head to toe, front and back, examination** of the patient is necessary – each region of the body is examined in detail and radiology requested as appropriate. The secondary survey has been described as 'tubes and fingers in every orifice'.

## HEAD AND FACE

- The conscious level is assessed using the Glasgow coma scale.
- The entire scalp and head is examined for lacerations, contusions and evidence of fractures.
- The eyes and pupils are carefully examined even in the presence of periorbital oedema.
- The presence of a basal skull fracture can be inferred from bleeding or CSF leakage from the nose and ears.
- **Battle's sign** (bruising around the mastoid processes) and **raccoon eyes** (bilateral circumorbital bruising) are also indications of an underlying basal skull fracture.
- If a serious head injury is suspected then arrangements must be made to obtain a **CT scan** of the head provided the patient is stable.

- **Scalp lacerations** are sutured when the patient is stable, except when they are a source of continuing blood loss. Suturing will invariably control any haemorrhage from scalp lacerations.
- The treatment of **maxillofacial trauma** can be delayed until the patient has been fully stabilized, provided it is not associated with airway obstruction.

## NECK

> It is assumed that all patients have an **unstable cervical spine** until proven otherwise, and the neck should be kept in a hard collar until a cervical injury has been excluded.

- Assessment of the neck includes palpating for cervical tenderness and arranging for cervical spine x-rays – AP and lateral views.
- Care must be taken that all seven cervical vertebrae and the first thoracic vertebra are adequately visualized on these x-rays; it may be necessary to repeat them with traction on the arms to get appropriate views.
- If there is a high index of suspicion of a cervical injury, the neck must be kept immobilized and expert opinion sought from orthopaedic or neurosurgeons.

## CHEST

- Life-threatening lesions will have been identified during the primary survey.
- The secondary survey will identify other possibly lethal conditions such as:

  Pneumothorax (Figure 7.1)
  Haemothorax
  Rib fractures
  Sternal fractures
  Flail segments
  Rupture of diaphragm
  Myocardial contusion
  Pulmonary contusion
  Tracheal injuries
  Aortic transection.

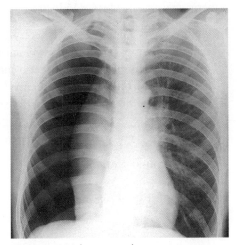

**Figure 7.1** Right pneumothorax

## ABDOMEN

**Penetrating injuries** are usually stab or bullet wounds (Figure 7.2). **Blunt injuries** usually result from assault or road traffic accidents (seat belt/steering wheel injury).

- The abdomen is initially assessed by **inspection**.
- Penetrating injury sites may be obvious but firearm injury **entry sites** may be overlooked.

- Bruising from seat belts or assault may be an indication of serious intra-abdominal injury.
- **Palpation** of the abdomen in the conscious patient may elicit the usual signs of tenderness, guarding and rigidity, but the clinical assessment of the unconscious patient is not as straightforward.

### Penetrating injuries

**Stab wounds** If possible, it is useful to have a history of the mechanism of injury and even to observe the offending weapon itself.
- A long thin 'stiletto' blade may cause considerable intraperitoneal damage.
- A wide carving knife may create only superficial injuries.
- If the patient is fully conscious and there is no clinical evidence of intraperitoneal injury, he/she may be treated conservatively and observed for changes in symptoms and vital signs.
- If there is evisceration of bowel or doubt about intra-abdominal injury, laparotomy should be performed and the damaged organs repaired.
- There is currently interest in the use of laparoscopy to assess intraperitoneal injury in both penetrating and blunt abdominal trauma.

**Ballistic injuries** The extent of damage caused by a missile or fragment (Figure 7.2) is dependent primarily on its speed and the track it takes through the body:

Kinetic energy = ½ Mass × Velocity²

- High velocity missile wounds (e.g. rifle, bomb fragment) cause extensive damage when compared with low velocity hand gun injuries. A high velocity missile imparts a much greater kinetic energy and causes tissue cavitation damage far removed from its track and entry/exit sites.
- In general, all firearm injuries to the abdomen require surgical exploration and laparotomy.

### Blunt injuries

Blunt abdominal trauma is much more common in the UK than penetrating injuries and usually results from RTAs. Crush or shearing injuries to the bowel, mesentery and solid organs are common.

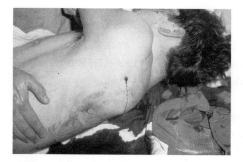

**Figure 7.2** Gunshot wound – left chest entering through the shoulder posteriorly. (Courtesy: Department of Military Surgery, Royal Army Medical College and Leonard Cheshire Department of Conflict Recovery at University College London)

- The presence of generalized or localized peritonism indicates intraperitoneal damage to hollow viscera or solid organs.
- If the patient is stable, further assessment by radiological means such as ultrasound or CT scanning may allow enough reassurance to manage the patient conservatively.
- **Repeated assessment** of the patient is required to look for changes that indicate the need for laparotomy, such as tachycardia, hypotension or altered abdominal signs.

In the unconscious patient it is more difficult to make a clinical assessment of the need for surgical intervention but various diagnostic aids are available **to assess the presence of intraperitoneal injury**:
- Diagnostic peritoneal lavage – blood; bowel contents
- Mini-laparotomy
- CT scanning
- Laparoscopy.

## PELVIS

**Major pelvic fracture** is often associated with **considerable retroperitoneal blood loss** and this needs to be taken into account in the fluid management of the patient. Unstable pelvic fractures need urgent stabilization.

The following checks lead to a diagnosis of pelvic injury:
- Pressing on both anterior superior iliac spines and the symphysis pubis – these structures should be absolutely stable. If there is any pain or evidence of mobility a major pelvic fracture should be considered.
- Blood at the external meatus of the penis is a sign of urethral injury which is often associated with serious pelvic damage.

**Radiological assessment** of the pelvis is by:
- Plain abdominal x-ray
  - Identifying disruption of the bony pelvic ring
  - Diastasis of the sacroiliac joints and symphysis pubis
- CT and MRI scanning.

## EXTREMITIES

The upper and lower limbs should be inspected for any signs of obvious fractures and wounds. The joints are also examined carefully.
- Vascular compromise must be excluded by **examining the pulse distal to any fracture.**
- Fractures of the lower limb may require **splinting** to reduce blood loss and pain.
- **Compound fractures** should be covered with Betadine-soaked dressings.
- **Antibiotics and tetanus prophylaxis** should be given immediately.

- **Radiological assessment** of any suspected fractures should be carried out once the patient has been resuscitated and more life-threatening injuries excluded or appropriately treated.
- Haemorrhage from wounds should be controlled by local pressure.

## SPINE AND BACK

At some point during the secondary survey it is essential that the patient is 'log rolled' such that the back can be examined along with digital examination of the rectum. The back is inspected for obvious wounds and injuries and the spine palpated for deformities, or tenderness in the conscious patient.

## PERINEUM

The perineum should be inspected for injury.
- The presence of **blood at the external urinary meatus is a sign of urethral damage.**
- Bleeding from the vagina may indicate menses, miscarriage or trauma.
- Pregnancy in a woman of child-bearing age must always be considered.
- **Digital examination** of the vagina, anus and rectum is mandatory. **Palpation of the anal sphincter and assessment of sphincter tone may give clues to spinal injury.** The presence of blood in the rectum is indicative of rectal trauma. Rectal and anal sphincter injuries often necessitate temporary defunctioning with a colostomy.
- In severe pelvic injuries the prostate gland may be dislocated, indicating rupture of the membranous urethra.

## NEUROLOGICAL

It is essential to perform a **thorough neurological examination** of the patient. This may have to be modified if the patient is unconscious. Tone, power and reflexes of the limbs should be assessed along with sensation. The cranial nerves should be examined and may reveal evidence of intracranial injury.

## DEFINITIVE TREATMENT

Following the primary survey and resuscitation, and the secondary survey and investigations, the patient will need definitive treatment. This will invariably involve surgery of some sort and many specialists will need to collaborate to ensure a successful outcome. Deciding 'where to begin' definitive treatment in a multiple trauma victim is determined by which is the most life-threatening injury. Throughout the period of definitive treatment, the patient must be constantly re-evaluated using the ABCs.

# TRAUMA SCORING SYSTEMS

- Glasgow coma scale – used in the assessment of head injuries.
- APACHE – acute physiology and chronic health evaluation. This is a complex scoring system, which is of little use in the acute situation, but can be useful for stratification of patients and audit.
- SAPS – simplified acute physiology score. This is a simplified version of the APACHE system.

---

**CRIB BOX – TRAUMA**

Trauma management includes:

- Patient safety
- Primary survey and resuscitation (**know your ABCs**)
- Secondary survey and subsequent management

**Look after the cervical spine!!**

Distinguish between **penetrating** and **blunt** injuries of the chest and abdomen

**Clinical and radiological** assessment of limb and spinal injuries is vital

**Scoring systems** are an aid in assessing severity of injury

# chapter 8

# BURNS AND RECONSTRUCTIVE SURGERY

## BURNS

Burn injury can be caused by flame, heat, electricity, radiation and exposure to chemicals.

> The primary pathology is destruction of skin, the body's protection against a hostile environment. This allows body fluids to evaporate and heat to be lost whilst presenting bacteria with a perfect medium for growth and a portal of entry to infect the victim.

Thus what looks like superficial trauma to the skin will have a far-reaching effect upon the whole patient. A major burn injury will require many visits to the operating room to restore skin cover by grafting. The patient will also need the support of specialists such as dietitians, physiotherapists, occupational therapists, psychiatrists, counsellors, social workers and many others. Treatment is therefore a team effort where each member is as important to success as the next.

### PRIMARY CARE

Major burn should be managed initially as in any other form of major trauma, i.e. **ABCs** (see Chapter 7). If a burn has occurred within 15 minutes, the extent of the injury may be lessened by removing the clothing and cooling the burn area with cold water. Chemicals and smoke may be absorbed into clothing and must be removed in these injuries. The patient is then wrapped warmly as body heat will be lost rapidly and a fall in core temperature will increase morbidity and mortality. Cling film, if available, can be placed over the burn. Damp or wet dressings will cause great heat loss and should be avoided in all but the smallest of injuries. The victim must be removed to safety if exposure to heat, smoke, chemicals or irradiation continues.

Rapid transport to a primary care facility should be organized. The commonest cause of death at this stage is hypoxia due to oxygen being used up in the combustion process, or by smoke inhalation and toxic fumes from combustible materials. Thus **airway management** is an important primary care consideration – Airway, Breathing, Circulation.

## DEFINITION OF A MAJOR BURN

A major burn is defined as:

'A burn of 20% total body surface area (TBSA) or more between the ages of 10 and 50 years. A burn greater than 10% TBSA under the age of 10 or over 50. Any burn with over 10% TBSA full thickness injury. Any burn associated with an inhalation injury or major trauma. Any electrical or chemical burn. Any burn involving the hands, feet, face or perineum.'

**Major burn**

- Greater than 20% TBSA
- Greater than 10% TBSA over 50 or under 10 years
- Greater than 10% TBSA full thickness injury
- Associated major trauma
- Associated inhalation injury
- Electrical or chemical injury
- Involving the hands, feet, face or perineum

- **The % TBSA** is estimated using the 'rule of nines' (Figure 8.1); alternatively, the patient's whole palm is roughly 1% of the body surface area and can be used as a guide.
- **Electrical and chemical burns** may involve deeper tissue structures and also cause metabolic disturbances.
- **Inhalation injury** may impair gaseous exchange and be life-threatening.
- **Major trauma** will complicate resuscitation and may require urgent surgery, blood replacement and other life-saving interventions.
- **Hands, feet, and face burns** are serious as they will limit function if not treated urgently.
- Burns to the **perineum** are easily infected by faecal contamination and are technically difficult to graft.

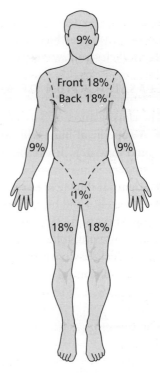

## THE SKIN

**Figure 8.1** Rule of nines

The skin is made up of layers. The outermost

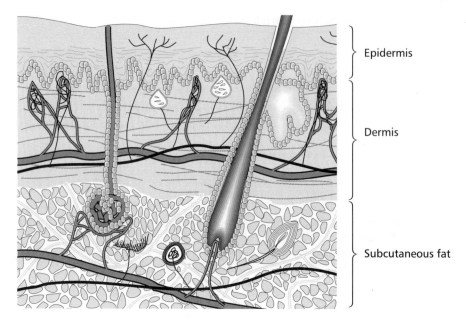

**Figure 8.2** Cross-section of the skin

layer is the epidermis being 20–1400 μm thick. Under this lies the dermis which is 400–2500 μm thick and contains downgrowths from the epidermis, such as hair follicles and sweat glands. A cross-section of the skin is shown in Figure 8.2.

## CLASSIFICATION OF BURNS

The classification of burns depends on their depth.

- **A superficial burn** will only involve the epidermis. It will be red and painful and may itch. It can be likened to a moderate sunburn and will not require surgery. It may also be called a **first degree** burn.
- **A partial thickness burn** involves the dermis. Some hair follicles and glands are damaged if the burn is not deep; this is a **second degree** or superficial partial thickness burn. If left, this wound will heal, without skin grafting, from cells in the surviving follicles and glands but will result in gross scarring. A deep partial thickness burn destroys most of the follicles and glands and will require skin grafting.

**Burn depth**

- Superficial or first degree – epidermis only
- Partial thickness or second degree – epidermis and dermis
- Deep partial thickness – dermis with sweat glands and hair follicles
- Full thickness or third degree – all layers to fat
- Fourth degree – underlying viscera or organs

- **A full thickness burn** will reach the subcutaneous tissue and fat and destroy all layers of skin. This is also called a **third degree burn**.
- **Fourth degree burns** involve underlying viscera or other organs (e.g. bone, liver).

## PATHOPHYSIOLOGY OF BURNS

On sustaining a burn injury, the body is presented with an interface between live, healthy tissue and dead and dying tissue. This interface will allow products from the wound to be transported by blood to all parts of the body. These products are very active and consist of **cytokines, denatured proteins** and many other **vasoactive substances**. In a massive burn they may cause immediate cardiovascular collapse and death. However, more commonly, there is a fall in cardiac output and a loss of vascular integrity, resulting in a **decreased circulating volume** and increased extracellular volume. Fluid is also lost into the burn wound and evaporation from this will accentuate the loss from the intravascular space.

If the patient survives, a rise in endogenous catecholamines will produce a **tachycardia** to compensate for the decreased intravascular volume and fall in peripheral resistance. This will also counteract the negative inotropic effects of the burn wound upon the heart and restore contractile power.

If no fluid is replaced, the haematocrit will rise, the circulating volume will fall and the patient will die. Survival depends on replacing the lost fluid and maintaining the intravascular volume. This is called fluid resuscitation. **Immediate survival depends on fluid resuscitation to maintain the intravascular volume.**

Satisfactory resuscitation will result in the vital signs bottoming out at approximately 2 hours and then improving. Cardiac output will return to normal at about 8 hours. It may double by 24 hours and may treble by 36 hours. Victims with ischaemic heart disease may not survive this initial period.

Core temperature will be reset to 38.5°C towards the end of resuscitation and oxygen consumption will be increased until skin coverage is complete. The patient must be kept warm to decrease the adverse effects of the injury. The victim will need extra calories to sustain the rise in core temperature and the increased heat loss through the burn wound. Muscle wasting will occur but can be limited by adequate nutrition. The high catecholamine output may result in an insulin-resistant hyperglycaemia and increased urine output caused by the osmotic effects of the ensuing glycosuria.

## FLUID RESUSCITATION

The initial treatment for burn injuries is to replace the intravascular fluid. This may be achieved using:

- Colloids such as 4.5% Human Albumin solution
- Crystalloids such as Ringer's lactate solution or Hartmann's solution
- Hypertonic crystalloids such as lactated 0.9% saline.

Each fluid has a formula based upon body weight, % total body surface area burned and time (Table 8.1).

In the United Kingdom the commonest regimen used is the **Muir and Barclay formula**. This uses 4.5% Human Albumin solution. From the time of the injury the resuscitation is split into six periods. The same amount of fluid is given in each period and is calculated as:

$$\frac{\text{Weight in kilograms} \times \% \text{ TBSA}}{2} = \text{ml of 4.5\% albumin}$$

From the time of the burn there are three periods of 4 hours, followed by two periods of 6 hours and finally one period of 12 hours. In addition, the normal daily requirements must be given.

The **Parkland formula** uses Ringer's lactate and is the commonest throughout the world. The amount of fluid to be given over 24 hours is calculated as:

$$\text{Weight in kilograms} \times \% \text{ TBSA} \times 4 = \text{ml Ringer's solution}$$

Half this amount is to be given in the first 8 hours; a quarter in the next 8 hours and the final quarter in the last 8 hours. This gives a 24-hour resuscitation period. No additional fluids need be given as each litre of Hartmann's has approximately 100 ml free water to act as the daily requirement.

**Table 8.1** Resuscitation formulae

| Formula | Fluid | Amount | Time period |
|---|---|---|---|
| Muir & Barclay | 4.5% Albumin | Wt × %TBSA/2 | Per period<br>3 × 4-hour periods<br>2 × 6-hour periods<br>1 × 12-hour period |
| Parkland | Hartmann's | Wt × %TBSA × 4 | 24 hours<br>Half in 8 hours<br>Quarter in 8 hours<br>Quarter in 8 hours |
| Hypertonic saline | 0.9% Saline plus 100 mmol sodium lactate per litre | 0.3 ml per kg × %TBSA | Per hour and review |

Finally, there is a hypertonic formula based on that suggested by **Monafo**. A solution is made up by adding 100 mmol sodium lactate to 0.9% saline solution. This is given at 0.3 ml/kg body weight per % TBSA over 1 hour. The plasma sodium is monitored and not allowed to exceed 160 mmol/l and the urine output must be greater than 0.5 ml/kg body weight per hour. The fluid is adjusted to maintain these parameters.

These formulae are only a guide. The response to resuscitation should be monitored and the fluids adjusted accordingly. The cardiac output and vascular filling are measured indirectly **by monitoring the urine output which must be maintained at >0.5 ml/kg/h.**

## INHALATION INJURY

A burn to the face can be superficial and cause dramatic swelling but will not compromise the airway. However, it may be associated with damage within the mouth and this can extend to lung tissue through the larynx and down the trachea and bronchi. Damage can also be sustained without facial injury by the inhalation of hot gases and particulate matter, superheated steam, noxious fumes or products of combustion. These may cause swelling in the upper airways and obstruction (Figure 8.3), or they may cause irritation to the lung tissue which will greatly decrease the efficiency of lung function.

**Any sign of inhalation of heat or smoke such as burned nasal hairs, intra-oral burns, cough or voice change, carbonaceous sputum or a suggestive history must be treated as a matter of urgency** and a tracheal tube inserted to avoid obstruction at a later time.

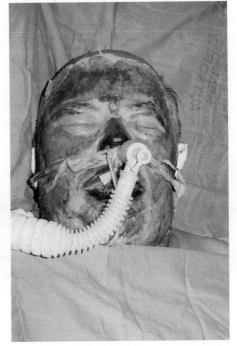

**Figure 8.3** Facial swelling during resuscitation

### Diagnosis and treatment of inhalation injury
- Inhalation injury is not a single entity.
- Treatment (Table 8.2) must be directed to maintaining a patent airway; adequate oxygenation with or without mechanical ventilation; and excretion of carbon dioxide.
- Inhaled poisons from burning materials may need specific treatments (cyanide and thiocyanate; carbon monoxide and hyperbaric oxygen).

**Table 8.2** Diagnosis and treatment of inhalation injury

| Site of injury | Treatment | Reason |
| --- | --- | --- |
| Superficial facial | None | Swelling will be gross but no airway obstruction |
| Lips to larynx | Intubate ± mechanical ventilation | Swelling may cause obstruction of airway |
| Below larynx | Intubate, sedate and mechanical ventilation | Obstruction risk and lung damage; poor gas diffusion |
| Inhalation of noxious substances | Intubate, sedate, oxygen therapy, mechanical ventilation | Pneumonitis; parenchymal damage; diffusion problems |

## PROGNOSIS OF BURN INJURY

There may be occasions when a burn injury is too severe and resuscitation would be unsuccessful. These cases must be discussed fully with the staff treating the patient and the patient's relatives, taking into account hospital guidelines, policies and current legislation.

A rough guideline to chances of survival can be obtained by **adding the age to % TBSA burned and subtracting this from 100.** This will give the percentage chance of survival, i.e. a 45-year-old with a 35% TBSA burn will have a 20% survival rate. However, very young victims have a higher mortality rate. Mortality risk is increased if the victim has a concurrent medical condition, by approximately 11% per illness. Current intensive care techniques increase survival chances, giving 80% TBSA burns a possible 50% chance of survival in some units.

## TREATMENT OF BURN INJURY

Historically, burns were treated without surgical intervention. The burned tissue was allowed to dry and separate from the living tissue; the underlying granulations were treated with tannin solutions as in the leather making industry, resulting in a hard, highly scarred, contracted surface. Today, the burn is left to separate in only those patients who would not survive a surgical procedure due to other concurrent illnesses, or when the burn is superficial enough that it will heal without intervention.

- **Surgical excision** of burns is the treatment of choice. The burn wound is excised tangentially to the surface, layer by layer until viable non-burned tissue is exposed. If very superficial, no other treatment is necessary. However, the majority of burns will require a skin graft to give adequate coverage of the wound and a satisfactory cosmetic result.

- **Wound coverage** is achieved by taking a tangential slice of epidermis (**a split skin graft**) from a non-burned area, commonly the thighs, and placing this over the wound. This graft will take very quickly and the donor site will heal within a week. Another harvest can then be taken. In big burns it is wise not to excise more than 20% TBSA burn at one visit to the operating theatre. Skin grafts can be meshed and stretched over larger areas. The more the stretch ratio, the greater the scarring as the wound has to heal from the edges of the mesh. Commonest ratios are 1:2 or 1:3 but if unburned areas are scarce a 1:9 mesh can be used.
- **Functional areas** are grafted first as delay will increase morbidity. However, if venous access is limited and has to be obtained through burned tissue, access sites will have priority to allow venous access through clean, grafted sites.

## COMPLICATIONS OF BURNS

### Infection
After leaving the site of injury alive, **the major cause of death is infection.** Early excision of the burn wound after resuscitation decreases this risk, as does quick and adequate wound coverage. The wound can be covered with an antimicrobial agent, such as silver sulphadiazine cream, or the excised site covered with xenograft or a synthetic covering such as Biobrane.

**Complications of burns**

- Infection
- Circulation, especially hands & feet
- Renal failure
- Abdominal crises
- Blood loss
- Nutritional
- Respiratory

### Circulation
The eschar is burned tissue which has lost its elasticity and becomes dry. **Eschar formation in circumferential burns will constrict the underlying tissues** and thus must be released with escharotomies. The escharotomy must reach underlying healthy tissue to be effective. Hands and feet are very vulnerable.

### Renal
Inadequate resuscitation will result in decreased renal function, or acute tubular necrosis and **renal failure.** A period of haemofiltration or dialysis may be required. If blood pressure or intravascular volume has not been maintained the patient may suffer from myocardial ischaemia or a cerebral vascular accident.

### Abdominal
Other complications include gastric ulceration (**Curling's ulcer**), which has become rare since the introduction of H$_2$ antagonists, and acalculous cholecystitis. Superior mesenteric artery syndrome and acute pancreatitis may present as an acute abdominal event.

### Haematological

Blood loss may be massive during excision of the burn wound. Normal erythropoeisis is suppressed and makes transfusion an inevitable event. Most commonly after excision of the wound, bleeding will be profuse and a consumption coagulation defect will occur, made worse by dilution with plasma expanders. These conditions can be reversed with fresh frozen plasma and platelets. The patient may exhibit hypercoagulability if allowed to become dehydrated.

### Nutrition

Adequate nutrition is difficult to maintain and burns that have a deficit of over 10 000 kcal have a greater mortality. Enteral nutrition is preferred as sufficient calories may be impossible to give parenterally. There is always the possibility of infection when using the parenteral route and dedicated central venous lines may be a luxury that cannot be afforded.

### Respiratory

Tracheostomy is associated with a greatly increased mortality and is only performed when oral or nasal endotracheal tubes are impossible to place or manage. Chest burns may constrict the thoracic cavity and limit respiratory excursion and may necessitate escharotomy.

## RECONSTRUCTIVE SURGERY

Reconstructive surgery is concerned with the restoration of form and function of damaged tissues. Primarily this means skin grafts to cover burned areas. At a later stage it will mean dealing with contractures that may have formed, especially those across joints, as these will limit movement.

However, reconstructive surgery is not limited to burns alone. Hand trauma may require extensive reconstruction to produce satisfactory function. This may involve grafting, tendon transfers, digit transplants and microvascular surgery. These techniques may be used at other sites where trauma has disrupted form and function. Reconstruction may be necessary to correct birth defects such as cleft lip (Figure 8.4) and palate deformity.

Deficits of tissue left after trauma or extensive surgery may be filled using tissue transfer. An example of **free tissue transfer** is the use of a myocutaneous flap from latissimus dorsi placed over a tibial wound, usually the result of a motor cycle accident; or a radial forearm flap (bone and muscle) used to reconstruct the mandible after a resection for an invasive malignant growth. If the tissue maintains its original blood supply, it can be rotated or transposed to a nearby region (**rotation flap**). This technique is used in breast reconstruction after a total mastectomy to restore some of the original body contour.

These techniques are being used more and more outside the realms of a single speciality (plastic surgery), i.e. by maxillofacial surgeons, trauma surgeons, and breast surgeons. Thus the techniques used by plastic surgeons have become important to all branches of surgery.

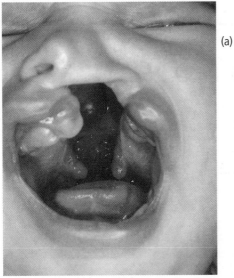
(a)

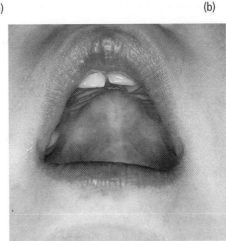
(b)

**Figure 8.4** (a) Cleft lip; (b) Result after repair

## COSMETIC SURGERY

The altering of form to satisfy the request of the individual is a branch of plastic surgery called cosmetic or aesthetic surgery. These operations are performed for various reasons. They may be used to remove excess tissue or fat, e.g. liposuction of the abdomen, face lifts; or to change shape as in rhinoplasty or breast augmentation or reduction. Some have sound psychological reasons whilst at the other end of the spectrum they are performed to satisfy a whim.

---

**CRIB BOX – BURNS AND RECONSTRUCTIVE SURGERY**

Learn definition of major burn

Burn classification according to depth

- Superficial
- Partial
- Deep partial
- Full
- Fourth degree

**Burn survival depends on fluid resuscitation** to maintain circulation

Inhalation injury is always serious

Prognosis is a function of age, fitness and %TBSA burn

Burns have **local** and **general** effects

Complications:

- Infection
- Circulation, especially hands and feet
- Renal failure
- Abdominal crises
- Blood loss
- Nutritional
- Respiratory

# chapter 9

# MALIGNANT DISEASE

## NATURE OF TUMOURS

### DEFINITION OF TUMOUR

A tumour (syn: neoplasm; new growth [NG]) is an abnormal mass of tissue, the growth of which exceeds and is unco-ordinated with that of normal tissues, and persists in the same excessive manner after cessation of the stimulus which evoked the change.

Tumours may be **benign** or **malignant** (Table 9.1).

**Table 9.1** Characteristics of benign and malignant tumours

| Benign | Malignant |
|---|---|
| Resembles tissue of origin | Often atypical, incomplete differentiation |
| Grows by expansion | Grows by expansion and infiltration |
| Forms a capsule (compressed adjacent normal cells) | Infiltrates adjacent tissues, so rarely forms a capsule |
| Growth remains localized | Ability for distant spread via lymphatic and blood vessels (metastasis) |
| Typically slow growing | Variable growth rates; tumour growth rates are log normally distributed |
| Histologically, few mitotic cells | Frequent mitotic cells seen |
| Cells of tumour look normal | Malignant cytological features: cellular atypia and pleomorphism; hyperchromatic cells; increased nuclear:cytoplasmic ratio |
| Usually harmless (depending on site of tumour but meningioma may compress brain tissue; pituitary adenoma may secrete hormones) | Endangers life by progressive spread, causing weight loss, cachexia. Spread to: liver = liver failure; brain = raised intracranial pressure |

## MALIGNANT TUMOURS

- Tumours arising from **epithelium** are known as **carcinomas** or **cancers**.
- Those arising from **mesothelium** (connective tissue) are known as **sarcomas** (Gk. flesh).
- The ability of the tumour cells to pass through the basement membrane is known as **infiltration**.
- Tumours that are *in situ* are those whose cells have the cytological appearances of malignant cells, but have not yet infiltrated the basement membrane.

### GRADING OF MALIGNANT TUMOURS

- The spectrum of grading ranges from **well differentiated** (those tumours that resemble their parent tissue histologically), through **poorly differentiated,** to **anaplastic** (in which the tumour bears no resemblance to its parent tissue).
- Anaplastic tumours have a rapid growth rate, metastasize early, and have a poor prognosis.

## PATHOGENESIS OF CANCER

Tumours develop because of a series of mutations in the genes that control cell growth. Some mutations can be inherited, others caused by high energy irradiation or chemical **carcinogens**.
- **Proto-oncogenes** encode for proteins that encourage cell growth and division.
- **Tumour suppressor genes** encode proteins that retard cell growth and division.

### ONCOGENES

**Mutations** in proto-oncogenes result in **oncogenes** which produce either:
- Too much growth stimulatory protein (e.g. platelet derived growth factor, PDGF)
- Overactive cell membrane receptors (e.g. *erb*-B, *erb*-B2) for growth factors
- A more active form of the cytoplasmic relay (*ras*) protein (e.g. Ki-*ras*, N-*ras*).

### SUPPRESSOR GENES

- halt cell growth (e.g. Rb, p53)
- or induce apoptosis (abnormal cells killing themselves) in abnormal cells (e.g. p53).
- Suppressor genes contribute to cancer when they are inactivated by mutations, depriving the cell of growth suppressing proteins.

Genetic mutations will typically have occurred decades before a tumour becomes palpable. They cause:
- Hyperplasia – a genetically altered cell may divide at a higher rate than its neighbouring cells

- Dysplasia – one in a million of these hyperplastic cells may suffer an additional mutation which loosens the control of cell growth still further, causing the cell to have an abnormal (**dysplastic**) appearance (Figure 9.1)

- *In-situ* cancer – if a group of dysplastic cells have not invaded through the basement membrane the lesion is said to be an *in-situ* cancer

- Invasive cancer – local invasion of cancer cells

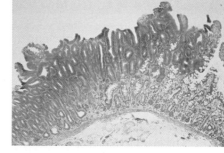

**Figure 9.1** Colonic dysplasia

- Metastasis – further mutations allow dysplastic cells to invade through the basement membrane into lymphatics and veins which carry the cancer cells to distant organs where they can establish new tumour deposits.

## INHERITANCE

A tendency to develop certain cancers may be inherited, e.g. women who inherit the mutated **BRCA1** and **BRCA2** genes have a high chance of developing breast cancer (85% if there is a positive family history). Genetic testing using gene probes may help to identify those families at high risk, so that appropriate surveillance can be undertaken.

### IMPLICATIONS OF GENETIC TESTING

A negative test may give a false sense of reassurance, e.g. 90% of breast cancers are **not** inherited.

A positive test poses other problems. Methods of surveillance are not sensitive enough to pick up tumours before they have metastasized; bilateral mastectomy is therefore no guarantee that a tumour will not have already metastasized. Patients may also have difficulty in obtaining life insurance.

## PATHOLOGY OF CANCER

This is described under the following headings:
- Incidence
- Age
- Sex
- Geography
- Predisposing factors
- Macroscopical features
- Microscopical features
- Spread
- Prognosis.

# INCIDENCE

Malignant tumours account for 30% of deaths in the Western world. The top ten solid cancers are shown in Table 9.2. This table excludes leukaemia, lymphoma and skin cancers which, apart from malignant melanoma, have an excellent 5-year survival.

Table 9.2 The top ten solid cancers*

| | | Total | Male (UK rank) | Female (UK rank) | % 5-year survival Overall |
|---|---|---|---|---|---|
| 1 | Lung | 40 223 | 27 968 (1) | 12 255 (2) | 8 |
| 2 | Colorectal | 19 452 | 9420 (2) | 10 032 (3) | 36 |
| 3 | Breast | 15 381 | 81 | 15 300 (1) | 64 |
| 4 | Stomach | 10 612 | 6322 (4) | 4290 (4) | 10 |
| 5 | Prostate | 8234 | 8234 (3) | | 43 |
| 6 | Pancreas | 6795 | 3282 (7) | 3513 (6) | 4 |
| 7 | Oesophagus | 5591 | 3357 (6) | 2234 (7) | 8 |
| 8 | Bladder | 5358 | 3665 (5) | 1693 (8) | 60 |
| 9 | Ovary | 4275 | | 4275 (5) | 25 |
| 10 | Brain | 2940 | 1660 (8) | 1280 (9) | |

*Mortality in UK, 1989. CRC Factsheet.

## AGE

Generally the incidence of a particular tumour increases with the age of the patient – two-thirds of those dying from cancer are over 60 years of age.

## SEX

Some tumours have a predisposition for certain sexes. Carcinomas of the lung, oesophagus and stomach are more common in men whereas women are more frequently affected by cancer of the breast (men make up 1% of all breast cancers), thyroid and gall bladder.

## GEOGRAPHY

Breast cancer is common in north European countries, but rare in the Orient. Colonic cancer is common in the Western world and rare in Africa. Carcinoma of the cervix is rare in Jewish women, possibly related to the custom of male circumcision. Carcinoma of the **oesophagus** has a high incidence in northern Iran, China and South Africa.

## PREDISPOSING FACTORS

### Genetic
Breast cancer is more common in women who have a first degree relative affected by the disease, particularly if the relative developed the tumour at a young age (BRCA1 and BRCA2).

The colonic polyps of familial adenomatous polyposis (an inherited autosomal dominant) will undergo malignant transformation.

### Environmental (chemical and radiation)
More than half the cancer deaths in the Western world can be attributed to smoking and diet.

- Smoking causes 30% of cancer deaths, being implicated in tumours of the lung, oesophagus, bladder, pancreas and probably tumours of the stomach, liver and kidney.
- Diets rich in saturated animal fats have been strongly associated with cancers of the colon and prostate.
- Diets deficient in fresh fruit and vegetables contribute to cancer because the 'cancer protective' effect of these foodstuffs is lacking.
- Ultraviolet B rays damage DNA and cause more than 90% of skin cancers, including malignant melanoma.

Recognized carcinogens together with occupations associated with cancer are shown in Table 9.3.

**Table 9.3** Recognized carcinogens and occupations associated with cancer

| Tumour | Carcinogen | Risk/Occupation |
|---|---|---|
| Lung | 3,4-benzpyrene, chrome, nickel ore, asbestos | Cigarette smoke, hot tar, mining |
| Mesothelioma | Asbestos | Asbestos workers |
| Bladder | β-Naphthylamine | Dyestuffs (aniline), rubber and plastics industry |
| Angiosarcoma of liver | Vinyl chloride | PVC plastics |
| Nasal sinuses | Unknown | Hardwood furniture and leather workers |
| Skin | Arsenic | Fowler's solution |
| | Soot, coal tar | Chimney sweep's tumour of scrotum (Percival Pott) |
| | Radiation: UV, x-rays | Exposure to sunlight |

## MACROSCOPIC APPEARANCE

A breast tumour infiltrates the surrounding stroma in a radial fashion, akin to the legs of a crab. On bisecting the tumour, its cut edges retract so that the plane is concave; microcalcification within the tumour gives it a 'gritty feeling', similar to cutting an unripe pear.

Malignant tumours arising on the surface of a viscus (e.g. skin or bowel) tend to have a **rolled or everted edge,** and appear **polypoid.** The polypoid region of the tumour may necrose, leaving a central **ulcer.**

Bowel cancers may cause a thickening of the bowel wall, reducing its lumen (annular stenosing) and causing obstruction.

## MICROSCOPIC APPEARANCE

- **Invasion** of malignant epithelial cells through the basement membrane into the submucosa, muscularis propria and beyond.
- If glandular in origin, the invading cells may attempt to form glands (well differentiated).
- Malignant cells will be seen invading nerve sheaths, blood vessels and lymphatics (neurovascular invasion).
- The individual malignant cells have an altered **cytological** (dysplastic) appearance:
  Hyperchromatic (dark blue)
  Pleomorphic (different shapes)
  Increased nuclear:cytoplasmic ratio (large nucleus, small cytoplasm)
  Frequent mitotic figures.

## SPREAD

Spread can be local, lymphatic, blood-borne or trans-coelomic.

### Local spread

Cancers infiltrate through the wall or stroma of the organ to involve neighbouring structures:

- Parotid tumours (Figure 9.2) may compress the facial nerve, causing facial paralysis.
- Thyroid tumours can infiltrate the recurrent laryngeal nerve, resulting in a hoarse voice.
- Breast cancer may spread to the chest wall or to the overlying skin and present as a cutaneous ulcer.
- A cancer in one organ may grow into a neighbouring organ, producing a fistula.

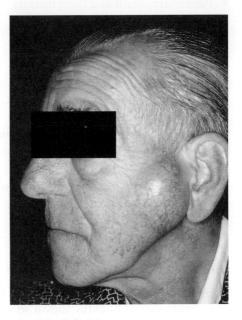

**Figure 9.2** Parotid tumour

### Lymphatic spread

- Lymphatic spread is a common feature of carcinomas but is rare in sarcomas.
- Tumour cells invade lymphatic channels, accumulate and grow in the regional lymph nodes, producing **metastatic**, or **secondary**, deposits of tumour.
- Malignant permeation of cutaneous lymphatic channels by an underlying breast cancer may cause the skin of the breast to resemble an orange rind (*peau d'orange*).
- A malignant mass of axillary lymph nodes (**malignant lymphadenopathy**) may be the presenting feature of an impalpable breast cancer.
- Malignant nodes palpated in the left supraclavicular region (**Virchow's node**) may represent metastatic deposits from an intra-abdominal cancer.
- Lymphatic spread from testicular tumours will involve the **pre-aortic** lymph nodes, whereas cancers arising in the anus, penis or skin of the leg will metastasize to the **inguinal** lymph nodes.

### Haematogenous spread

- Haematogenous spread is common to both carcinomas and sarcomas.
- Malignant cells from bowel cancer may invade the draining veins and be transported to the liver, via the portal vein (Figure 9.3).
- Renal cell cancers classically grow in continuity along the renal vein into the inferior vena cava and even into the right atrium.
- Pulmonary, brain and bone metastatic deposits may develop by blood-borne spread.

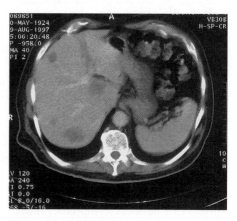

**Figure 9.3** Hepatic metastases

### Trans-coelomic spread

Trans-coelomic spread is common in intra-abdominal malignancies:

- Gastric and colonic tumours can spread widely in the peritoneal cavity, resulting in multiple peritoneal deposits.
- These deposits exude fluid, and present as a malignant **ascites**.
- Tumour deposits on the pleural membranes produce malignant **pleural effusions**.
- Gastric cancers that spread trans-coelomically and seed in the ovaries are known as **Krukenberg's tumour**.

## PROGNOSIS

The prognosis depends on the stage and grade of the tumour.

### Staging of tumours – Clinical extent of the tumour

The 5-year survival figures shown in Table 9.2 represent the percentage of all patients presenting with a particular tumour who are alive 5 years from diagnosis. This is an oversimplification since some patients will present with a localized tumour, whilst others will present after the tumour has already metastasized.

One of the simplest staging classifications in use is Dukes', for colorectal cancer:
- Stage A – the tumour is confined to the bowel wall
- Stage B – the tumour has penetrated the muscularis propria of the bowel
- Stage C – the tumour has spread to the lymph nodes.
The 5-year survival of groups A, B and C are 90%, 70% and 30%, respectively.

All cancers can be staged using the TNM classification:
- T – the characteristics (size/position) of the primary tumour
- N – whether or not there is lymph node involvement
- M – whether or not there are distant metastases in other organs.

### Grading of tumours – the degree of cellular atypia
Tumours are graded depending on cytological and histological features as:
- Well differentiated
- Moderately differentiated
- Poorly differentiated.

Despite advances in diagnosis, surgical technique and oncology, the death rate from common solid tumours has not reduced significantly over the last 50 years. It is hoped that cancer **screening programmes** and the use of **adjuvant therapy** will improve the mortality statistics.

## SCREENING

The objectives of screening are:
- To detect the tumour at an earlier stage before it becomes symptomatic
- To excise the tumour before it has metastasized.

There is a theoretical opportunity to cure a patient of cancer by surgery – by detection and excision prior to dissemination. This is known as the cancer control window (CCW) (Figure 9.4 line A).

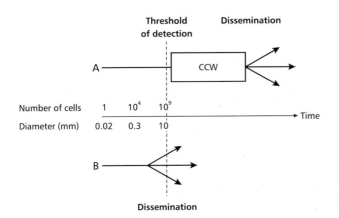

**Figure 9.4** Diagrammatic representation of the cancer control window (CCW)

If the cancer has already disseminated by the time it reaches the threshold of detection (line B), clearly only effective **systemic therapy** (i.e. chemotherapy or hormone treatment) will cure the patient. The current threshold of detection is typically a tumour of 1 cm diameter, which represents $10^9$ cells, and is the result of 30 tumour doublings (Figure 9.5).

An ideal screening programme should meet the following criteria:

- The screening test should be able to detect the cancer, and exclude benign disease, i.e. have a **high sensitivity** (ability to diagnose malignant disease) and **high specificity** (ability to exclude benign disease).
- Once detected at a preclinical stage, the disease should be curable with current therapy.
- The test should be easy to perform and interpret, and be minimally invasive.
- Screening tests should be considered for common conditions, where early diagnosis improves the survival.
- The cost should be considered; it may well be very expensive (screening mammogram = £25.00).

There are various screening programmes, as follows:
- Breast cancer – screening mammogram every 3 years, women between 50 and 64 years
- Cervical cancer – cervical smear every 3 years until 60 years

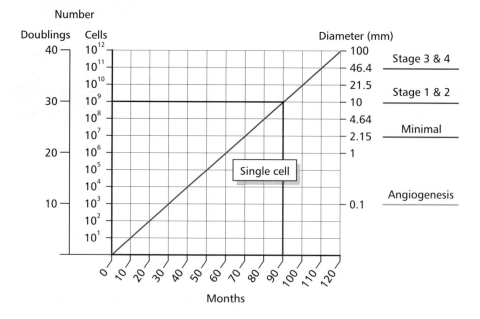

**Figure 9.5** A diagrammatic representation of the growth rate of a breast cancer with a tumour doubling time of 90 days. At the time of detection (10 mm lump) most of the tumour's biological life will already have passed

- Gastric cancer – in Japan, by endoscopic examination of stomach
- Colorectal cancer – registry of patients with familial adenomatous polyposis. Use of faecal occult blood test; if test positive, then colonoscopy
- Prostate cancer – serum prostate specific antigen (PSA)
- Genetic screening – for mutations that predispose to certain cancers.

## CLINICAL PRESENTATION OF CANCER

Symptomatic cancers can present due to:
- The effects of the primary tumour
- The effects of metastatic tumour
- General effects of cancer.

### EFFECTS OF THE PRIMARY TUMOUR

#### Pain
Pain is due to pressure or destruction of tissues containing nerve fibres for pain. The core of many solid organs lack such fibres, so a tumour may grow for some time, e.g. within the **liver**, and only produce pain when the richly innervated peritoneal capsule is invaded. Tumour occluding a hollow viscus (e.g. the **colon**) causes colic. For tumours arising in the tail of the **pancreas**, pain (felt in the back) may be the only symptom.

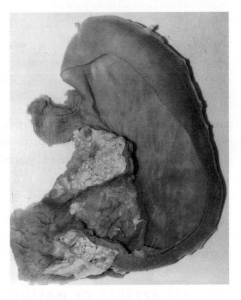

#### Bleeding
A tumour that ulcerates and causes necrosis of an underlying blood vessel may present with bleeding (Figure 9.6). Tumours typically present with a slight, but prolonged blood loss (Fe-deficient anaemia).

#### A lump
Frequently a lump is the presenting symptom. This is true for breast tumours, and not an uncommon presentation in renal and colonic tumours.

**Figure 9.6** Carcinoma of gastric antrum

#### An emergency
Cancer may present due to bleeding, obstruction or perforation.

### EFFECTS OF SECONDARY TUMOUR (METASTATIC DEPOSITS)

#### Lymph nodes
Malignant lymph nodes typically feel 'hard or craggy', may be 'matted' together and 'fixed' either to skin or underlying tissue.

### Bone

Metastatic tumour that has spread to bone may present with **bone pain,** or a **pathological fracture** (a fracture caused by minimal force) (Figure 9.7). A pathological fracture in a vertebral body may cause spinal compression and paraplegia. Tumours that typically spread to bone are: **breast, bronchus, kidney, thyroid and prostate.**

### Brain

Cerebral metastases may present with symptoms of raised intracranial pressure (headaches), focal neurological signs or epilepsy (typically late onset).

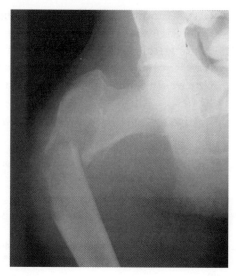

**Figure 9.7** Pathological fracture of femur

### Liver

Hepatic metastases may present as pain felt in the right upper quadrant, hepatomegaly, or liver failure and jaundice.

### Peritoneal or pleural

Metastases present as an accumulation of fluid in the cavity, either as ascites with abdominal distension, or as a pleural effusion causing shortness of breath.

### Skin

Cutaneous metastases typically occur in the scar of the operation performed to remove or diagnose (porthole recurrences post-diagnostic laparoscopy) the cancer. There are also often 'satellite lesions' around a malignant melanoma.

### Local recurrence

Tumour can recur at the site where the primary tumour was excised, due to seeding of tumour cells at the time of excision, or failure to excise the tumour *in toto.* Local recurrence of breast cancer is usually visible; local recurrence of rectal cancer following an anterior resection may be palpable per rectum as a 'rectal shelf'.

## GENERAL EFFECTS OF MALIGNANCY

### General features

Features common to most disseminated tumours include anorexia, weight loss, lethargy, nausea and vomiting, sweats especially at night, weakness and muscle wasting.

### Paraneoplastic syndromes

In addition to the physical effects of the primary or secondary tumour, general systemic symptoms are shared by many tumours:

- Hypercalcaemia – breast, lung, renal, prostate and myeloma; **parathyroid related protein** (PTH rP)
- Cushing's syndrome – lung and adrenal carcinoma; **ACTH**
- Inappropriate ADH – lung
- Polycythaemia – kidney; **erythropoietin**
- Fever – lymphoma, kidney
- Dermatomyositis – lung, breast, pancreas
- Thrombophlebitis – breast, prostate, pancreas (Troisier's syndrome)
- Immunodeficiency – myeloma, lymphoma, thymoma
- Hypertrophic osteoarthropathy – lung.

## DIAGNOSIS OF CANCER

When discussing the diagnosis of any cancer it is often easier to construct an answer using Table 9.4, considering the history, examination, and special investigations of the primary tumour, secondary tumour and the general features of the tumour. The example given is for a **rectal cancer;** the diagnostic features of the other common cancers are found in the appropriate chapters.

**Table 9.4** Example of cancer diagnosis using history, examination and tests

|  | Primary | Secondary | General |
|---|---|---|---|
| History | Routine: altered bowel habit, blood/mucus PR, tenesmus, palpable lump Emergency: perforation/peritonitis, obstruction | Pain: liver, bone Pleural effusion: SOB Ascitic distension Neurological signs Lump: lymph node metastases | Anorexia, weight loss, weakness, lethargy, fever, sweats, nausea Paraneoplastic syndromes |
| Exam | Routine: abdominal mass, tumour felt PR Emergency: obstruction/peritonitis | Liver: palpable, jaundice Umbilicus: Sister Joseph's nodule Moving: dullness/pleural effusion PR: rectal shelf (local recurrence) Supraclavicular lymph node | Anaemia, cachexia |
| Tests | Blood: FBC, U&E Sigmoidoscopy Barium enema Colonoscopy/biopsy | Blood: LFTs, alkaline phosphatase X-ray: chest, bones Liver: ultrasound/CT scan Bone scan Biopsy: lymph nodes Cytology: ascitic/pleural fluid | Nutritional status: weight, BMI Blood tests: serum protein, serum calcium |

# TREATMENT OF CANCER

Treatment of cancer may be either 'curative' or 'palliative'. Current methods of treatment employ:
- Surgery
- Radiotherapy
- Chemotherapy
- Hormone manipulation (for hormonally sensitive tumours).

Combination of these modalities is called **adjuvant therapy**.

## SURGERY

### Curative surgery
- The best hope of curing a patient with a solid cancer is to excise the tumour *in toto* at an early stage before it has metastasized.
- The lymph nodes draining the tumour are excised (*en bloc*) with the specimen, in the hope of reducing the incidence of **local recurrence**, and accurately **staging** the tumour assess the need for adjuvant therapy.

'Curative' surgical excisions include oesophagectomy for oesophageal cancer, total gastrectomy for gastric cancer, and hemicolectomy for tumours of the colon.

### Palliative surgery
If excision of the tumour is not possible or if the tumour has widely disseminated, the remainder of the patient's life may be improved by palliative procedures. These include:
- Stenting an obstructing tumour – the lumen of a viscus may be kept patent by use of stents, e.g. oesophagus, bile duct, ureter
- Surgical bypass – bowel proximal to a tumour is anastomosed to bowel beyond the tumour to relieve an obstruction (entero-enterostomy); or proximal bowel can be exteriorized (colostomy)
- Stabilizing secondary tumours in bone – secondary tumours in bone are liable to pathological fracture. If detected, they may be stabilized and unnecessary morbidity avoided, e.g. intramedullary nailing of long bones and fixation of vertebrae to prevent collapse (and paraplegia)
- Drainage of malignant effusions – malignant pleural effusions can be tapped by pleural aspiration, prevention of reaccumulation of the fluid can be achieved by instilling tetracycline or bleomycin into the pleural space. Drainage of malignant ascites either externally (paracentesis), or into the venous circulation using a shunt is possible.
- Debulking the tumour load – cancer of the ovary spreads widely in the peritoneal cavity and omentum. Excision of the ovary and omentum reduces the tumour load, reduces the degree of malignant ascites and improves the efficacy of chemotherapy.

## RADIOTHERAPY

Ionizing radiation damages nuclear DNA. This damage remains latent until the cell attempts division at which time the cell dies. The effects of radiation on the cytoplasm are usually readily reversible. Adequate oxygenation of the tissue is essential for effective radiotherapy, however many tumours are relatively anoxic.

Radiotherapy does not distinguish between normal cells and tumour cells but the following reasons explain why radiotherapy can be used to treat tumours:

- Because tumour cells undergo frequent mitosis they are more radio-sensitive. Cells which do not undergo mitosis (neurones and muscle cells) are radio-resistant.
- Since normal cells have a greater ability to repair damage than tumour cells, doses of radiotherapy are **fractionated** (small doses given over a prolonged period to achieve the required dose), allowing normal cells to repair damage between treatments.
- Radiation damage to the CNS, lungs, kidneys and gastrointestinal tract results from damage to the endothelial cells of the arteries, producing endarteritis obliterans, rather than damage to the cells of the organ itself.

The chance of tumour control rises exponentially with doses over 4000 cGy (1 cGy = 1 rad). Above 6000 cGy there is a rapidly rising risk of complications and this imposes the maximum dose limit.

Radiotherapy may be 'curative' (typically tumours of the larynx, prostate) or 'palliative' (to inoperable tumours or metastatic deposits).

### Curative (radical) radiotherapy:

- Uses maximum doses.
- Minimizes collateral damage to surrounding organs by planning how the radiotherapy is delivered at successive treatments.
- By altering the angle at which the beam arrives surrounding tissues can be spared, but large doses can be targeted on the tumour.

Surgical excision of tumours may be inadvisable because the tumour is situated in such a position that excision is not technically possible or because excision would result in a mutilating procedure with unacceptable side-effects. Such tumours may be 'cured' by radical radiotherapy. The crude 5-year survival for tumours treated by radical radiotherapy alone are shown in Table 9.5.

### Palliative radiotherapy

Palliative radiotherapy uses the smallest dose, over the shortest period of time, that is necessary to relieve symptoms.

**Table 9.5** Crude 5-year survival rates of tumours treated by radical radiotherapy

| Tumour | 5-year survival (%) |
|---|---|
| Skin (basal & squamous cancer) | 95 |
| Head & neck | |
|     Oral cavity | 50 |
|     Glottis | 80 |
|     Nasopharynx | 50 |
|     Paranasal sinuses | 40 |
| Bladder | 50 |
| Prostate | 60 |
| Malignant gliomas | 30 |
| Oesophagus | 15 |
| Cervix | 70 |

Indications include:

- Pain from bony metastases (Figure 9.8)
- Mediastinal obstruction from bronchial carcinoma
- Haemorrhage and pain from cancers of cervix, bladder and rectum.

**Adjuvant radiotherapy**

Surgery is the best method of removing the primary tumour; however, microscopic deposits in the periphery of the sample and in the surrounding lymph nodes may lead to loco-regional recurrence of the tumour.

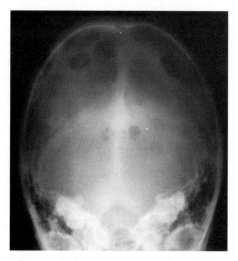

**Figure 9.8** Secondary deposits in skull

- Radiotherapy may not be successful in treating large anoxic tumour masses, but is ideally suited in treating a large volume of tissue containing peripheral micrometastases.
- Hence radiotherapy either **before** (to shrink the tumour size) or **after** surgery is used to reduce the incidence of local recurrence and hopefully improve survival.
- Radiotherapy given prior to surgery reduces the healing properties of an organ, predisposing to anastomotic and wound dehiscence. To minimize this complication, surgery should be performed 3–6 weeks after preoperative radiotherapy.

- For breast cancer, treated by wide local excision, post-operative radiotherapy reduces the risk of local recurrence by 24%.
- The combination of wide local excision and radiotherapy for breast cancer achieves survival rates similar to those for mastectomy, but allows the woman to preserve her breast.
- Pre- and post-operative radiotherapy is also useful in preventing local recurrence of rectal cancers following excision by anterior resection.

### Methods of administering radiotherapy

**Teletherapy** uses an external beam of ionizing radiation. The degree of tissue penetration is dependent on the beam energy, measured in electron volts (eV). Historically, hot-filament tubes generated x-rays with energies of 300 keV. Megavoltage beams can be delivered using:

- Cobalt-60 – decays by emitting $\gamma$-rays with energies of 1.3 MeV
- Linear accelerators – generate beams of x-rays with energies of 2–20 MeV
- Cyclotrons – generate fast neutrons, have a much greater ionizing potential than megavoltage x-rays or $\gamma$-rays and may be useful in treating cells in anoxic tissue.

The advantages of high energy irradiation include:

- Greater penetration, allowing treatment of deeply placed tumours
- Skin sparing – reduced erythema, desquamation, and telangictasia
- Sharper beams of greater accuracy, reducing collateral damage.

**Brachytherapy** is the use of interstitial or intracavity radioactive sources. The damage to normal tissue is reduced by delivering a radioactive source directly to the tumour site. Radioactive sources of caesium-137 or cobalt-60 can be placed in tubes and inserted into the uterus. Iridium-192 wire is used to treat tumours of the tongue.

**Unsealed radioactive sources** – iodine-131 is selectively taken up by thyroid cells to treat metastases of follicular and papillary thyroid cancers.

## SYSTEMIC THERAPY

A systemic therapy offers the only hope of treating tumours that are dispersed widely in the body. Systemic therapy uses:

- Chemotherapy (use of cytotoxic agents)
- Hormone therapy.

Both these modalities can be used in combination with surgery (**adjuvant therapy**).

### Chemotherapy

- Ideally, a chemotherapeutic drug should exhibit selective toxicity to cancer cells.
- No **qualitative** metabolic differences have been demonstrated between normal and neoplastic cells.
- Chemotherapy utilizes **quantitative** differences in the proliferative kinetics of normal and tumour cells, killing cells which are actively dividing.

## Chemotherapeutic agents can be divided into:

- Phase specific agents which act on a specific phase of the cell cycle (e.g. 6-mercaptopurine, vincristine, methotrexate which act on the S phase of DNA synthesis)
- Cycle specific agents which act on all phases of the cell cycle, except the resting G0 phase (e.g. 5-fluorouracil, cyclophosphamide and actinomycin D).

Complications of chemotherapy include:

- Damage to rapidly multiplying cells in the bone marrow leads to anaemia, infection and bleeding (thrombocytopenia).
- Other common side-effects include diarrhoea, nausea, vomiting and hair loss.
- Tumours may also become resistant to chemotherapeutic drugs. Leukaemia, lymphomas and testicular cancers are successfully treated by combination chemotherapy.

**Adjuvant chemotherapy** is the administration of chemotherapy **after** surgery. Since many patients who have had an apparently 'localized' tumour excised will ultimately die from that tumour, it is assumed that undetectable **micrometastases** are present at the time of surgery. Adjuvant chemotherapy is aimed at destroying these micrometastases and improving survival.

Examples of adjuvant chemotherapy include:

- The use of cyclophosphamide, methotrexate and 5-fluorouracil (CMF) in treating an early breast cancer in a pre-menopausal woman (given in pulses over 12 months, following wide local excision and post-operative radiotherapy)
- The use of cisplatin, bleomycin and vinblastine following orchidectomy for testicular tumours.

**Neoadjuvant chemotherapy** is the administration of chemotherapy **before** surgery. This allows:

- The destruction of systemic micrometastases as early as possible
- Tumour shrinkage enabling excision of an 'inoperable tumour'
- The degree of tumour shrinkage to indicate efficacy of a cytotoxic regimen.

Classification of chemotherapeutic drugs

- Antimetabolites – block biochemical pathways in the cell. Methotrexate binds to an enzyme that normally converts folic acid to adenine and guanine (building blocks of DNA).
- Alkylating agents – cyclophosphamide and chlorambucil bind to DNA, causing fragmentation or cross-linking of the strands. If not repaired this leads to cell death.
- Plant alkaloids – vincristine and vinblastine cause polymerization of the protein tubulin which is necessary in the formation of the mitotic spindle during cell division.
- Cytotoxic antibiotics – dactinomycin, doxorubicin and bleomycin interfere with the transcription of DNA.

## Hormone therapy

The growth of **breast** and **prostatic** cells is regulated by circulating sex hormones and tumours arising from these tissues may also express sex hormone receptors. By **blocking these receptors** or by **reducing the level of circulating sex hormone**, tumour growth may be retarded:

- Tamoxifen is a widely used oestrogen antagonist useful in treating breast cancer.
- Oestrogen levels can be reduced by oophorectomy or administering an aromatase inhibitor which blocks oestrogen production.
- Prostate cancer may be treated by reducing testosterone production by either orchidectomy or administration of the LHRH agonist goserilin.
- Following thyroidectomy, metastatic thyroid cancer can be treated by administering a large dose of thyroxine, thereby inhibiting release of TSH and preventing it from stimulating the growth of thyroid cancer cells.

# FUTURE PROSPECTS

## GENE THERAPY

Recent understanding of the genetic mechanisms of tumour development have led to gene therapy. In many cases this involves inserting genetic material directly into tumour cells using attenuated viruses as couriers.

### Antisense strategy

Transcription of double stranded oncogene DNA produces a single strand of mRNA that binds to the ribosomes and synthesizes (translates) the proteins necessary for cell division. Strands of antisense mRNA (mRNA whose bases are complementary to the oncogene mRNA) inserted into tumour cells will specifically bind to the oncogene mRNA and prevent translation of the oncogenes into growth stimulating proteins.

### Triplex strategy

New short strands of DNA (oligonucleotides) that specifically bind oncogenes are inserted into cancer cells, preventing transcription of oncogenes and preventing the production of the proteins necessary for cell division. This is known as triplex strategy because the oligonucleotide winds around the double strand of DNA to produce a three-strand helix.

### Tumour suppressor genes

Many cancer cells lack tumour suppressor genes; inserting DNA that codes for p53 and pRB suppressor genes into cancer cells may result in a cessation of tumour growth.

### Inhibiting the Ras proteins

Mutated Ras proteins are found in up to 30% of tumours. Ras relay proteins behave as a switch which is 'turned on' by stimuli transmitted to it from outside the cell. These activated proteins stimulate transcription of DNA and cell division. In the absence of external stimuli the Ras proteins remain 'switched off'. The mutated Ras proteins behave as a switch stuck in the 'on' position, constantly instructing the cell to divide. By inhibiting the enzymes necessary for maturation of the Ras protein, it is hoped to selectively inhibit tumour growth.

## IMMUNOTHERAPY

Despite many important developments in immunology, treatment of cancer by immunotherapy has been disappointing. Bolstering the immune response in a general manner with the use of cytokines (interferons, interleukins and tumour necrosis factor) should be therapeutic. Unfortunately, despite extensive trials relatively few patients benefit from this general approach.

The development of specific monoclonal antibodies (MCA) to tumour antigens has also been tried. They are generally obtained from mice immunized with human cancers. It was hoped that MCA (either alone or tagged with radioactive isotopes or cytotoxic drugs) would act as **magic bullets**, homing in on tumour cells and destroying them.

Unfortunately, if a patient is treated repeatedly with MCA, he will mount his own immune response to the MCA, and destroy it. Work is now under way to disguise or 'humanize' murine MCA so that it is no longer destroyed by the human immune system.

## PUBLIC HEALTH

**Prevention is better than cure**. It is estimated that 50% of cancer deaths could be prevented by **stopping smoking, eating a healthy diet and preventing obesity**. Occupational health measures are also important in preventing the small numbers of cancers associated with particular industries.

## MULTIDISCIPLINARY TEAMS

Although a patient with cancer may present primarily to a **surgeon**, the effective diagnosis and treatment of cancer requires the combined skills of different medical disciplines, usually working in teams:
- Radiologists, histopathologists and cytologists confirm the diagnosis of cancer.
- Surgeons and oncologists jointly plan the treatment.
- Specialist nurses are able to explain to the patient the nature of the illness and treatment. They can also provide considerable psychological support to the patient and their family through the illness and during the convalescent period.

Despite best endeavours, many tumours will recur and there is a need to help the patient through the terminal stages of his/her disease.
- The palliative care team provide medical relief of symptoms and manage analgesia, allowing the patient to maximize the amount of time spent at home with the family.
- In the final stages of the disease it may no longer be possible for the patient to remain at home and admission to a hospice (a hospital specializing in terminal care) can be arranged.

In order to maximize and standardize the delivery of cancer treatment in the United Kingdom, is has been proposed that specialized **cancer centres** and units are established, so that the necessary expertise is concentrated and readily available.

---

**CRIB BOX – MALIGNANT DISEASE**

Learn the definition of a tumour

Appreciate the difference between benign and malignant

Epithelium = carcinoma; mesothelium = sarcoma

**Malignant spread is:**

- Local
- By lymph
- By blood
- Trans-coelomic

**Prognosis depends on:**

- Stage
- Grade

You need to know Dukes' staging (colorectal) and understand TNM

Screening for disease (including cancer) is a common question – learn it!

**Effects of malignancy:**

- Local
- Metastatic
- General (inc. paraneoplastic syndromes)

**Diagnose on:**

- History
- Examination
- Special investigations

**Treat cancer with:**

- Surgery
- Radiotherapy
- Chemotherapy
- Hormone manipulation
- Nursing, symptomatic and psychological support

Treatment is **curative** or **palliative**

**Future**

- Gene therapy
- Immunotherapy
- Better public health
- Cancer centres

chapter 10

# THE BRAIN, SPINE AND NERVES

## THE BRAIN

### RAISED INTRACRANIAL PRESSURE

The cranium is an enclosed rigid space containing brain, blood and cerebrospinal fluid (CSF). Any 'space occupying' lesion (e.g. tumour, blood clot), brain swelling or excess CSF within this space will cause a rise in intracranial pressure.

Symptoms and signs are:

- Headache – becomes progressively more severe, is worse in the mornings and intensifies with coughing or exertion.
- Vomiting – often during the night or early morning when the headache is most severe.
- Papilloedema – may lead to blurred vision and blindness.

**The triad of headache, vomiting and papilloedema is almost pathognomonic of a space occupying lesion within the skull.** In addition there may be other signs:

- Mental disorders – personality change, drowsiness, dementia, reduced conscious level, coma.
- Pulse, blood pressure, respiration – a rapid increase in intracranial pressure raises the blood pressure (to maintain cerebral blood flow) and lowers the heart rate (Cushing's reflex). Respiratory depression also occurs.
- Head enlargement – occurs in children before the sutures have fused.

The onset of symptoms and signs equates to the speed of onset of raised intracranial pressure. Tumours produce symptoms slowly. Rapid haematoma formation (trauma, spontaneous intracranial bleed) causes more or less instantaneous symptoms with rapid progression to coma.

### HEAD INJURIES

- Head injury is extremely common and as such is relatively trivial, although substantial blood loss can occur from scalp lacerations which can also become infected.
- **Associated brain injury is serious** and, if suspected or probable, is an indication for hospital admission and observation.

## Skull fractures

Most skull fractures are simple closed linear cracks (Figure 10.1) which in themselves are harmless. However, with a fracture and impaired consciousness there is a **high chance of an intracranial haematoma** developing.

- **Compound fractures carry the risk of meningitis or abscess** and need antibiotics. They may involve the anterior fossa and cribriform plate (periorbital haematoma and CSF rhinorrhoea) or middle fossa (CSF otorrhoea and bleeding from the ear). Basal fractures are commonly compound through the paranasal sinuses and may allow air into the cranium (aerocele).
- Cranial nerves can be damaged if the fracture involves their exit foramina, notably the olfactory and facial nerves.
- Depressed fractures can be closed or compound and need exploration for debridement and repair of the dura.

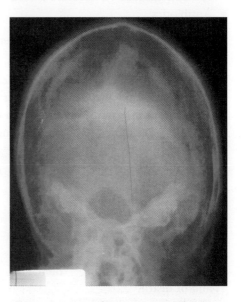

**Figure 10.1** Linear fracture in occipital region

### Brain injury

Brain injury occurs due to the **primary effect** of the head injury and to **secondary events**. Primary brain injury is difficult to classify but can usefully be regarded as **focal** (sharp injury) or **general** (blunt injury), although in the clinical setting it is often a mixture of both.

**Focal brain injury** This results from a blow to the head with an object of small surface area – a 'sharp' injury (Figure 10.2). The patient may remain conscious if there is no general brain damage. This type of injury typically produces:

- Depressed skull fracture – often compound due to scalp laceration
- Focal brain damage – due to cerebral contusion
- Epilepsy – secondary to the focal damage
- Infection – leading to brain abscess if untreated.

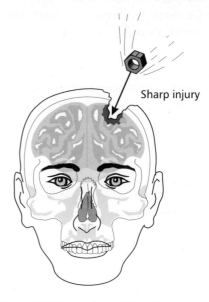

Sharp injury

**Figure 10.2** Mechanism of 'sharp' injury

### Investigations
Skull x-ray and CT scanning will show the depressed fragment well.

### Treatment
- Local debridement and elevation of the depressed fragment
- Anticonvulsants – if the dura is torn or if there is focal contusion
- Antibiotics.

The prognosis of a 'sharp' injury is generally extremely good.

**General brain injury** This results from a rapid acceleration/deceleration injury, e.g. traffic accidents and falls. The head comes to an abrupt halt on impact but the brain continues to move within the cranium – a 'blunt' injury (Figure 10.3). Movement and rotation of brain within the skull causes:

- Diffuse brain injury – occurring principally in the white matter. Mild injury produces the clinical syndrome of concussion, i.e. short loss of consciousness with good recovery, no residual deficit, amnesia for the event and post-traumatic amnesia of variable length, depending upon the degree of injury. Severe injury produces devastating damage and/or death.

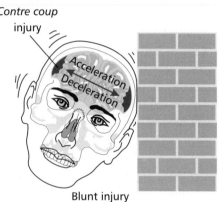
Figure 10.3 Mechanism of 'blunt' injury

- Cerebral contusions – bruising of the cortex at the site of impact and/or on the opposite side of the brain (*contre coup* injury), producing focal neurological signs.
- Cerebral lacerations – fractures and tears in the brain substance.

> **Primary brain damage caused at the time of injury is irreversible. Treatment is aimed at preventing secondary brain damage.**

Causes of secondary brain damage are:
- Hypoxia – chest trauma or airway obstruction
- Hypotension – blood loss from external or internal injuries
- Cerebral oedema – common in children
- Intracranial haematoma – extradural, subdural, intracerebral
- Meningitis.

Head injury patients often have other injuries requiring **more urgent treatment:**
- Hypoxia and $CO_2$ retention occurs in chest injuries or airway obstruction and causes secondary brain damage

- Bleeding from intra-abdominal injuries or fractures causes hypotension and reduced cerebral perfusion
- Spinal injuries should be excluded with radiology
- Brain CT scan is needed in any unconscious or deteriorating patient or when brain injury is suspected.

**Management of the airway, breathing and circulation always comes first!**

### Management of brain injury

The extent of **recovery depends on the severity of the primary brain injury.** The primary injury may be complicated by secondary events and these avoidable and treatable factors may be responsible for a poor outcome or death. The most common avoidable cause of death is failure to recognize an intracranial haematoma – heralded by a decline in conscious level. It should be noted that a previously drowsy patient who becomes restless is exhibiting a decline in conscious level. After initial resuscitation, management consists of careful observation and general medical support/treatment.

> **Secondary brain damage is treatable/avoidable**
>
> - Hypoxia
> - Hypotension
> - Cerebral oedema
> - Intracranial haematoma
> - Meningitis

**Observation** consists of the following:
- Glasgow coma scale – an observation chart recording eye opening, verbal and motor responses (Figure 10.4)
- Focal signs – development of new focal neurological signs such as unilateral weakness indicate a developing haematoma
- Pupil dilatation – this is a late sign of ipsilateral intracranial haematoma or oedema sufficient to cause herniation of the temporal lobe through the tentorial hiatus and compress the third cranial nerve. The pupil on the affected side dilates and fails to react to light. By the time both pupils dilate a fatal outcome is almost inevitable
- Pulse and blood pressure – rising blood pressure and falling heart rate (Cushing's reflex) may indicate rising intracranial pressure; particularly sensitive in children.

**Medical management** of a head injury not requiring surgery consists of general nursing, attention to fluid and electrolyte balance and nutrition as well as any or all of the following:
- Mechanical ventilation – to optimize the arterial blood gases
- Dehydration – diuretics (mannitol, frusemide) and fluid restriction helps to prevent and treat cerebral oedema
- Antibiotics – for compound fractures
- Anticonvulsants – for fits.

| Ward | | Consultant | | | NEUROLOGICAL OBSERVATION CHART | | | | | | | | | | | | |
|---|---|---|---|---|---|---|---|---|---|---|---|---|---|---|---|---|---|

Surname      Unit No.
First Name
Date Of Birth
Address      Sex

Sheet No:

| Bed No. | | Date: | | | | | | | | | | | | | | | | |
|---|---|---|---|---|---|---|---|---|---|---|---|---|---|---|---|---|---|---|
| | | Time: | | | | | | | | | | | | | | | | |
| **C** | EYES OPEN (Eyes closed by swelling= C) | Spontaneously | | | | | | | | | | | | | | | | |
| | | To speech | | | | | | | | | | | | | | | | |
| | | To pain | | | | | | | | | | | | | | | | |
| **O** | | None | | | | | | | | | | | | | | | | |
| **M** | BEST VERBAL RESPONSE (Intubated = T) | Orientated | | | | | | | | | | | | | | | | |
| **A** | | Confused | | | | | | | | | | | | | | | | |
| | | Inappropriate words | | | | | | | | | | | | | | | | |
| **S** | | Incomprehensible sounds | | | | | | | | | | | | | | | | |
| **C** | | None | | | | | | | | | | | | | | | | |
| **A** | BEST MOTOR RESPONSE (Better arm) | Obey commands | | | | | | | | | | | | | | | | |
| **L** | | Localize pain | | | | | | | | | | | | | | | | |
| **E** | | Flexion to pain | | | | | | | | | | | | | | | | |
| | | Extension to pain | | | | | | | | | | | | | | | | |
| | | None | | | | | | | | | | | | | | | | |

**Figure 10.4** Glasgow coma scale

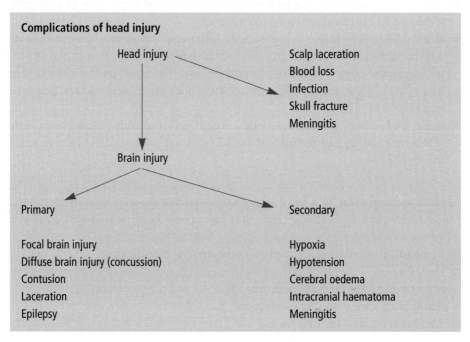

**Complications of head injury**

Head injury → Scalp laceration
Blood loss
Infection
Skull fracture
Meningitis

↓

Brain injury

Primary

Focal brain injury
Diffuse brain injury (concussion)
Contusion
Laceration
Epilepsy

Secondary

Hypoxia
Hypotension
Cerebral oedema
Intracranial haematoma
Meningitis

**Surgery** may consist of:

- Craniotomy for intracranial haematoma
- Craniotomy for repair of dural tear, e.g. CSF rhinorrhoea
- Insertion of intracranial pressure monitor – to warn of impending intracranial haematomas or swelling.

### Extradural haemorrhage

This is the quintessential neurosurgical emergency (Figure 10.5). **It classically results from a skull fracture in the temporal region which tears the middle meningeal artery.** Brisk bleeding strips the dura off the inside of the skull and the ensuing haematoma compresses the brain. There is usually no primary brain injury but the resulting compression may be fatal due to a rapid increase in intracranial pressure. Extradural haemorrhage may also develop from a torn venous sinus or bleeding from within a fracture.

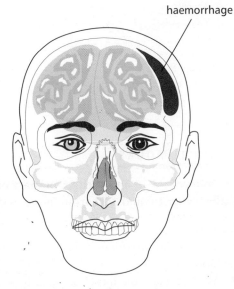

Extradural haemorrhage

**Figure 10.5** Extradural haemorrhage – note dilated pupil

### Symptoms and signs

- Commonly the injury is relatively mild with a brief period of unconsciousness.
- The patient then recovers (**the lucid period**) for a variable interval – usually hours.
- Progressive symptoms of raised intracranial pressure supervene as the extradural clot enlarges.
- Reduced level of consciousness, coma, contralateral hemiparesis and dilated ipsilateral pupil then develop.
- A haematoma may be felt over the fracture site.

**Investigation and treatment** consist of x-rays and CT scanning. X-rays show a fracture in 80% of cases. CT scanning confirms the diagnosis. The haematoma is evacuated urgently via a craniotomy and the bleeding point controlled.

### Acute subdural haematoma

This is usually associated with a serious primary brain injury and other injuries. The patient is often in a deep coma from the time of the injury.

**Treatment** consists of craniotomy and evacuation of the haematoma, when practicable, which offers the only hope of survival.

## Chronic subdural haematoma

Slow subdural bleeding may follow minor trauma which is often forgotten. It occurs most commonly in the elderly, alcoholics, or patients with clotting disorders and is caused by disruption of a bridging vein between the cerebral cortex and dura.

**Signs and symptoms** are:

- Slowly progressive raised intracranial pressure with lateralizing signs
- Often mistaken for a rapidly developing intracerebral tumour
- Confusion in the elderly.

**Treatment**
Diagnosis is usually made by CT scanning. The haematoma is liquefied and can be evacuated through burr holes.

# BRAIN TUMOURS

Tumours of the brain are either **primary** or **secondary**. Primary tumours are generally malignant and arise from the connective tissue or glial cells.

## Gliomas
Account for approximately 50% of all intracranial tumours. They are subclassified into:

- Astrocytoma – the most common. In adults they occur in the cerebrum and are usually malignant. In children they occur in the cerebellum and may well be benign.
- Ependymoma – occurs mainly in children, arising in the ventricles, especially the fourth.
- Oligodendroglioma – found in the cerebral cortex in adults; slow growing and often calcified on x-ray.
- Medulloblastoma – typically occurs in children as a very malignant tumour of the cerebellum in the midline. It is prone to disseminate throughout the nervous system and frequently presents with blockage of the fourth ventricle, producing obstructive hydrocephalus.

## Secondary tumours

Metastases constitute 20% of all cerebral tumours and commonly derive from primary tumours in the bronchus, kidney, breast, gastrointestinal tract or malignant melanoma.

## Other intracranial tumours
Derive from the structures surrounding the brain – meninges, cranial nerves, pituitary gland, blood vessels and skull.

## Meningioma
Account for 20% of intracranial tumours and are found typically in middle-aged women. They arise from the arachnoid and occur at both the base and vertex of

the cranium. Although benign, they can cause pressure symptoms. A hyperostosis of the skull with a characteristic radiological appearance may be present. Surgery to remove the tumour is usually successful.

## Neuromas
These are tumours of nerves and nerve roots arising from Schwann cells. The most common example is the **acoustic neuroma** arising from the sheath of the VIIIth cranial nerve in the cerebellopontine angle, causing deafness, facial numbness and weakness followed by cerebellar hemisphere signs and eventually features of raised intracranial pressure. Neurofibromatosis patients may develop bilateral acoustic neuromas.

## Pituitary tumours
These tumours (see also Chapter 15) present with endocrine problems, raised intracranial pressure, or visual disturbance due to pressure on the optic chiasma – classically a bitemporal hemianopia.
   Pituitary adenomas are classified by the type of hormone they secrete:
- Prolactin – amenorrhoea and infertility in women and impotence in men
- Growth hormone – acromegaly in adults and gigantism in children
- ACTH – Cushing's disease
- Non-functioning adenomas – hypopituitarism and visual disturbance due to their large size.

## Craniopharyngioma
These are benign tumours arising from embryological cell rests in Rathke's pouch. They are suprasellar in situation and often present in childhood but may occur in adults. They usually present with visual disturbance and endocrine dysfunction.

## Skull
Primary tumours are extremely rare; they include benign osteoma and malignant sarcoma. Sarcoma may complicate Paget's disease. Many tumours metastasize to bone, including the skull – lung, thyroid, breast, kidney and prostate.

### Symptoms and signs of intracranial tumours
- Raised intracranial pressure
- Hydrocephalus – tumours may compress the ventricles and obstruct the normal flow of CSF
- Localizing signs – depend on the position of the tumour and its effect on the brain – they are many and varied: hemiparesis, hemianopia, cranial nerve palsy, endocrine dysfunction, epilepsy, personality change, etc.

### Diagnosis
The diagnosis of intracerebral tumour requires a full **history** (which may have to be taken from relatives), **clinical examination** and **special investigations**:
- Imaging – MRI and/or CT scanning.
- Cerebral angiography – useful for vascular tumours and in the differential diagnoses of arteriovenous malformations and aneurysms.

- Histology – obtained by biopsy either via a burr hole or craniotomy. Benign tumours are often excised thereby obtaining pathological information and cure.
- Chest x-ray – to exclude a symptomless primary lung cancer.

### Management

- Curative management usually involves craniotomy with surgical excision of a benign tumour.
- Palliative management
  - Symptoms of raised intracranial pressure – steroids, debulking operations, ventricular shunts, aspiration of cysts
  - Symptoms of local brain dysfunction – anticonvulsants.

Symptoms such as hemiparesis and hemianopia respond less reliably to surgery but it is often very gratifying to remove tumours in the cerebellar hemispheres even if they are malignant.

### Adjuvant therapy

- Radiotherapy – used extensively in malignant tumours and is the only mode of treatment known to prolong life in malignant gliomas
- Chemotherapy – routine in cerebral lymphomas but confined to research trials with other malignant brain tumours.

## CEREBRAL ABSCESS

### Aetiology

- Compound fractures – head injury
- Direct – more than 50% result from middle ear or mastoid infection spreading either directly, or via blood vessels, to the temporal lobe or cerebellum. Frontal or ethmoid sinus infection involves the frontal lobe. Septic thrombosis of the venous sinuses may occur – notably cavernous sinus thrombosis caused by infection on the face
- Bloodstream – from lung infection (bronchiectasis; abscess) or septic endocarditis.

### Symptoms and signs

Symptoms and signs are usually those of the underlying condition, such as middle ear infection or frontal sinusitis, with relatively fast onset of symptoms of a space occupying lesion with appropriate localizing signs. Epilepsy is particularly common. Diagnosis is by CT or MRI scanning.

### Treatment

The abscess is aspirated via a burr hole and the pus cultured; antibiotics are given depending on the microbiology. The primary focus of infection must also be treated.

## SPONTANEOUS INTRACRANIAL HAEMORRHAGE

There are two main causes which are treated surgically:

1 Congenital saccular aneurysms of the circle of Willis (Figure 10.6)
2 Arteriovenous malformations of the brain.

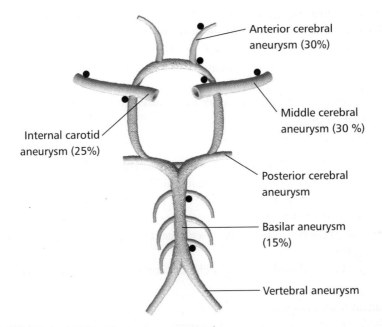

**Figure 10.6** Circle of Willis with common aneurysm sites

### Aneurysms
### Pathology
Aneurysms are caused almost exclusively by a congenital weakness of the arterial wall, producing a pea-sized saccular aneurysm (often called a 'berry' aneurysm because of its appearance), usually in relation to a bifurcation – 85% occur in the anterior half of the circle of Willis and 15% are multiple. Women are affected more than men.

### Clinical features
- **Subarachnoid haemorrhage** into the cerebrospinal fluid, often after strenuous activity, heralded by a rapid rise in intracranial pressure leading to sudden severe headache with nausea and vomiting, and loss or depressed level of consciousness. There may be an associated intracerebral haemorrhage or subdural haemorrhage with focal neurological signs. Blood in the CSF causes meningeal irritation with neck rigidity and a positive Kernig's sign (resistance to passive straight leg raising). **Approximately one-third of patients die without recovering consciousness.**
- **Pressure symptoms.** The III (oculomotor) nerve is especially **prone to pressure** caused by a large internal carotid artery aneurysm (ptosis or paralysis of eye movements) but others can be affected.

### Complications
- **Rebleeding.** The risk of further bleeding is highest within the first 2 weeks and remains high for approximately 6 weeks (up to 20%). After this the risk reduces but remains present indefinitely.

- Delayed cerebral ischaemia may occur at any time between the third and twenty-first day post-bleed. Arterial spasm causes cerebral infarction and is an extremely serious cause of morbidity and mortality. The use of selective cerebral calcium antagonists such as nimodipine reduces this complication.
- Hydrocephalus can occur, secondary to impaired absorption of CSF due to the presence of blood.

## Treatment

If the patient makes a reasonable recovery from the initial haemorrhage, then cerebral angiography is performed to locate the site of the aneurysm which is then **clipped via a craniotomy in order to prevent re-bleeding**. Conservative management is used when the angiogram is negative, indicating probable thrombosis within a small aneurysm. There have been **recent advances in endovascular obliteration** of aneurysms.

Prognosis is related to the patient's clinical condition and presentation.

### Arteriovenous malformations

Also called cerebral angiomas, these comprise a mass of fragile abnormal arteries, veins and capillaries which are developmental in origin. They are a less frequent and less disastrous cause of subarachnoid haemorrhage than aneurysms, often presenting with epilepsy because they usually lie near or on the cerebral cortex. Some malformations occur in recognized patterns – **von Hippel–Lindau disease** (retino-cerebellar angiomatosis) and **Sturge–Weber syndrome** (encephalo-trigeminal angiomatosis); the latter characterized by a port wine cutaneous angioma on the face. It is sometimes possible to hear intracranial bruits with a stethoscope.

The diagnosis and extent of the malformation requires angiography. Treatment is often multimodal, involving a combination of surgery, embolization, and stereotactic radiotherapy.

## HYDROCEPHALUS

Hydrocephalus (see Figure 10.8) literally means 'water on the brain' and is a condition characterized by **excess intracranial CSF and dilated ventricles**. CSF is a clear low protein fluid in which the brain and spinal cord float. The total volume is around 150 ml and 600 ml is produced daily by the choroid plexi in the lateral, third and fourth ventricles. Flow is from the lateral ventricles to the third ventricle (via the foramina of Monro), and then to the fourth ventricle (via the aqueduct of Sylvius) from where it enters the subarachnoid space (via the foramina of Magendie and Lushka) (Figure 10.7). It is absorbed into the venous system through the arachnoid granulations of the superior sagittal sinus. **Obstruction along the ventricular pathway or failure of reabsorption produces a rise in pressure, dilatation of the ventricles and thinning of the cerebral cortex.** There are two types of hydrocephalus:

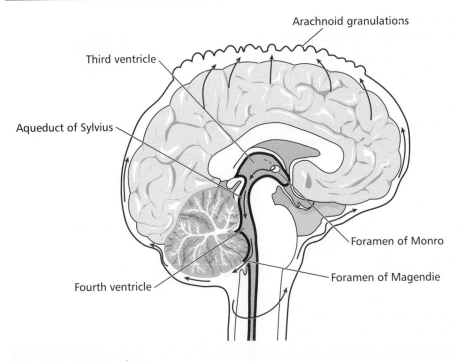

Third ventricle

Arachnoid granulations

Aqueduct of Sylvius

Foramen of Monro

Foramen of Magendie

Fourth ventricle

**Figure 10.7** Circulation of CSF

- **Obstructive hydrocephalus** – CSF cannot escape into the subarachnoid space due to a mechanical obstruction by tumour, infection or congenital stenosis of the aqueduct of Sylvius
- **Communicating hydrocephalus** – CSF escapes into the subarachnoid space but there is a failure or abnormality of absorption due to adhesions or obliteration of the subarachnoid space secondary to subarachnoid haemorrhage, meningitis or surgery.

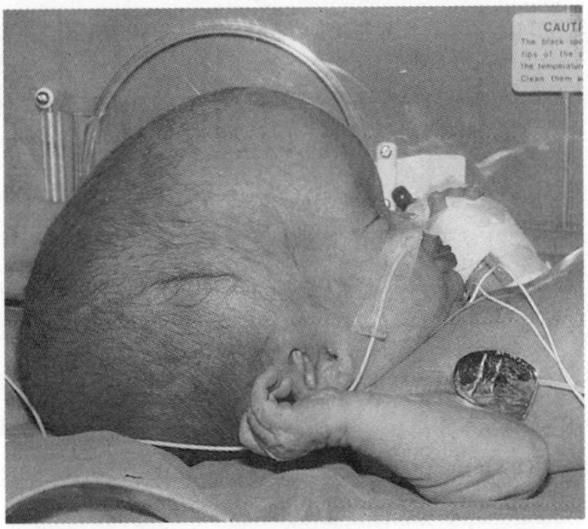

**Figure 10.8** Hydrocephalus

### Clinical features

In adults there is raised intracranial pressure.

In children, the fontanelles have not fused and the head enlarges (Figure 10.8). The eyes are pushed downward and have a distinct 'sunsetting' appearance. Mental retardation is usual and there may be optic atrophy.

## Treatment

In obstructive hydrocephalus secondary to tumour, it is desirable to remove the obstruction if possible. Otherwise a ventricular shunt is performed (Figure 10.9), diverting the CSF through a subcutaneous tube, usually, into the peritoneum.

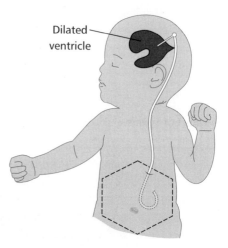

Dilated ventricle

**Figure 10.9** Ventriculoperitoneal shunt

## THE SPINE

Neurosurgical disease affecting the spine gives symptoms due to pressure on:
- The spinal cord (myelopathy)
- Nerve roots (radiculopathy).

At the junction of the spinal cord and the lumbosacral plexus (conus medullaris) there may be both myelopathy and radiculopathy. Lesions below L1/2 (adults) and L2/3 (children) can only affect nerve roots.

### Symptoms of spinal lesions

Symptoms are usually chronic except for trauma and infection:
- Pain – usually the first complaint and is often referred to the distribution of a nerve root which may spread around the trunk or down a limb. It is often made worse by coughing or sneezing which raises the intrathecal pressure. Movement of the spine often causes acute pain. **Pain caused by spinal tumour is often worse at night when lying flat.**
- Weakness and wasting – in the form of an upper motorneurone or lower motorneurone distribution, depending on whether it is due to compression of the spinal cord or nerve roots.
- Sensory impairment – according to the position of the lesion.
- Compression from lateral lesions may produce the **Brown–Séquard** (cord hemisection) syndrome with spastic weakness and loss of vibration sense on the same side as the lesion (due to involvement of the long pyramidal tracts) and loss of pain and temperature sensation on the opposite side (due to involvement of the lateral spinothalamic tract).
- Sphincter disturbance – usually a late occurrence.

## Investigation of spinal disease
- Plain x-rays remain extremely useful in the investigation of spinal injuries, degenerative conditions and tumours.
- Magnetic resonance imaging (MRI) is now the mainstay of special investigations of the spine due to its sensitivity in detecting soft tissue abnormalities.
- CT myelography is useful in some cases where MRI cannot be performed either due to the presence of a pacemaker or small metal objects within the body.

## Pathology
Spinal disease can be congenital (**spina bifida**) or acquired:
- Traumatic – fracture-dislocation of spine
- Infective – tuberculosis; staphylococcus
- Neoplastic – benign and malignant
- Degenerative: spondylosis; disc herniation.

## SPINA BIFIDA

Spina bifida (Figure 10.10) is caused by an embryonic failure of fusion in the midline of the structures which cover and protect the spinal cord. It is related to maternal **folic acid** deficiency and is seen less frequently nowadays due to antenatal diagnosis and termination. There are different degrees of severity:

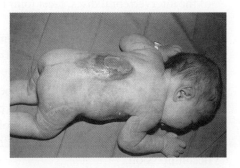

**Figure 10.10** Spina bifida

- Spina bifida occulta – i.e. 'hidden'. This is the mildest form, consisting of a gap in the bony neural arches of one or more vertebrae seen incidentally on x-rays. There may be an overlying dimple, sinus, tuft of hair or haemangioma.
- Meningocele – a cystic swelling of meninges containing CSF overlying the vertebral neural arch defect. Despite its name there is often a degree of cord or nerve root deformity.
- Meningomyelocele – in this case the spinal cord and roots are adherent to the meningeal sac and can be demonstrated by transillumination. The lower limbs, bladder and anal sphincter have varying degrees of paralysis.
- Myelocele (spina bifida aperta) – complete failure of fusion with the neural groove exposed and leaking CSF.

## Clinical features
Spina bifida is particularly common in the lumbosacral area (90%). Meningomyelocele is nearly always associated with **hydrocephalus** secondary to an **Arnold–Chiari malformation** – the brain stem and cerebellar tonsils prolapse

through the foramen magnum obstructing the CSF pathway through the fourth ventricle. There may be other congenital deformities.

### Treatment
- Minor degrees of spina bifida need no treatment.
- Meningocele and meningomyelocele should be repaired early to prevent progressive neurological damage. This is done by raising lateral skin flaps to cover and protect the neural tissue.
- Associated hydrocephalus requires a ventriculoperitoneal shunt.
- Meningitis is prevented by early surgical treatment and antibiotics.
- Long-term physiotherapy for the lower limbs is necessary.
- Urinary and faecal diversion may be required in later life.
- Severe deformities may be better left untreated.

## DEGENERATIVE CONDITIONS

- Cervical spondylosis – 'wear and tear' in the cervical spine – results in bulging of the intervertebral discs, facet joint hypertrophy and instability. It is common in the middle aged and elderly.
- Cervical disc herniation is more common in the younger age group and causes radiculopathy and/or myelopathy.
- Lumbar disc herniation is extremely common in young adults, resulting in symptoms attributable to the trapped lumbosacral plexus. Classically, this gives rise to **sciatica due to a lateral prolapse**. A **central prolapse** is rarer and causes the more serious syndrome of **cauda equina compression**, leading to 'saddle anaesthesia' and sphincter disturbance requiring emergency surgical decompression.

The mainstay of treatment is conservative with NSAIDs, analgesics and physiotherapy. Failure of conservative measures or neurological complications requires surgery.

## SPINAL EXTRADURAL ABSCESS

Spinal extradural abscess is uncommon and usually results from staphylococcal septicaemia. It is rapidly progressive, requiring urgent treatment, usually via laminectomy with drainage and antibiotic therapy. The risk of delayed treatment is that of permanent neurological deficit due to venous infarction of the spinal cord.

## SPINAL TUMOURS

- **Extradural** – present with symptoms of root irritation in the same manner as prolapsed discs. Metastatic deposits are by far the most common. Primary tumours are rare – sarcoma, chordoma, neurofibroma.
- **Intradural extramedullary** – meningioma; neurofibroma. Apart from metastases, these are the commonest spinal tumours and, happily, are benign.

- **Intramedullary** – astrocytoma; ependyonoma. Astrocytomas are commonly malignant and fairly fast growing tumours with a poor prognosis. Ependymomas are much slower growing and often amenable to surgery.

### Treatment
Laminectomy is usually required to confirm the nature of the tumour and to decompress the cord. Wherever possible, the tumour is completely excised, this generally being the case with benign tumours. With malignant tumours, radio-therapy is the mainstay of treatment.

## NERVES

### PERIPHERAL NERVE INJURIES

#### Classification
There are three types of peripheral nerve inujury:
- Neuropraxia (pressure injury) – light pressure applied for a considerable time, leading to loss of conduction along the nerve fibres. Wallerian degeneration does not occur. Rapid, complete recovery is expected within 2–3 weeks of the injury.
- Axonotmesis (crush injury) – associated with Wallerian degeneration of the axons distal to the site of the lesion. The supporting Schwann tubes remain intact and regeneration occurs and is usually complete, albeit slow.
- Neurotmesis (cutting injury) – severance with attempted regeneration of nerve fibres into inappropriate Schwann tubes; the fibres reach different endings from those to which they were originally connected. Recovery under these cir-cumstances is always incomplete but function may still be useful.

#### Clinical features
- Motor – paralysis, wasting, deformity, absent reflex jerks
- Sensory – anaesthesia/paraesthesia in the distribution of the affected nerve; neurogenic ulceration/damage, e.g. Charcot's joint
- Vasomotor – reduced blood supply with atrophy of the skin; reduced sweating.

#### Treatment
- Primary suture of nerve ends – only if there is a clean cut such as by glass or a sharp blade
- Secondary suture – after 2–3 weeks following debridement of the wound and treatment of infection.

### SPECIFIC NERVE LESIONS

#### Radial nerve
The radial nerve is usually injured in fractures as it winds around the spiral groove in the humerus, resulting in **wrist drop** due to paralysis of the wrist exten-sors and loss of sensation over a small area of the dorsum of the hand at the base of the thumb and index finger (Figure 10.11).

## Median nerve

The median nerve is often damaged in elbow fractures or lacerations of the wrist. In high lesions the pronators of the forearm and the majority of the flexors of the wrist and fingers are all paralysed. There is paralysis of the opponens pollicis, abductor pollicis, part of the flexor pollicis brevis and the outer two lumbricals. There is **wasting of the thenar eminence** and sensation is lost on the thumb, index and middle fingers and half of the fourth finger (Figure 10.12). The loss of sensation is a serious disability.

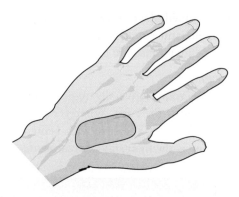

Figure 10.11 Radial nerve sensory loss

## Carpal tunnel syndrome

This syndrome is due to pressure on the median nerve as it passes under the flexor retinaculum and results in pain, numbness and weakness in the median nerve distribution, especially at night. Relief is often obtained by cooling the hand or hanging it in a dependent position. It can be treated by night splints holding the wrist in a neutral position, injections of hydrocortisone around the carpal ligament, or surgery to divide the flexor retinaculum.

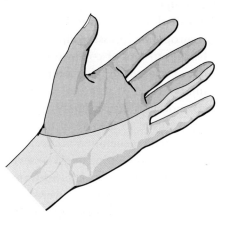

Figure 10.12 Median nerve sensory loss

## Ulnar nerve

The ulnar nerve is most commonly injured at the elbow and occasionally at the wrist. There is paralysis of the interossei, the inner two lumbricals, adductor pollicis and hypothenar muscles. This is associated with wasting, particularly between the metacarpal bones and of the hypothenar eminence. The fingers assume the position of hyperextension proximally and flexion distally. This position is called *main en griffe* or clawing of the hand. Injuries above the elbow affect flexor carpi ulnaris and part of the flexor digitorum profundus. Sensory changes occur over

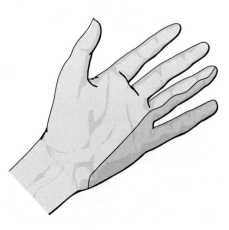

Figure 10.13 Ulnar nerve sensory loss

the medial half of the hand, including the whole of the little finger and half the ring finger (Figure 10.13).

### Brachial plexus

The majority of these lesions are due to traction.

- Upper arm type (**Erb–Duchenne**) (C5 and C6) – occurs as an obstetric or motor cycle injury where the head is forced away from the shoulder. Paralysis of the deltoid, biceps, brachialis, brachioradialis and most of the rotators of the shoulder produces a 'waiters tip' position of the arm.
- Lower arm type (**Klumpke's**) (C8 and T1) – occurs with dislocation or forcible abduction of the shoulder or a cervical rib. There is paralysis of the flexors of the wrist and fingers and of the **intrinsic muscles of the hand** with anaesthesia on the inner side of the forearm and hand.

### Sciatic nerve

The sciatic nerve is injured by stab wounds around the buttock or dislocation of the hip and results in paralysis of the hamstrings and all muscles below the knee. Below the knee is also anaesthetized except for the medial calf and foot supplied by the saphenous branch of the femoral nerve. The resulting disability is severe and amputation may be considered.

### Lateral popliteal nerve

This nerve is injured as it winds around the neck of the fibula. The classic injury is from a car bumper resulting in a fractured fibula, but is seen with tight splints, plaster casts or the lithotomy position (urology). Foot drop and inversion of the foot follows with anaesthesia over the anterior and lateral aspects of the lower leg and foot.

---

**CRIB BOX – BRAIN, SPINE AND NERVES**

**Raised intracranial pressure** – headache, vomiting, papilloedema, mental disorders, Cushing's reflex, large head in children

**Brain tumours** – primary are gliomas; secondary from lung, breast, melanoma, etc.

**Other intracranial tumours** – meningioma, neuroma, pituitary, craniopharyngioma

**Cerebral abscess** – most from middle ear

**Subarachnoid haemorrhage** – berry aneurysms and A-V malformations

**Hydrocephalus** – obstructive and communicating

**Head injury** – see complications diagram:
- Primary brain damage is irreversible
- Secondary brain damage is preventable

**Extradural haemorrhage** – knocked out; recovers (**lucid interval**); unconsciousness; lateralizing signs (pupil dilates on same side)

**Chronic subdural** – elderly, drunks, bleeding disorders; presents like a tumour

**Spina bifida** – Arnold–Chiari malformation common; maternal folic acid deficiency

**Spinal tumours** – secondary metastases are the most common

**Nerve lesions** – pressure (neuropraxia); crush (axonotmesis); cut (neurotmesis)

chapter 11

# DISEASES OF ARTERIES

## ATHEROSCLEROSIS

Atherosclerotic arterial disease affects everyone with increasing age and, together with ischaemic heart disease and strokes, accounts for half of all deaths.
- Arteries can be classified anatomically and functionally into:
  - Large – elastic **capacitance** vessels; the aorta and major branches
  - Medium – **distribution** vessels, e.g. femoral, carotid
  - Small – **supply** vessels within the substance of tissue.
- **Atherosclerosis primarily affects large and medium sized vessels.**
- The condition is characterized by subintimal deposits of fatty material (**atheroma**, Figure 11.1) which eventually becomes fibrotic, calcified and hard (**sclerosis**).
- Atheroma **narrows** the arterial lumen and may also ulcerate through the intima to produce overlying thrombus which can **embolize** distally or propagate locally to **occlude** the vessel.
- Bleeding within an atheromatous plaque will elevate the intima to cause occlusion.
- Rarely, the atheroma 'splits', allowing blood to flow into the subintimal plane which occludes the artery by 'dissection'.

Although the condition is generalized, there are specific sites where atheroma tends to be more pronounced, producing recognized disease patterns (Figure 11.2).
- Such sites are characteristically at **points of arterial bifurcation** or branching where mechanical shear stresses may predispose to atheroma deposition, e.g. carotid bifurcation, proximal coronary arteries, renal artery origin.
- In the lower limb the aortic bifurcation (**aorto-iliac disease**) and the superficial femoral artery in the thigh (**femoro-popliteal disease**) are commonly affected.

### Aetiology
The cause of atherosclerosis is unknown but several factors are recognized:

- Age – increases with increasing age
- Sex – pre-menopausal women seem protected
- Smoking – majority of symptomatic patients smoke
- Metabolic – diabetes mellitus, familial hyperlipidaemias, high cholesterol
- Hypertension – increased incidence of atheroma
- Alcohol – moderate intake seems to protect
- Racial – differences may be dietary and/or genetic
- Job – sedentary job more at risk.

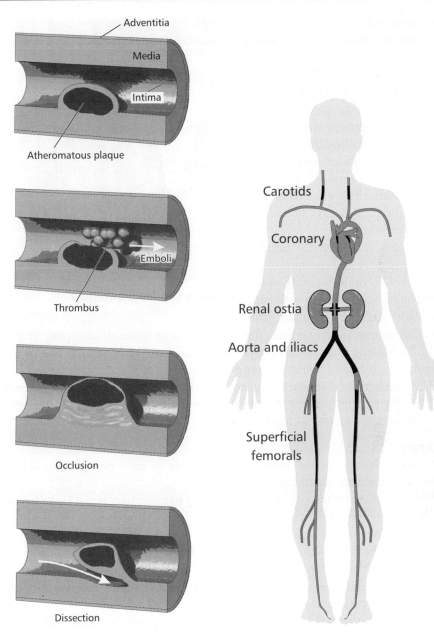

**Figure 11.1** Atheroma and possible consequences

**Figure 11.2** Common sites of atheroma deposition

## ATHEROSCLEROSIS OF THE LEGS

Next to coronary and carotid disease, the lower limbs are most commonly affected. Decreased blood flow caused by arterial stenosis or thrombotic occlusion produces three classic problems related to the severity of ischaemia, i.e. **intermittent claudication, rest pain, and gangrene.**

### Intermittent claudication

- A modest reduction in blood flow causes cramp in affected muscle groups on exercise. **The pain disappears with rest and returns with further exercise.**
- The muscle groups affected are typically those immediately below the arterial stenosis or occlusion – thus superficial femoral disease produces calf claudication whereas aorto-iliac occlusion produces buttock and thigh claudication.
- The pain is caused by insufficient blood supply and accumulation of metabolites in the working muscles.
- Having to stop walking in the middle of the street because of pain is

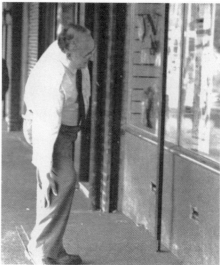

**Figure 11.3** 'Window-shopping'

embarrassing, so the patient often pretends to be 'window-shopping' (Figure 11.3), walking from one shop front to another until pain requires him to stop and rest – so-called 'window-shoppers' disease'.
- The **claudication distance** is a measure of the **severity** of arterial insufficiency. Typically patients present to their doctor when they can walk no further than a few hundred metres without resting.

### Rest pain

- Severe reduction in the blood supply results in pain even at rest due to ischaemia of nerves and skin.
- The patient complains of extreme permanent nagging pain in the lower leg and particularly the forefoot and toes which 'feel trapped in a vice'.
- **The pain is worse at night** in bed when sleep lowers the pulse and blood pressure, thereby diminishing further the poor blood flow. Some relief is obtained by dangling the affected leg out of bed or by rising to sit or stand. Lowering the leg in this manner eases the pain, perhaps by a gravitational increase in hydrostatic blood pressure.
- Eventually the patient is forced to abandon his bed entirely and spend both day and night in a chair with both legs dependent. The consequent venous engorgement tends to produce a swollen, blue foot which can be mistaken for injury or deep vein thrombosis (DVT) if the clinical history is discounted.

### Gangrene

- Death (necrosis) of tissue in bulk occurs when the blood supply is sufficiently impaired.
- Patches of black **dry gangrene** appear commonly on the dorsum of the foot, the toes, the ankle and shin. Whole toes or the complete forefoot may demarcate and mummify (Figure 11.4).

- Added infection results in **wet gangrene** with dripping smelly pus, spreading cellulitis, toxaemia and death if untreated.

### Differential diagnosis of leg pain

Approximately 10% of patients referred with leg pain to a vascular surgeon will have a non-vascular cause for their problem, e.g.:

- Bones and joints – arthritis, metatarsalgia, gout
- Nerves – peripheral neuropathy, sciatica
- Muscles – myopathy, tendonitis
- Veins – deep venous thrombosis.

### Natural history of leg atherosclerosis

It is logical to imagine progressive ischaemia of the leg causing the progressively worsening symptoms of claudication, rest pain and gangrene outlined above. However, the reduction in blood flow caused by atherosclerosis is not always relentlessly progressive because of **collateral circulation** in smaller vessels which bypasses any obstruction in larger arteries and tends to increase with time (Figure 11.5).

- Thus 40% of claudicants will spontaneously improve in the first year.
- Conversely, a sudden arterial occlusion allows no time for a collateral circulation to develop and asymptomatic individuals or patients with mild claudication can present with acute ischaemia.

It is important to remember that atherosclerosis is a systemic disease – 50% of patients presenting with intermittent claudication will die of **ischaemic heart disease** or **stroke** within 5 years.

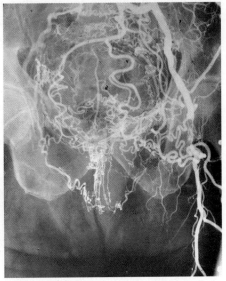

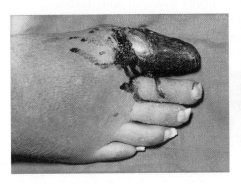

**Figure 11.4** Gangrenous toe

**Figure 11.5** Angiogram showing gross collateral circulation across the pelvis

## CLINICAL ASSESSMENT

### HISTORY

- Risk factors – smoking, diabetes, job, etc.
- Severity – claudication distance, sleep disturbance, continuous rest pain
- Onset – sudden onset suggests embolism or thrombosis
- Atherosclerosis elsewhere – angina, previous myocardial infarction, strokes
- Drugs – beta-blockers cause peripheral vasoconstriction.

> The degree of disability is important; for example, job-threatening intermittent claudication at 200 metres in a 50-year-old postman with a family to feed, is a different treatment problem from an obese 75-year-old woman with the same disability, but which bothers her only on rare occasions when she walks far enough.

### EXAMINATION

**Observation** – examine the whole patient, i.e. completely undressed apart from underwear. Look particularly for **nicotine stains**, lung and heart disease (can the patient lie flat?), cyanosis, abdominal pulsation (aneurysm), xanthelasma (lipid disease), scars (previous surgery). In the legs look for pallor (particularly on elevation), loss of hair, oedema, infection, cellulitis, ulcers, gangrenous patches, collapsed veins (venous guttering). When there is doubt regarding the cause of leg pain, it is essential to observe the patient walking.

**Palpation** – feel and compare the temperature of both feet (is one side cold?). Palpate all the **pulses** in a fixed and logical order and check paired pulses synchronously, where possible, to detect any comparative difference in volume or a delay between one side and the other, indicating a unilateral stenosis. The usual sequence is both radials, both brachials, both subclavians, carotids separately, the precordium and heart for thrills (aneurysm, cardiac enlargement), abdominal aorta (aneurysm; pulse present or not), both femorals, popliteals separately, both posterior tibials at the ankle and both dorsalis pedis pulses. Finally, the radial and femoral pulses are simultaneously felt to check for radiofemoral delay.

**Auscultation** – the objective is to locate bruits which indicate turbulent flow and stenosis. Listen to the carotids, the heart (valve disease), the abdominal aorta, the iliac fossae (iliac vessels), the common femorals in the groin and the superficial femorals in the thigh.

> **HELPFUL HINTS**
> Throughout the examination, bear in mind what you might expect to find taking account of the patient's symptoms. Thus in left calf claudication, absent left popliteal and left foot pulses would be usual and confirms the validity of the history obtained. Likewise, in buttock and thigh claudication, one would expect to find the femoral and distal pulses absent. Nothing is more irksome to an examiner than being given a beautiful history which is subsequently marred by inconsistent clinical findings! Remember also the **Leriche syndrome**, caused by bilateral aorto-iliac occlusion, i.e. bilateral buttock and thigh claudication, impotence in men, and absent femoral pulses.

It is useful to draw a simple diagram to record the clinical findings (Figure 11.6). This will ensure that nothing is forgotten and clearly illustrates all the salient findings. The ankle/brachial systolic pressure index (see below) is usefully incorporated.

## SPECIAL INVESTIGATIONS

Numerous techniques are available to further assess lower limb atherosclerosis but the simple tests, such as checking for diabetes and anaemia, should be done before embarking on extensive invasive investigations such as the following:

- **Doppler ultrasound** – Doppler systolic arterial pressure can be measured in the clinic with a hand-held probe and a blood pressure cuff (Figure 11.7). Placing the probe over an artery gives an audible blood flow signal which ceases when the cuff is inflated to systolic pressure. By measuring the normal brachial systolic pressure and comparing it to the ankle pressure, an **ankle/brachial systolic pressure index** is calculated, e.g.:

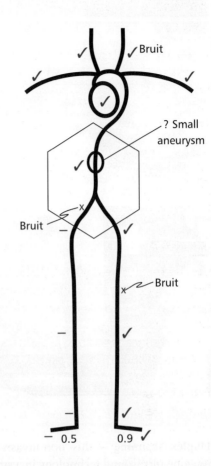

**Figure 11.6** Example of clinical findings

$$\frac{\text{Ankle pressure} = 100}{\text{Brachial pressure} = 120} = \text{ABSPI of } 0.8$$

The ankle systolic pressure is usually the same or slightly higher than the brachial, giving an ABSPI of 1 or greater, which is normal and excludes significant vascular disease. An **index of <0.4 is usually seen with rest pain** and/or gangrene whereas higher figures correlate with severity of claudication. Using a **treadmill** (Figure 11.8) the claudication distance can be measured accurately and compared to the pre- and post-exercise pressure indices, thereby giving a measure of the collateral circulation. The Doppler signal can be displayed graphically as a flow velocity waveform to give information on upstream or downstream stenosis or occlusion. Such non-invasive investigations are usually conducted in a dedicated **Vascular Laboratory**.

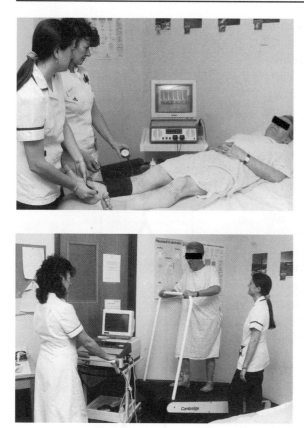

**Figure 11.7** Measuring ankle systolic pressure with cuff and Doppler probe

**Figure 11.8** Exercising on a treadmill

- **Duplex scanning** – this non-invasive investigation combines Doppler and imaging ultrasound technology in a single device (hence duplex). A two-dimensional image of a blood vessel is obtained and blood flow velocity can be measured to give further information (Figure 11.9). The image can be colour coded to show forward and reverse flow and enable visualization of atheromatous plaques and stenoses. Although particularly helpful in assessing carotid disease, it is increasingly used elsewhere.
- **Angiography** – two-dimensional x-ray images are obtained during intra-arterial injection of contrast medium to produce films of the arterial tree (Figure 11.10). Flexible catheters introduced via the femoral, brachial or axillary arteries allow placement of dye and visualization of any part of the arterial network. **Digital subtraction imaging (DSI)** uses computer enhancement of the radiographic image to give very clear pictures with minimal use of contrast medium. **All angiography is presently invasive and carries risks of serious haemorrhage, thrombosis and arterial damage.** It should not be undertaken lightly and is used only when surgery or other invasive treatment is considered necessary. Other ingenious methods to visualize blood vessels are continually being developed using spiral computerized tomography (CT) and magnetic resonance imaging (MRI).

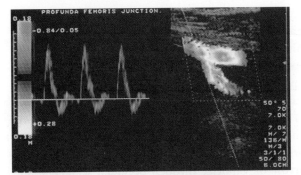

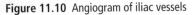

**Figure 11.9** Duplex scan of femoral artery

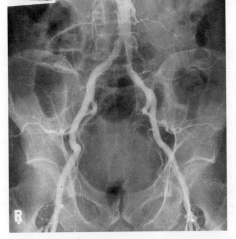

**Figure 11.10** Angiogram of iliac vessels

## TREATMENT

The treatment options for lower limb atherosclerosis are:
- Conservative management
- Angioplasty
- Reconstructive arterial surgery
- Lumbar sympathectomy
- Amputation.

In all patients, attention to general health is important (e.g. stop smoking, diabetic control, obesity, heart failure, hyperlipidaemia). Foot care is important, particularly in diabetics with peripheral neuropathy. The treatment chosen for any individual depends on the severity of symptoms, the general health of the patient and finally the angiographic picture.

### Conservative management

This is used primarily for patients with mild to moderate intermittent claudication, the vast majority of whom will improve spontaneously by **cessation of smoking, losing weight** and **exercising regularly**. It is usual to recommend low-dose **aspirin** for its anti-platelet/anti-thrombotic effect and moderate alcohol intake is thought to be beneficial.

## Angioplasty

This is used when symptoms are severe enough to warrant active treatment, i.e. crippling claudication, rest pain and gangrene. At angiography, if the atherosclerotic lesion is suitable, a balloon catheter can be passed along a guidewire into the lumen of the artery and positioned appropriately. Inflation of the sausage-shaped balloon dilates the narrowed segment to restore full patency and blood flow. Such a procedure carries the full title of **percutaneous transluminal balloon angioplasty** and is usually done via the femoral artery in the groin. Other transluminal techniques for restoring arterial continuity employ guided drills and thermal laser catheters to burrow or vaporize through occluded segments, and expandable **stents** can be inserted to maintain patency once achieved.

Radiological skills have advanced to the point where angioplasty has superseded traditional surgery in many cases. However, the **complications of arterial rupture, bleeding and acute thrombosis** mean that such treatment is undertaken with a vascular surgeon immediately available, and **patients undergoing angioplasty must be prepared for open surgery if complications ensue or the technique fails.** Long segment occlusion (>10 cm) or extreme tortuosity of the artery can render transluminal angioplasty impossible.

## Reconstructive arterial surgery

**Arterial surgery** restores blood flow either by:

- Directly removing atheroma from within an artery (**endarterectomy**)
- Using a bypass graft to channel blood around an obstruction and direct flow into a healthy distal artery.

Endarterectomy is of limited use in the lower limb but is used extensively in carotid disease. The success of bypass surgery is dependent largely on the patency of the distal vessels or run-off as viewed on angiography. A **good run-off** implies that below the blocked segment of artery there are healthy vessels with a low resistance to forward flow of blood through the planned bypass graft. Conversely, a **poor run-off** means diseased or completely blocked distal vessels with a high resistance to flow. The run-off may be so poor that bypass surgery is not possible.

Bypass grafts are either **anatomical** (following the anatomical route of the occluded vessel) or **extra-anatomical**.

Aorto-iliac disease can be bypassed with an **aorto-bifemoral** or an **aorto-biliac** 'Trouser' graft (Figure 11.11). In patients unfit for major abdominal surgery, an extra-anatomical **axillo-bifemoral** subcutaneous graft is used. If only one iliac artery is blocked, the patent femoral artery on the unaffected side is used to supply blood to the ischaemic leg through a **femoro-femoral** graft.

Femoro-popliteal disease, i.e. occlusion of the superficial femoral artery, is bypassed with a **femoro-popliteal** or a longer **femoro-distal** graft to a patent artery in the calf or ankle (Figure 11.11).

The ideal graft material is the patient's own long saphenous vein (**autogenous vein graft**) because it is lined by endothelium and has a high long-term patency rate (around 50% at 5 years). Because of its size, use is limited to femoro-

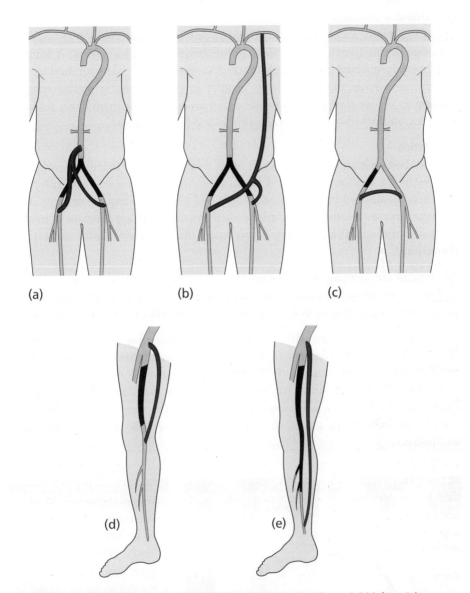

**Figure 11.11** Types of bypass grafts: (a) aorto-bifemoral; (b) axillo-bifemoral; (c) left-to-right femoro-femoral; (d) femoro-popliteal; (e) femoro-distal

popliteal or distal grafts, and the venous valves must be broken down with a special valve stripper to allow flow, or alternatively the vein is completely removed and reversed before grafting. Prosthetic grafts are made of **Dacron** or **Teflon (PTFE)** and come in all shapes and sizes. They remain patent for many years when used for large calibre aorto-iliac bypass, but are prone to thrombosis in smaller diameters and are a poor substitute for saphenous vein in the lower leg.

## Phenol lumbar sympathectomy

Used for patients with rest pain in whom angioplasty or reconstructive surgery is not possible due to extensive atherosclerosis or severe medical illness. A solution of phenol is injected through the back into the lumbar paravertebral gutter, thereby destroying the sympathetic ganglia in this region. Sympathectomy is thought to reduce rest pain by blocking afferent sympathetic pain fibres from the lower leg and possibly by increasing skin blood flow.

## Amputation

Used for rest pain and gangrene when other treatments have failed, are not possible, or the leg cannot be salvaged because of extensive gangrene and infection. Gangrenous toes can be amputated if the blood supply is adequate or after arterial reconstruction. Other amputations used in ischaemia are **forefoot** (Lisfranc; Chopart), **through-ankle** (Syme), **below-knee, through-knee** (Gritti–Stokes) and **above-knee**.

The type of amputation depends on:
- The tissue viability and likelihood of healing at the chosen level of amputation
- The potential of the patient to mobilize and rehabilitate on a prosthetic limb.

Preservation of the knee with a below-knee amputation is the operation of choice since it allows excellent rehabilitation and mobilization on a below-knee **patella tendon weight bearing (PTB)** prosthesis (Figure 11.12). The above-knee amputation requires a more cumbersome prosthesis with a mechanical locking knee and rehabilitation is consequently poorer. A through-knee amputation is often suited best to the infirm chairbound patient because it gives good power and balance.

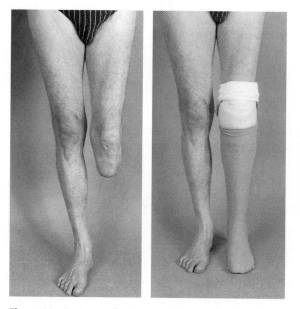

Ischaemia acounts for 85% of all lower limb amputations in the UK. Most are elderly (60–75) and half will be dead within 5 years; many will also lose their second leg. Despite intensive physiotherapy and support from prosthetists, the majority never become independent of a wheelchair.

**Figure 11.12** Picture of amputee with and without prosthesis

# ACUTE LIMB ISCHAEMIA

This is a surgical emergency which is most often seen in the leg and rarely in the arm. It is caused by:

- Acute thrombosis – in pre-existing atherosclerotic disease
- Embolus – of thrombus from the heart (post-infarct; atrial fibrillation)
- Trauma – long bone fractures with angulation; direct injury (often iatrogenic).

The history may help to confirm the aetiology. Trauma is obvious but differentiating between thrombosis and embolus may be difficult since atherosclerosis and heart disease often coexist. Enquire about previous claudication and heart disease. Classically, patients with emboli are referred from the coronary care unit a few days post-infarction when mural thrombi within the left ventricle detach and embolize to the leg.

The **clinical examination** reveals the classic 'P' signs:

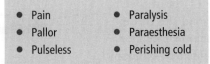

- Pain
- Pallor
- Pulseless
- Paralysis
- Paraesthesia
- Perishing cold

- Pulses are absent below the site of the occlusion.
- **Embolus** tends to lodge at sites of arterial branching where the internal lumen of the artery decreases in size and traps it.
- **Saddle embolus** is the term for an embolus at the aortic bifurcation with bilateral ischaemic legs and absent femoral pulses.
- Emboli cause stasis of blood flow, resulting in proximal and distal propagation of thrombus which in turn blocks other arteries and causes further ischaemia.
- **Acute thrombosis** secondary to atherosclerosis may be clinically indistinguishable from embolus.

If left untreated, irreversible ischaemic necrosis of muscle and skin occurs within 12–24 hours, resulting in fixed flexion contractures and spreading purple livedo.

**Special investigations** include ECG and echocardiogram to determine a cardiac embolic source, e.g. myocardial infarction, atrial fibrillation, valve disease, atrial thrombus. **Angiography** is usually necessary to differentiate between embolus and atherosclerotic thrombosis, or to visualize the site of arterial injury in trauma.

## Treatment

The aim is to restore circulation to the limb before gangrene develops.

**General measures** include the prevention of further thrombosis by **intravenous heparin**. Heart disease and other medical problems such as diabetes are treated. In trauma, resuscitation and other injuries will take precedence but a severely angulated fracture or dislocation should be reduced as soon as possible to 'unkink' the blood vessels and restore flow.

**Specific treatment** consists of the following:

- **Acute thrombosis** is treated by **intra-arterial thrombolysis**. At angiography the diagnosis is confirmed and an intra-arterial catheter positioned within the thrombus. A thrombolytic agent (e.g. streptokinase) is infused and dispersion of the thrombus monitored with further angiograms and repositioning of the catheter as required. Circulation is restored following complete lysis of the thrombus. Additional measures such as balloon angioplasty or arterial reconstructive surgery will be needed to treat the underlying atherosclerotic disease.

- **Embolus** to small peripheral arteries may be dissolved with thrombolysis. Large emboli are usually removed with surgery using a **Fogarty balloon catheter** (Figure 11.13). In the leg the femoral artery is exposed in the groin and opened (arteriotomy) to enable insertion of the catheter which is passed beyond the thrombus and the balloon inflated. Withdrawing the inflated balloon extracts the thrombus to restore blood flow and the arteriotomy is

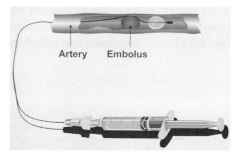

**Figure 11.13** Fogarty catheter

then repaired. The technique of **embolectomy** is simple, can be done under local anaesthetic, and is effective. However, the majority of these patients are already extremely ill with heart disease and **post-operative mortality due to cardiac complications is high (30–40%)**.

- **Trauma** is treated by direct repair or reconstructive arterial surgery as necessary.

## ARTERIAL ANEURYSM

An aneurysm is an abnormal localized dilatation of an artery. The vascular surgeon deals with acquired aneurysms which occur in large and medium sized vessels, most commonly the infra-renal abdominal aorta. Congenital aneurysms occur in the circle of Willis in the skull ('berry' aneurysm – see subarachnoid haemorrhage, Chapter 10), or as part of arteriovenous malformations. Aneurysms can be classified according to shape (Figure 11.14) as:

- Fusiform – circumferential dilatation
- Saccular – asymmetric bulge.

### Pathology

Acquired aneurysms occur as a result of weakness of the arterial wall due to degeneration of collagen and elastin in the media. The exact cause of the degeneration is unknown but may be linked to **atheromatous disease** (occlusion of the vasa vasorum), or be part of the normal **ageing process**. Aneurysms are seen in certain diseases of **connective tissue** synthesis (Marfan's syndrome). Anatomically they develop commonly in sites just proximal to bifurcations, suggesting that **reflected pressure waves** (standing waves) are important in aetiology. **Hypertension** and **smoking** are also implicated. Blood flow within an aneurysm is turbulent and in large arteries the blood usually clots to form layers of laminated thrombus (Figure 11.15) surrounding a central patent core through which flow is maintained.

- In smaller arteries the blood may **thrombose** and completely occlude the lumen.
- Thrombus may also **embolize** distally to cause acute limb ischaemia or patchy small infarcts.
- If the aneurysm grows sufficiently large, it may **rupture** and produce catastrophic haemorrhage.

The **abdominal aorta is the commonest site** for aneurysm formation (Figure 11.16), but they may occur in any artery.

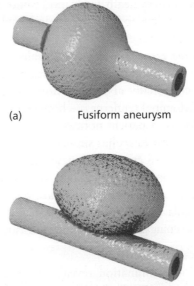

(a)    Fusiform aneurysm

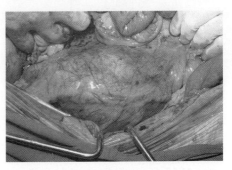

(b)    Saccular aneurysm

**Figure 11.14** Types of aneurysm: (a) fusiform – circumferential dilatation; (b) saccular – asymmetric bulge

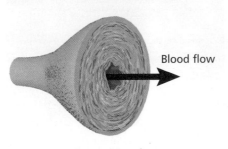

Blood flow

**Figure 11.15** Cross-section of aneurysm to show laminated intraluminal thrombus

**Figure 11.16** Abdominal aortic aneurysm

## ABDOMINAL AORTIC ANEURYSM

- Aneurysm of the infra-renal aorta occurs in **2% of men over the age of 60** and is less common in women.
- There is a **familial tendency** to aneurysm formation, particularly in male siblings of known patients.
- The normal abdominal aorta is approximately 2 cm in diameter.
- Aneurysms grow at an average rate of 0.5 cm annually and there is a **significant risk of rupture beyond 6 cm diameter** with few aneurysms attaining 8 cm.

- Immediate death from intra-abdominal bleeding occurs in 90% of ruptured aneurysms and of the remainder who survive to hospital, half will also perish despite surgery.
- **Most aneurysms are symptomless**, being discovered coincidentally on routine examination or ultrasound scanning for other reasons.
- Occasionally abdominal aortic aneurysms present with lumbar backache or abdominal tenderness – both signs of impending rupture.
- Rarely, a patient notices a pulsatile abdominal lump him/herself – 'Doctor, I think my heart has slipped into my tummy'.
- Large (>6 cm) aortic aneurysms are likely to rupture eventually if the patient lives long enough and does not die of other problems.
- Small aneurysms (<6 cm) are relatively safe but their size should be checked regularly with ultrasound scans.
- Screening programmes using ultrasound scanning may be introduced in the future.

### Clinical examination

Clinical examination reveals an **expansile pulsatile mass** above the umbilicus (Figure 11.17). The aneurysm size can be measured accurately with ultrasound scanning (Figure 11.18).

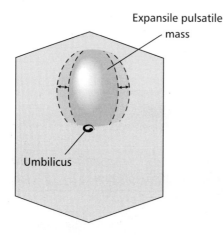

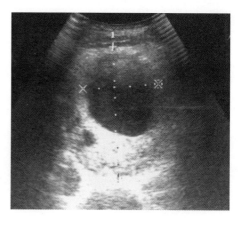

**Figure 11.17** Clinical findings – abdominal aortic aneurysm

**Figure 11.18** Ultrasound of abdominal aneurysm

### Treatment

Treatment consists of surgically replacing the aneurysmal segment with a Dacron graft and should be offered to patients with large or symptomatic aneurysms who are fit enough to withstand major surgery (Figure 11.19). At operation the aorta above and below the aneurysm is controlled with clamps and the sac opened. The graft is then sewn into the lumen and the aneurysm sac closed over the graft. **The operation carries a mortality of 5%.**

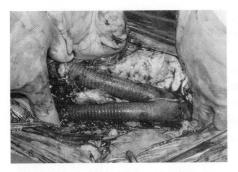

Figure 11.19 Aneurysm repair – graft *in situ*

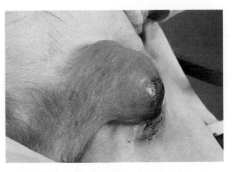

Figure 11.20 False aneurysm in groin

A new technique of **endoluminal repair** may be used in selected cases where the anatomy of the aneurysm is suitable. A graft is inserted into the aneurysm via the femoral artery in the groin, thereby avoiding the need for abdominal surgery.

## SPECIAL ANEURYSMS

### False aneurysm in groin

False aneurysm (Figure 11.20) is simply a pulsating haematoma surrounding a perforated artery which bleeds into surrounding tissue dense enough to contain the haematoma. They are increasingly common due to needle and catheter puncture wounds necessary during angiography or interventional radiology and seen usually in the groin (femoral artery) or elbow (brachial artery). Often they resolve spontaneously but surgical repair may be necessary.

### Dissecting aneurysm

Dissecting aneurysm occurs in atheromatous hypertensives or patients with medial degeneration (e.g. Marfan's syndrome) and starts usually in the proximal thoracic aorta or arch. The aortic wall splits, allowing blood to flow into the subintimal plane and 'dissect' the arterial wall distally, producing a false second lumen within the media. A 'twin-barrelled' aorta is formed, which ends usually with fatal rupture externally into the pleural space (see Chapter 19).

## CAROTID ATHEROSCLEROSIS

Atherosclerotic plaques are found commonly at the carotid bifurcation and may cause problems by embolization of platelet aggregates, cholesterol or thrombus into carotid cerebral territory to produce:

- **Transient ischaemic attacks (TIAs)** – 'little strokes', defined as **a focal neurological deficit of abrupt onset lasting up to 24 hours and leaving no residual neurological signs**. Usually they manifest as unilateral weakness of the face, arm or leg with or without speech disturbance and caused by microemboli producing transient reversible ischaemia of the cerebral cortex.

- **Amaurosis fugax** – fleeting blindness caused by transient ischaemia of the retina due to emboli to the retinal artery. The history is of a 'curtain or shutter' crossing the visual field. With an ophthalmoscope, refractile crystals of cholesterol can sometimes be observed traversing the retinal vessels.
- **Complete stroke** – infarction of an area of the brain, leaving the patient with permanent residual neurological deficit which may be mild to severe depending on the extent of brain damage. A stroke is usually sudden but may evolve slowly over a period of hours or days ('stroke in evolution'). Strokes are the third most common cause of death after ischaemic heart disease and cancer. Many victims survive in a severely crippled and dependent state whereas only a minority recover almost full function.

### Investigation of carotid disease
- The history is usually quite clear but other causes of neurological symptoms, e.g. migraine, multiple sclerosis, hypoglycaemia, cardiac dysrhythmias, should be excluded.
- Record which is the dominant hemisphere and any risk factors for atherosclerotic disease.
- Neurological signs vary, depending on how the patient presents; often there is nothing to find unless a full stroke has developed.
- **Listen to the carotid arteries for bruits**. They are best heard at the angle of the jaw and indicate stenosis >50% or more but the bruit will disappear with very tight stenosis simply because the blood flow is insufficient to generate noise.

Specific investigations are **carotid duplex scan** (Figure 11.21) to visualize ulcerated plaques and measure stenosis, **brain CT** (Figure 11.22) or **MRI scan** to detect infarcts and **carotid angiography**, if necessary, to show accurately the extent of disease.

### Treatment of carotid disease
Treatment of carotid atherosclerosis is aimed specifically at **prevention of permanent neurological disability due to stroke**. The risk of major stroke or death following a TIA is around 6% per year.

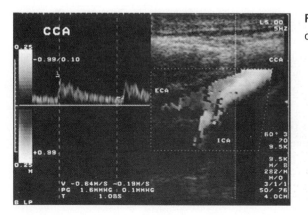

**Figure 11.21** Duplex scan of carotid artery

**Medical treatment** is indicated in all patients and essentially is the treatment of risk factors such as diabetes, obesity, smoking, hyperlipidaemia and, particularly, **hypertension. Anti-platelet therapy** such as low-dose aspirin is instituted.

**Surgery** comprises carotid endarterectomy to remove ulcerated atheromatous plaques and stenosis. Unfortunately, manipulation of the carotid artery during surgery causes a stroke in about 4% of cases. Thus **the risk of stroke due to surgery must be balanced against the risk of stroke with medical treatment alone.** Large controlled studies have so far concluded that surgery should be offered to symptomatic patients with carotid stenoses >70%. Carotid balloon angioplasty rather than surgery is presently the subject of trials.

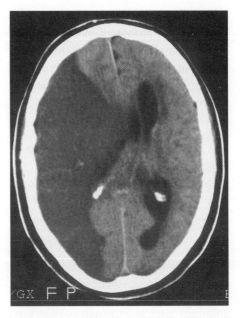

**Figure 11.22** Brain scan showing cerebral infarct

## MISCELLANEOUS ARTERIAL DISEASES

This section outlines some arterial diseases which come to the attention of the surgeon less frequently than aneurysms or atherosclerosis of the legs and carotids, or have an aetiology which is not strictly atheromatous in origin. **This does not imply that they are uncommon or unimportant.**

### THE DIABETIC FOOT

A diabetic patient presenting with gangrene and infection in the foot is depressingly common. The 'diabetic foot' (Figure 11.23) is caused by a combination of three factors:

1  Atherosclerosis – diabetes is a risk factor for atherosclerotic ischaemia
2  Small vessel disease – in simple terms diabetics develop a type of small vessel arteritis which occludes small arterioles and leads to ischaemia in the presence of normal proximal pulses
3  Peripheral neuropathy – diabetic peripheral neuropathy causes numbness and paraesthesia of the feet. Consequently, minor trauma or blistering due commonly to poorly fitting shoes goes unnoticed and unheeded until severe ulceration or infection ensues. Infection, once present, is difficult to treat due to coincidental poor blood supply.

Although diabetics do present with classical symptoms of pure proximal atherosclerosis amenable to angioplasty or reconstructive surgery, commonly all three problems coexist to a greater or lesser degree.

A typical clinical presentation is a **painless** deep infected ulcer on a pressure area (heel, ball of foot) with spreading cellulitis, wet gangrene and bounding palpable foot pulses.

Treatment includes diabetic control, antibiotics, debridement of dead tissue, drainage of pus and arterial reconstruction/angioplasty if needed. Below-knee amputation is often required.

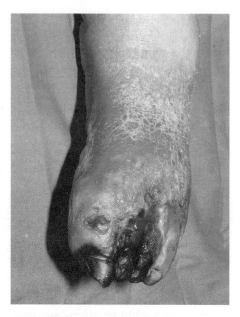

**Figure 11.23** Diabetic foot

## THROMBOANGIITIS OBLITERANS (BUERGER'S DISEASE)

This is a clinical syndrome of occlusive arterial ischaemia presenting almost exclusively in men 20–40 years old who are **heavy smokers**. All small arteries may be affected but presentation typically is with lower limb ischaemic claudication or rest pain and gangrene. As the name implies, **the condition is thought to be inflammatory** rather than simply atherosclerotic and produces thrombotic occlusion of the smaller arteries below the knee, with a characteristic fine network of 'corkscrew' collaterals seen on angiography. Reconstructive arterial surgery is often impossible and treatment is limited to sympathectomy, amputation and cessation of smoking.

## RAYNAUD'S PHENOMENON

- This is a common condition, affecting women most often and characterized by episodes of spasm of the digital arteries in response to cold.
- Patients complain of fingers and toes becoming white and numb when exposed to decreases in temperature.
- On rewarming, the digits become first **blue** as spasm decreases and returning blood is deoxygenated, and finally **red**, painful and hyperaemic as full blood flow returns.
- Attacks last from minutes to hours and are **symmetrical**, affecting both hands and/or both feet.
- In the majority, the condition is a benign inconvenience and is termed **primary Raynaud's**.

Its importance is that the phenomenon can be a symptom of underlying disease, when it is termed **secondary Raynaud's** and is then associated with trophic skin changes and tissue loss due to digital gangrene. Secondary Raynaud's phenomenon is seen most commonly in **autoimmune and connective tissue disorders**, for example:

- Systemic sclerosis
- Systemic lupus
- Mixed connective tissue disease
- Rheumatoid arthritis
- Primary biliary cirrhosis
- Generalized vasculitis.

**Occupational Raynaud's** occurs following prolonged use of vibrating tools such as grinders and chain saws. The aetiology is trauma to the vessels or nerves. It is recognized as an industrial disease termed **vibration white finger (VWF)**.

**Blood diseases** causing **hyperviscosity** and sluggish flow also produce Raynaud's phenomenon, e.g. leukaemia, polycythaemia, cold agglutinins, myeloma, cryo-globulinaemia.

Proximal obstruction to blood flow will reduce arterial pressure in the digital arteries and give rise to symptoms similar to Raynaud's phenomenon but not necessarily symmetrical. Thus **cervical rib, thoracic outlet syndrome, atherosclerosis, Buerger's disease and emboli** must be considered in patients with unilateral symptoms.

### Investigation
Investigation of Raynaud's phenomenon is aimed at eliminating any possible underlying cause, particularly autoimmune disease. **Thus an auto-antibody screen is mandatory as well as routine haematology and chest x-ray for cervical rib.**

### Treatment
Treatment of primary Raynaud's is symptomatic, e.g. wearing gloves and avoiding cold. Vasodilator drugs such as nifedipine may help. **Cervical sympathectomy** for upper limb Raynaud's was used extensively in the past but is now largely abandoned because of poor long-term results. Conversely, in the lower limb, lumbar sympathectomy is often successful. In secondary Raynaud's phenomenon, appropriate therapy is aimed at the underlying disease process.

## SUBCLAVIAN STEAL SYNDROME

- This condition (Figure 11.24) is caused by atherosclerotic occlusion or stenosis of the subclavian or innominate artery proximal to the origin of the vertebral artery.
- Consequently, blood flow in the vertebral artery is reversed and the arm on the affected side 'steals' blood from the brain stem, particularly when the arm is exercised.
- Patients are usually elderly and present with episodes of vertigo, unsteadiness and falling over.
- Auscultation reveals a bruit at the base of the neck and the blood pressure is reduced in the arm on the same side.
- Correction is achieved by angioplasty, endarterectomy or bypass surgery.

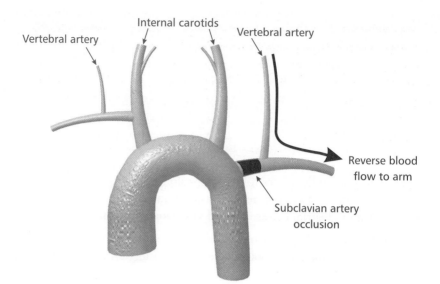

Figure 11.24 Diagram of subclavian steal syndrome

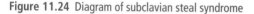

**CRIB BOX – DISEASES OF ARTERIES**

**Atherosclerosis**

- Risk factors – smoking, diabetes, obesity, sedentary lifestyle, male, hypertension
- Leg symptoms – claudication, rest pain, gangrene
- Investigation – Doppler ABSPI, duplex, angiogram
- Treatment – conservative, angioplasty, reconstruction, sympathectomy, amputation

**Acute ischaemia**

Remember the 'P' signs. Is it embolus or thrombosis?

Caused by:

- Acute thrombosis; previous history of claudication?
- Embolus; heart disease, recent infarct, on CCU?
- Trauma; treat the patient first, straighten the limb if bent/dislocated

Treatment:

- Thrombosis needs thrombolysis ± reconstruction
- Embolus needs embolectomy with Fogarty balloon catheter
- Trauma needs appropriate repair/reconstruction/amputation

**Aneurysm**

- Congenital or acquired. Fusiform or saccular
- Commonest is infra-renal AAA – 2% men over 60. Asymptomatic until leak/rupture
- Investigation – measure diameter with ultrasound
- Treatment – repair with Dacron graft when large
- Remember false and dissecting aneurysm

## Carotid disease

- Symptoms – none, TIA, amaurosis fugax, full stroke. Remember definition of TIA
- Investigate – listen for bruits, duplex, angiogram
- Treatment – is to prevent stroke; medical mainly and aspirin. Surgery when >70% stenosis

## Miscellaneous

- Diabetic foot – atherosclerosis, small vessel disease, and neuropathy
- Buerger's – young men, heavy smokers, usually need amputation
- Raynaud's – mainly women, primary and secondary; connective tissue disease, VWF
- Subclavian steal – arm steals blood from brain via reverse vertebral flow

# chapter 12

# DISEASES OF LEG VEINS

## ANATOMY

Normal venous flow is from the superficial veins via perforators through the deep fascia into the deep veins that drain in turn into the femoral vein, iliac vein, inferior vena cava (IVC) and thus back to the heart (Figure 12.1). The venous valves ensure flow in the correct direction and the **calf muscle pump** provides the driving force. The plexus of deep veins in the calf muscles converge to form the popliteal vein behind the knee.

The superficial veins comprise the **long and short saphenous veins** and their tributaries:

- The long saphenous vein perforates the deep fascia and joins the femoral vein in the groin.
- The short saphenous vein joins the popliteal vein in the popliteal fossa.
- Large perforating or communicating veins tend to occur at recognized sites in the lower, middle and upper calf and the lower and middle thigh.

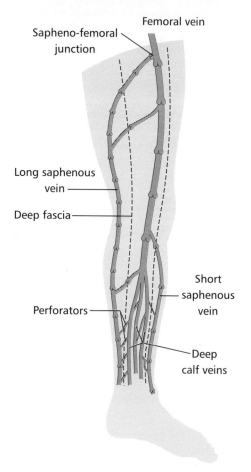

Figure 12.1 Anatomy of leg veins

## PHYSIOLOGY

In the upright position venous return from the leg is reliant on the efficacy of the calf muscle pump and the venous valves (Figure 12.2). Resting venous pressure in the superficial veins of the foot is around 100 mmHg and this falls to 20 mmHg when the calf is exercised.

- Thus the deep system is high pressure and the superficial veins low pressure when functioning normally.
- Valvular incompetence in the deep or perforating veins will allow high pressure blood to reflux into the superficial veins and cause dilatation and varicosity.

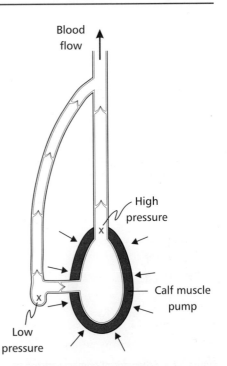

**Figure 12.2** Physiology of leg veins

## VARICOSE VEINS

Varicose veins are **irregularly dilated, tortuous and lengthened.** Varicose veins of the leg occur in 20% of the population and are more common in women (ratio 5:1) and people with a standing job. They are common in the Western world and rare in native Africans. There is a strong familial tendency to develop varicose veins.

### Aetiology
Varicose veins can be either **primary or secondary.**

- **Primary** or idiopathic represent the vast majority (Figure 12.3). The true pathology is unclear but is probably an inherited weakness of the vein wall which causes dilatation and this in turn leads to parting of the valve cusps with consequent valvular incompetence and reflux or retrograde flow of blood. Women are afflicted more than men and this may be due to hormonal influences or pregnancy. The term primary by implication means that the deep system is normal.
- **Secondary** varicose veins (Figure 12.4) occur due to:
  - **Previous deep vein thrombosis** (DVT). DVT destroys the deep and perforating venous valves allowing venous reflux and raised pressure.
  - **Pelvic tumour** causing venous obstruction and raised venous pressure. The pregnant uterus is the commonest example.
  - **Congenital arteriovenous fistulae**, causing venous hypertension. Such disorders are rare (e.g. Klippel–Trenaunay syndrome).

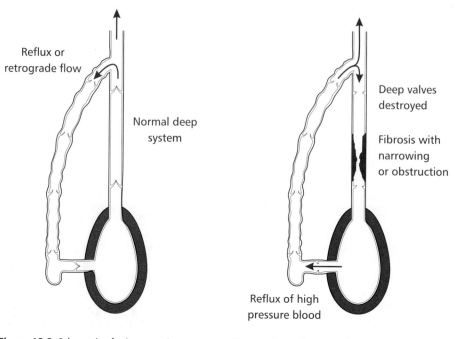

**Figure 12.3** Schematic of primary varicose veins

**Figure 12.4** Schematic of secondary varicose veins

## Clinical features

The majority are **asymptomatic** but unsightly. Varicose veins cause problems due to the increased venous pressure in the veins and tissues. Symptoms increase in number and severity with time to produce a clinical picture of **chronic venous insufficiency** (Figure 12.5):

- **Aching** – a 'bursting' discomfort after prolonged standing relieved by elevation of the leg or a compression stocking
- **Ankle swelling** – caused by increased hydrostatic pressure transmitted to the venules and capillaries with consequent oedema of the lower leg
- **Venous flares** – fan-shaped dilatation of superficial venules spreading around the ankle and particularly below the medial malleolus
- **Venous eczema** – an itchy scaly erythematous rash of the lower calf, usually centred above the medial malleolus
- **Pigmentation** – a brown discoloration of the skin in the 'gaiter' area caused by deposition of haemosiderin in the tissues
- **Thrombophlebitis** – superficial thrombosis due to stasis can occur in large varicosities. The vein becomes hard, inflamed and tender, resembling a thick cord of variable length beneath the skin. Resolution can take many weeks and often the vein is destroyed, thus curing the varicosity
- **Lipodermatosclerosis** – fibrosis of the skin and subcutaneous fat caused by long-term venous hypertension, fibrin deposition and inflammation. The calf and lower leg is said to resemble an inverted champagne bottle

- **Ulceration** – venous ulcers occur typically in relation to the medial malleolus and can be extensive. Venous stasis/hypertension is the underlying cause but at cellular level interference with tissue oxygen diffusion and capillary thrombosis are probably responsible for skin necrosis

- **Bleeding** – erosion through poor quality skin of a varicosity, or minor trauma, can occasionally produce substantial blood loss if not controlled with pressure and elevation.

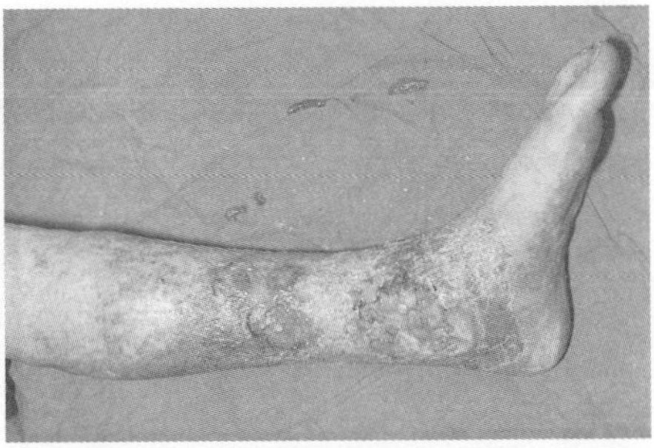

**Figure 12.5** Leg with ulceration and late changes of chronic venous insufficiency

### Clinical examination

- Examine the patient **standing** and look for varicose (Figure 12.6) veins in the distribution of the long saphenous (groin to medial malleolus) and short saphenous (popliteal fossa to lateral malleolus) systems.

- At sites of incompetent perforators the varicosities tend to be large and are termed 'blow-outs'.

- In the groin overlying the saphenofemoral junction a blow-out is called a **saphena varix** and may be confused with a femoral hernia.

- The patient should also be checked for oedema, skin changes and ulcers.

- The leg should be felt for varicosities that cannot be seen. A saphena varix may be felt rather than seen in the groin and a fluid thrill is felt if the patient coughs or the varicosities lower in the leg are tapped (**tap test**).

- Lying the patient supine and elevating the leg will cause the veins to collapse and a saphena varix to disappear.

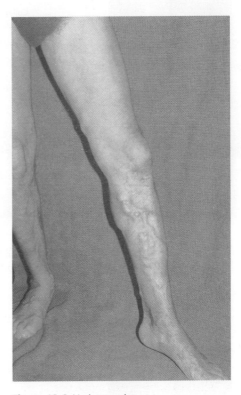

**Figure 12.6** Varicose veins

## The Trendelenburg test

The patient lies supine and the leg is elevated to collapse the veins. The long saphenous vein is now occluded in the groin by pressure with a finger (Figure 12.7a, c), and the patient asked to stand. The finger is now removed (Figure 12.7b, d). The test is **positive** when the varicose veins can be seen to fill from the groin downwards due to **incompetence at the sapheno-femoral junction**. Similar, though exhaustive, application of pressure at various points along the course of the varicose vein will determine other sites of perforator incompetence; this can be done with intelligent use of two rubber tube tourniquets. Accuracy is improved by using a Doppler probe or duplex scanning to determine sites of reverse flow, the objective being to decide on appropriate treatment and surgery.

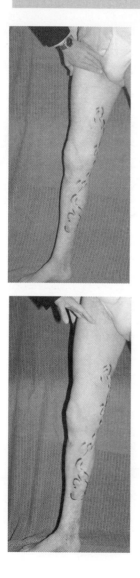

(a)

(b)

Collapsed
vein

(c)

Hand
removed

Retrograde
filling
of varicose
vein

(d)

**Figure 12.7** The Trendelenburg test

## Treatment of varicose veins

Treatment is directed at relieving symptoms such as aching, but cosmesis is an important consideration, particularly in women.

### 1 Elastic support

Graduated compression support stockings (Figure 12.8) are manufactured to provide decreasing levels of compression from the foot and ankle proximally to the upper leg. This increases calf muscle pump efficiency, aids venous return, reduces oedema and compresses distended superficial varicosities to alleviate aching. The pressure exerted by stockings can exceed 40 mmHg and, in patients with coexisting reduced arterial pressure due to atherosclerosis, may produce ischaemia and are contraindicated.

### 2 Sclerotherapy

Sclerosant injections are indicated for tortuous venous tributaries in the absence of main long or short saphenous trunk varicosity. Hence only minor varicose veins or those left following surgery to the main trunks are suitable generally, although some spe-

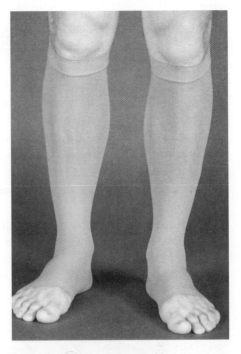

**Figure 12.8** Elastic support stocking

cialists advocate sclerotherapy (Figure 12.9) as primary treatment for larger veins. Sclerosants work by inducing a chemical phlebitis, thereby damaging the intima and occluding the lumen. The most commonly used is sodium tetradecyl sulphate (STD) at concentrations up to 3%, but other solutions such as hypertonic saline or glucose are available. In practice the patient lies flat and up to 2 ml of sclerosant is injected into the vein at various sites. Compression is then applied with

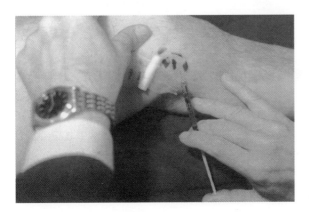

**Figure 12.9** Sclerotherapy

bandages or a stocking for up to 6 weeks, during which time the vein occludes (compression sclerotherapy). Common side-effects are pigmentation of the skin and small superficial ulcers at the injection sites where the sclerosant leaks and causes necrosis. Rarely, the sclerosant enters the deep venous system and causes a DVT.

### 3 Surgery

Surgery is indicated in symptomatic large varicose veins with sapheno-femoral and/or sapheno-popliteal incompetence. Through a small groin incision the long saphenous vein is disconnected from the femoral vein and tied off. Numerous other small tributaries are also divided and tied. It is usual to 'strip' the long saphenous vein down to the knee by use of a flexible wire or plastic cord passed retrogradely down the lumen; other varicosities are avulsed through tiny stab incisions.

- The operation is commonly designated **groin tie (or high tie)** (Figure 12.10), **strip and avulsions**.
- Short saphenous varicosities are treated similarly with surgery to the sapheno-popliteal junction.
- If appropriate, incompetent perforating veins can be divided in the subfascial plane using 'laparoscopic' equipment inserted through a small incision in the upper calf.

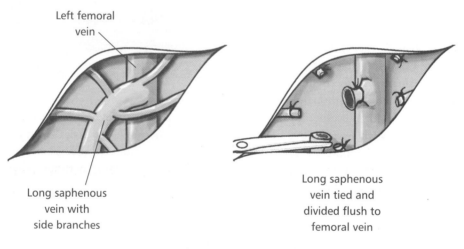

Left femoral vein

Long saphenous vein with side branches

Long saphenous vein tied and divided flush to femoral vein

**Figure 12.10** Groin tie

## LEG ULCERS

Chronic ulceration of the lower leg affects about **1%** of the population and is a large social and economic problem. The majority are venous but it is important to be able to recognize those of other aetiology. In broad terms ulcers can be classified into **venous, ischaemic and neuropathic** (Figure 12.11). The diagnosis is made from the site of ulceration, the history, clinical examination, and the ankle Doppler arterial pressure.

## VENOUS

- Sometimes improperly called stasis or varicose ulcers, this group represent the majority of lower leg ulcers.
- They occur **in relation to the medial malleolus** though they often spread and become circumferential around the lower calf and ankle.
- The surrounding skin shows other signs of venous disease such as **varicosity, oedema, pigmentation, eczema and lipodermatosclerosis.**
- Around **70% have a previous history of DVT** or circumstances associated with DVT (e.g. lower limb fracture, major surgery).
- The remainder give no such history and may be due to severe primary varicose veins with ankle perforator incompetence, or may have suffered a 'silent' DVT.

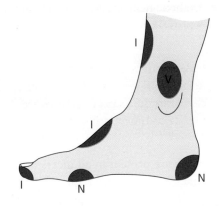

**Figure 12.11** Foot ulcers: V, venous; I, ischaemic; N, neuropathic

## ISCHAEMIC

These occur at sites of naturally poor arterial supply, i.e. **the shin, dorsum of foot and toes.** Ischaemic ulcers can be macro- or microvascular in origin:

- **Macrovascular** implies atherosclerotic or thrombotic disease in the proximal leg arteries. **Foot pulses are absent** with other signs and symptoms of arterial disease (see Chapter 11). Doppler pressures are reduced and usually there is rest pain.
- **Microvascular** implies occlusive thrombotic or embolic disease at the arteriolar level. **The foot pulses and Doppler pressures are usually normal** but the site of ulceration is clearly ischaemic. The usual problem is a **vasculitis** associated with an underlying disorder such as diabetes, rheumatoid arthritis, inflammatory bowel disease or autoimmune disease. Microemboli from the heart or proximal atheromatous plaques typically produce toe lesions. Hyperviscous blood disorders such as polythycaemia, leukaemia, or sickle cell crises cause microvascular sludging and occlusion, resulting in ischaemic necrosis and ulceration.

## NEUROPATHIC

- These occur at pressure points such as the heel or ball of the foot and are associated with a peripheral neuropathy, producing numbness and paraesthesia.
- The patient cannot feel minor trauma or friction causing damage to the skin and quite simply 'wears' a hole into the foot as if it were shoe leather.

- Friction from ill-fitting shoes produces damage where they rub.
- **Diabetic neuropathy** is the most common problem but any nerve damage (e.g. leprosy) or appropriate neurological disease has the same effect.

Many ulcers have a **mixed** aetiology; for example a diabetic patient may have neuropathy, ischaemia and venous problems. Despite careful nursing, immobile patients confined to bed can develop **pressure sores** on the heels and elsewhere which are essentially ischaemic (due to pressure) and neuropathic (inability to move).

Bacteria are present in all ulcers but this is usually coincidental rather than pathogenic. Antibiotics are required in the presence of cellulitis or spreading infection. Topical antibiotic (as opposed to antiseptic) use often causes skin irritation and is unnecessary.

Very rarely squamous carcinoma develops in a chronic leg ulcer – **Marjolin's ulcer**.

### Treatment of leg ulcers

Treatment in all cases is directed primarily at the underlying disease process. The ulcer itself needs to be managed with dressings that encourage healthy granulation and epithelial growth; these will vary depending upon the size, degree of exudate, slough, etc. Deep ulcers with much tissue loss may require **plastic surgery**. Gangrenous ulceration secondary to inoperable arterial disease needs major amputation.

In **venous ulceration the essential for healing is reduction in venous pressure**. This can be achieved with enforced bed rest and leg elevation, but is rarely appropriate. Improving calf muscle pump function whilst allowing normal activity is the ideal; it is accomplished with correctly applied pressure bandaging renewed on a once or twice weekly basis. Most ulcers will heal within 12 weeks and thereafter elastic stockings are worn indefinitely to keep the ulcer healed. **Surgery** to improve venous return and thereby lower venous pressure is usually considered after healing but may be done earlier. It is important to assess deep vein function and patency before planning surgery. Non-invasive vascular laboratory tests using plethysmography, Doppler and duplex scanning can provide information to determine whether surgery to superficial varicosities or perforators will improve the haemodynamics; venography may also be helpful. However, many patients are elderly and infirm and elastic compression stockings is often the most agreeable therapy.

## DEEP VEIN THROMBOSIS

Thrombosis in the deep leg veins (DVT) is a serious complication of surgery and prolonged immobility from whatever cause (medical illness, trauma, jet travel). It can also occur for no apparent reason in otherwise fit people. Preventing DVT and dealing with its sequelae form a major part of surgical practice.

## Pathology

Thrombosis is the formation of a solid mass (thrombus) from the constituents of the blood within the vascular system during life. **Virchow's triad** of postulates (1856) as to predisposing factors are:

1 **Intimal damage** – pressure from a pillow, sling, plaster cast; trauma from surgery, operating table, fracture
2 **Stasis** – slow circulation due to poor muscle pump; bed rest, anaesthesia, immobility
3 **Abnormal blood** – 'hypercoagulable state'; post-surgery, polycythaemia, splenectomy, malignancy, pregnancy, oestrogens, dehydration, congenital thrombophilia (deficiency of antithrombin III, protein C, protein S).

A thrombus begins as an aggregate of platelets adherent to the vein wall. Fibrin accumulates over the platelets and enmeshes red cells, white cells and further platelets. Thrombus may propagate as a long filament floating in the bloodstream, part of which can break off and embolize. After a few days a thrombus becomes organized by invasion of fibroblasts and capillaries from the vessel wall to which it then becomes fused. This fixed thrombus eventually becomes recanalized to restore flow but the whole process destroys the delicate valve cusps and damages the vein wall. Calcification can occur following resolution and shows on radiographs as phleboliths, particularly in the pelvic veins.

## Clinical signs

- The commonest site of DVT is in the soleal sinuses of the calf and the usual signs are heat, pain and tenderness on palpation but **many are asymptomatic**; low grade fever can be the only abnormality.
- Dorsiflexion of the foot may cause pain in the calf (**Homans' sign**).
- Thrombus extending to the popliteal vein obstructs venous return and produces **oedema** in the lower leg.
- Extensive spread from the calf to the femoral and iliac veins can produce gross venous obstruction, resulting in massive oedema and steely blue, painful, venous engorgement of the whole leg (phlegmasia cerulia dolens). Venous gangrene is rare and usually fatal.
- Other sites of DVT include the femoral, iliac and pelvic veins; in these the thrombus may not produce any clinical signs unless/until it embolizes to the lungs.

## Investigations

- Clinical suspicion of DVT should be confirmed with tests because around one-half of patients with calf tenderness post-operatively do not have a thrombosis.
- Duplex scanning and/or ascending venography (Figure 12.12) of the deep system using dye injected into a foot vein are readily available investigations.
- Confirmation of DVT prevents unnecessary and prolonged anticoagulation therapy in normal patients.

## Incidence and risk factors

- The true incidence of DVT in medical and surgical patients is difficult to estimate.
- The majority of thrombi start in the calf, remain localized and lyse spontaneously, whereas **20% extend to the popliteal and more proximal veins.**
- Research using highly sensitive radiolabelled fibrinogen scans shows evidence of **DVT in a third of post-operative patients.**
- Hip replacement surgery produces DVT in over 50%, and post-mortem studies of patients with fractured neck of femur reveals the majority to have DVT.
- Prolonged abdominal or pelvic surgery increases the risk compared to lesser operations.
- Many patients probably develop DVT in the preoperative period due to illness and enforced bed rest.

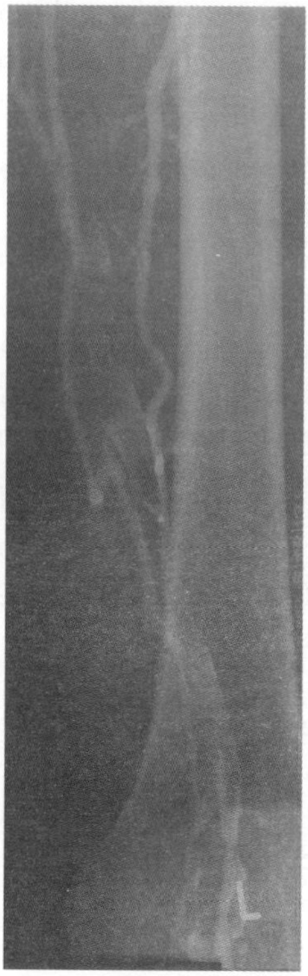

**Figure 12.12**
Venogram showing extensive superficial femoral vein thrombosis (thrombus outlined by dye within the vessel lumen)

## DVT prophylaxis

Unless contraindicated, it is usual to provide DVT prophylaxis to all adult surgical in-patients, and probably wise to continue for a few weeks after discharge if immobility is likely. Therapy is directed at reducing **stasis** and decreasing the **hypercoagulable state:**

- **Stasis** – elastic support stockings; mechanical calf pumps; early mobilization; leg exercises
- **Anticoagulation** – subcutaneous heparin 5000 units twice daily or subcutaneous low molecular weight heparin daily.

### Risk factors for DVT

- Previous thromboembolism
- Varicose veins
- Increasing age
- Obesity
- Pregnancy and post-partum
- Heart disease
- Cancer
- Immobility
- Size and site of operation
- Trauma and burns
- Oestrogens
- Thrombophilic disorders

**The simple measure of giving subcutaneous heparin and wearing stockings (Figure 12.13) reduces the rate of post-operative DVT by 80%.** Heparin has not been proven to substantially increase the risk of perioperative bleeding.

## Treatment of DVT

Treatment is aimed at alleviating symptoms and **preventing pulmonary embolus**. Elevation of the limb reduces swelling and analgesics are given for pain and fever. **Elastic stockings** should be worn. **Full anticoagulation** is started as soon as is practicable, bearing in mind potential bleeding problems in the post-operative period:

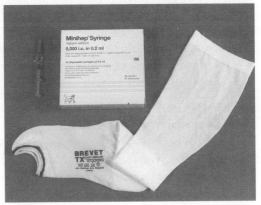

**Figure 12.13** Heparin and an anti-embolism stocking

- **Heparin** – intravenous heparin via a syringe pump is given in doses of 20 000–40 000 units per day following a loading dose of 5000 units. Efficacy of dose is monitored by maintaining the blood activated partial thromboplastin time (APTT) at twice normal. **Heparin prevents further thrombus formation** and significantly reduces the risk of pulmonary embolus. It is continued until oral anticoagulation is established – usually 5–10 days in post-operative patients.

- **Warfarin** – oral warfarin is started with loading doses of 10 mg on consecutive days followed by a reduced daily dosage of 2–10 mg. Dosage is monitored by maintaining the blood International Normalized Ratio (INR) at 3. Once oral coagulation is established, the heparin is stopped. **Warfarin is continued for 3–6 months to reduce the risk of further thrombosis or embolism.** Patients found to have thrombophilic disorders need warfarin indefinitely.

- **Thrombolysis** – fibrinolytic agents such as streptokinase can be given to lyse thrombus more quickly than natural processes. Use is limited in post-operative patients because of the risk of bleeding in fresh wounds. Such agents are usually given systemically by intravenous infusion, but direct infusion into the affected leg has also been used.

- **Thrombectomy** – in cases of severe ileo-femoral thrombosis, it is possible to operate on the femoral vein in the groin and extract the occluding thrombus but this procedure is rarely undertaken and only when the limb is threatened.

- **Caval filters** – considered in patients who have suffered pulmonary emboli despite anticoagulation, and in cases where venography shows large amounts of loose thrombi lying in the main veins and embolization seems likely. The device is fitted into the inferior vena cava just below the renal veins via a catheter in the internal jugular vein; radiology is needed for correct positioning. The most commonly used is a **Greenfield filter** which resembles an umbrella skeleton. The filter prevents emboli reaching the heart.

If untreated, 30% of calf DVT and 50% of more proximal DVT will produce pulmonary emboli, of which 30% will be fatal. Standard anticoagulation treatment reduces this figure almost to zero. Most patients with DVT will eventually suffer **post-thrombotic syndrome**.

# PULMONARY EMBOLUS

It is estimated that 21 000 patients die each year from pulmonary embolism (PE) and in many cases PE is the agonal event in a terminal disease process. However, it is also implicated in 5% of all post-operative deaths, and occurs perhaps in as many as 25% of all patients admitted to hospital.

## Clinical features

PE obstructs perfusion of the lungs with deoxygenated blood and puts a load on the right heart. Symptoms will vary depending on the size and number of emboli (one large or many small) and the health of the heart and lungs. There are therefore differing presentations:

1 Sudden chest pain, collapse and death in a previously well patient.
2 Sudden chest pain and collapse requiring emergency resuscitation followed by gradual improvement.
3 Sudden chest pain with shortness of breath and possible hypotension.
4 Mild episodes of pleuritic pain and gradually worsening shortness of breath with haemoptysis.

## Diagnosis

The most important differential diagnosis is myocardial infarction. Examination may show cyanosis, a rapid heart rate and raised jugular venous pressure.

- **Chest x-ray** may show diminished vascular markings.
- **Arterial blood gas** analysis shows reduced oxygen tension.

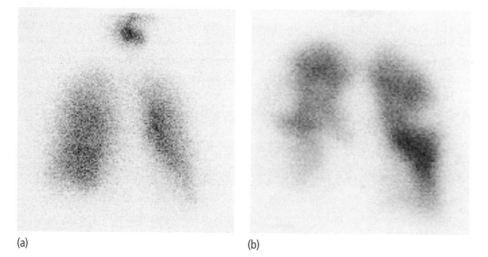

(a)    (b)

**Figure 12.14** Ventilation/perfusion scan showing mismatch between (a) ventilation (normal) and (b) perfusion (reduced)

- **Electrocardiogram** may show classic S1 Q3 T3 with right heart strain V1–3.
- **Lung ventilation/perfusion** scan will show reduction in perfusion (Figure 12.14).
- **Pulmonary arteriogram** provides radiological proof but is seldom required.

### Treatment

- Patients who suddenly collapse undergo cardiopulmonary resuscitation, external cardiac massage serving to break up a massive embolus within the main pulmonary trunk, pushing fragments to the lung periphery and restoring flow.
- **Full anticoagulation is given to all patients.**
- Thrombolysis via a catheter positioned in the pulmonary artery can be used.
- Pulmonary embolectomy is sometimes indicated.

## POST-THROMBOTIC SYNDROME

This is the term applied to venous disease of the leg following DVT. Thrombosis causes damage by destroying valve cusps and producing fibrosis which can narrow or occlude the deep veins; the calf muscle pump becomes less effective and venous hypertension ensues. **The symptoms are those of severe chronic venous insufficiency** outlined previously, i.e. eczema, lipodermatosclerosis, pigmentation, ulceration.

It is likely that all patients who suffer a DVT will eventually develop post-thrombotic syndrome, but it can take many years to present – probably because the calf muscle pump can compensate initially but eventually fails. At 10 years post-DVT, 75% will have symptoms.

Investigation and treatment is essentially as for varicose veins and ulcers. Surgical treatment depends on the severity and site of deep venous damage. Bypass operations are possible for proximal occlusions, as are plastic operations to repair or replace deep valves.

**CRIB BOX – DISEASES OF LEG VEINS**

**Anatomy**
- Long (groin) and short (popliteal fossa) saphenous veins
- Perforators
- Deep veins
- Calf pump

**Physiology**
- Calf pump reduces foot venous pressure from 100 to 20 mmHg
- Deep system is high pressure
- Valves important

**Varicose veins**
- Primary – majority
- Secondary – DVT, pelvic tumours, A-V fistulae
- Symptoms – mainly cosmetic, especially women; chronic venous insufficiency
- Examination – learn the Trendelenburg test
- Treatment – stockings, sclerotherapy, surgery

**Leg ulcers**
- Venous
- Ischaemic (macro and micro)
- Neuropathic

Remember Marjolin's ulcer.

**DVT**
- Virchow's triad
- Risk factors

You must know DVT prophylaxis.

**PE**
- Symptoms due to obstruction of right heart and decreased lung perfusion
- Best treatment is prevention

**Post-thrombotic syndrome**
- Venous disease of the legs following DVT
- Symptoms of severe chronic venous insufficiency

# chapter 13

# LYMPH NODES AND LYMPHATICS

The lymphatic system has two major functions:

- **Drainage** – tissue fluid returns to the bloodstream via a system of lymphatic vessels and filtering lymph nodes. The thoracic duct is the largest lymphatic vessel, arising from the cisterna chyli in the abdomen and ascending the thorax to join the left subclavian vein at its junction with the left internal jugular. It collects lymph from the whole body except the right chest, right arm and right head and neck; this drains via the smaller right lymphatic duct into the right subclavian vein. The volume of lymph entering the circulation is 2–4 litres a day, i.e. approximately equal to the total plasma volume.
- **Defence** – lymph nodes filter and trap bacteria and other particulate matter, and produce lymphocytes and antibodies.

## ENLARGED LYMPH NODES

Lymph node pathology invariably causes some degree of swelling and is a common clinical problem. Palpation for 'glands' in the neck, axillae and groins is part of routine clinical examination. Enlargement is either **local** or **generalized** and causes can be classified into **infective** and **neoplastic**.

### LOCAL ENLARGEMENT

- **Infective** – loco-regional nodes will enlarge in response to **acute** infections, so-called reactive nodes or lymphadenitis (e.g. an infected foot lesion will be associated with tender palpable glands in the groin). Reactive glands resolve as the infection is overcome but sometimes suppuration and abscess formation occurs. Lymphatic channels in the skin may be visible as red lines running from the septic focus – lymphangiitis – particularly with streptococcal infection. **Tuberculous** infection produces chronic lymphadenitis which is most commonly observed in the neck.
- **Neoplastic** – **secondary** local and distant node involvement is a characteristic of most cancers, e.g. breast, melanoma. Left supraclavicular nodes enlarge following malignant spread from within the abdomen (Troisier's sign) or chest. Malignant nodes are firm, non-tender and often fixed to surrounding tissue. **Primary** lymphatic malignancy (Hodgkin's disease, lymphoma) is less common but is seen particularly in the neck, axilla and groin as large discrete rubbery nodes.

## GENERALIZED ENLARGEMENT

- **Infective** – many viral and bacterial infections cause a generalized lymph-adenopathy, e.g. glandular fever, HIV, septicaemia, secondary syphilis. The nodes are usually small and numerous – 'shotty' – and splenic enlargement is common.
- **Neoplastic** – late stage lymphomas and leukaemias. The nodes tend to be large and rubbery with associated splenic and hepatic enlargement.

### Diagnosis

The diagnosis of enlarged lymph nodes (Figure 13.1) depends on **history, clinical examination** and **special investigations**. The history might indicate sites of septic foci (bad teeth, athlete's foot, tonsillitis, etc.), symptoms of systemic infection (fever), or malignancy (weight loss). **In all cases the clinical examination must be thorough:**

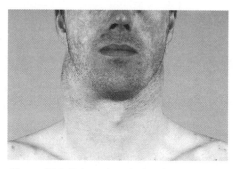

**Figure 13.1** Enlarged cervical nodes

- Look for pathology in the areas drained by the affected group of nodes. For example, groin nodes drain the whole leg, the buttocks, perineum and lower trunk – a small melanoma between the toes or an anal or penile carcinoma will be overlooked if not searched for. Left supraclavicular nodes may be secondary to **any** malignancy, anywhere in the body.
- Examine the other lymph nodes. Generalized enlargement means systemic disease.
- Feel for splenic and hepatic enlargement, or intra-abdominal malignancy.

Investigations will include chest x-ray to exclude tumours or show mediastinal lymphadenopathy. Haematology will confirm the likes of leukaemia or glandular fever. **Lymph node biopsy** is often necessary and can be done with open excision or fine needle aspiration cytology.

## INFLAMMATORY LYMPH NODE ENLARGEMENT

Some rare causes of lymph node enlargement do not fit the infective/neoplastic classification and are best described as purely inflammatory in origin. It is seen in diseases in which a generalized inflammatory process can involve the lymph nodes. The commonest examples are **sarcoidosis** and **rheumatoid arthritis** (Felty's syndrome).

## LYMPHOEDEMA

Oedema is defined as excessive accumulation of interstitial fluid in the tissues.

Oedema has many causes related to the physiological balance of hydrostatic and colloid osmotic pressures between the capillary and extracellular fluid space, and the removal of interstitial fluid and proteins by the lymphatics. **Lymphoedema is oedema caused by defective lymphatic drainage of interstitial fluid** and affects the limbs primarily.

## Clinical signs

When oedematous skin is compressed with the finger or thumb, for a few moments a depression or pit is produced due to a squeezing effect on the fluid-laden tissue. This effect is easily demonstrated on the swollen legs of heart failure patients. Lymphoedema, however, is classically described as **'brawny' and non-pitting**, a slightly false description since lymphoedema will pit under compression but not as readily as other forms. This is because chronic lymphoedema produces fibrosis and overgrowth of connective tissue which will not pit. Lymphoedema also renders a limb susceptible to infection and cellulitis, causing further swelling and scarring.

## Causes

Lymphoedema (Figure 13.2) can be **primary** or **secondary**. Secondary causes are by far the most common and are due to lymphatic damage or obstruction:

- Filariasis – a parasitic disease widespread in tropical and subtropical countries and spread by mosquito. The worms infest the lymphatics, particularly the legs and genitals, causing fibrosis and obstruction with subsequent gross lymphoedema (elephantiasis).
- Surgery – excision of lymph nodes *en bloc* can be a part of surgical treatment in many cancers (breast, utcrus, mclanoma).

**Causes of oedema**

Increased hydrostatic pressure

- Cardiac failure
- Venous obstruction

Increased capillary permeability

- Inflammatory response (injury; infection; allergy)
- Hypoxia

Hypoproteinaemia

- Starvation
- Malabsorption
- Albuminuria (nephrotic syndrome)
- Liver disease

Hypernatraemia

- Renal failure
- Steroids (Cushing's)
- Excess intake

Lymphatic

- Primary
- Secondary

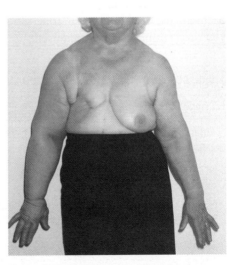

**Figure 13.2** Post-mastectomy lymphoedema

- Radiotherapy – fibrotic destruction of lymph nodes occurs following radiotherapy treatment and lymphoedema is the consequence; commonly seen in the arm following breast cancer treatment.
- Malignancy – lymphatics can become obstructed due to malignant invasion but lymphoedema is more common following surgery or radiotherapy to malignant nodes.
- Infection – severe cellulitis can damage lymphatics sufficiently to cause lymphoedema.

## PRIMARY LYMPHOEDEMA

Primary lymphoedema (Figure 13.3) is a relatively rare congenital condition affecting the lower limb which is more common in women (3:1). It is caused by imperfect development of lymphatics which may be absent, hypoplastic or varicose. One or both legs may be affected. The familial form is called **Milroy's** disease.

Treatment of lymphoedema is largely symptomatic; compression hosiery can control most cases and pneumatic compression devices worn at night are useful for more severe swelling.

Gross lymphoedema of the leg can be treated with surgical excision to reduce bulky subcutaneous swelling. It is important to control recurrent episodes of infection and cellulitis; patients should be instructed on skin care and long-term low-dose antibiotics are often used.

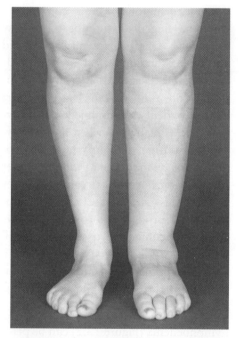

**Figure 13.3** Primary lymphoedema of the leg

---

**CRIB BOX – LYMPH NODES AND LYMPHATICS**

**Lymphatic system** – two functions, drainage and defence

**Enlarged nodes** – local or general; infective or neoplastic. Rarely inflammatory, e.g. sarcoidosis; rheumatoid arthritis

**Always feel for nodes**

**Oedema** – causes: hydrostatic, capillary permeability, low protein, high sodium, lymphatic obstruction

**Lymphoedema** – primary and secondary; secondary is by far the commonest and the most important

# chapter 14

# THE SKIN AND APPENDAGES

When examining skin lesions, it is important to do so under good lighting and use a magnifying lens to improve vision. Tumours or swellings related to the skin are described like any other in terms of site, size, surface, shape and special signs. **The regional nodes should always be examined.** Histology on all excised lesions is mandatory.

### Surgical techniques

- **Formal excision** with a scalpel may be performed under local or general anaesthesia and may vary from a small elliptical diagnostic skin biopsy, through excisional surgery of small lesions with primary closure, to reconstruction of large defects with flaps or grafts.
- **Shave excision** (Figure 14.1) is a simple technique performed under local anaesthesia, mainly for removing mature moles. The cosmetic result is generally much better than formal excision for this sort of lesion.
- **Punch biopsy** is readily performed in the outpatient clinic using a disposable skin biopsy punch. These come in various sizes, the most useful being 4 mm. The technique is particularly useful for biopsy of tumours.

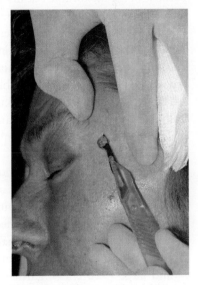

**Figure 14.1** Shave excision

- **Curettage and electro-desiccation** is also performed under local anaesthesia, usually in the outpatient clinic. It is a rapid, simple and effective technique for removal of seborrhoeic keratoses, some viral warts, selected small basal cell carcinomata, cutaneous horns and some kerato-acanthomata. The electro-desiccation can be undertaken with either electrocautery or diathermy.
- **Fulguration** with a monopolar diathermy machine (**Hyfrecator**) can be used to destroy numerous small lesions such as skin tags and spider naevi without anaesthesia.
- **Cryosurgery** using liquid nitrogen sprays and probes is invaluable for a whole variety of epidermal lesions, such as viral warts, seborrhoeic and solar keratoses.
- **Lasers** are used for vascular lesions such as port wine stains, certain types of pigmented lesions and skin resurfacing.

# COMMON SURGICAL DERMATOLOGY

## CONGENITAL DISORDERS

### Moles (melanocytic naevi)

Although only 10% of melanocytic naevi are actually present at birth, the word 'naevus' infers a circumscribed developmental anomaly (Figure 14.2) and so the potential for an individual to develop moles can be considered congenital. There is enormous public concern about any pigmented skin lesion, because of the inexorable rise in the incidence of malignant melanoma. **It is therefore important to feel reasonably confident about distinguishing between the common types of pigmented lesion (Table 14.1).** Not every pigmented skin lesion is a mole or malignant melanoma and those commonly encountered are listed.

- **Congenital** pigmented melanocytic naevi, i.e. those present at birth, form a special subgroup of moles, arbitrarily classified according to size into small (<1.5 cm), medium (1.5–20 cm) and large (>20 cm – 'garment'

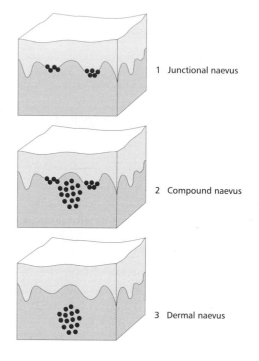

1  Junctional naevus

2  Compound naevus

3  Dermal naevus

**Figure 14.2** Melanocytic naevi

**Table 14.1** Common pigmented skin lesions

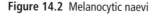

| Benign | Malignant |
| --- | --- |
| Melanocytic naevus | Melanoma |
| Ephelis (freckle) | Pigmented basal cell carcinoma |
| Lentigo | |
| Seborrhoeic keratosis | |
| Skin tag | |
| Histiocytoma | |

naevi). **The risk of malignant melanoma arising in congenital naevi is proportional to their size,** so small lesions carry virtually no risk, whereas garment naevi carry an appreciable risk and affected individuals should be kept under regular surveillance – unfortunately, their size prohibits prophylactic removal. Many congenital naevi develop a warty surface and can become quite hairy.

- **Acquired** melanocytic naevi, i.e. those arising after birth, mostly develop during childhood, but new moles may appear up to the age of 30–35 years, particularly during pregnancy. It is important to appreciate that moles may undergo gradual changes in their appearance as they, and the individual who possesses them, mature. Moles on the scalp, face and neck tend to mature most rapidly, whereas those on palms, soles and genitalia may remain immature. Immature moles are **'junctional naevi'**, i.e. naevus cells are distributed along the dermo-epidermal junction. They present clinically as uniformly pigmented macules, with a fairly regular border. The first step in the process of maturation is for some naevus cells to descend into the dermis whilst others remain at the junction – the mole is now called a **'compound naevus'** which clinically appears raised above the surrounding skin. Its surface may become slightly warty and its pattern of pigmentation variegated, though in a regular fashion. When all junctional activity ceases, the mole is called an **'intradermal naevus'**, the clinical correlate of which is a dome-shaped or sometimes fleshy lesion. Pigment production ceases when the naevus cells have descended so deep within the dermis that ultraviolet light can no longer penetrate and stimulate melanin production. The maturation process may arrest at any stage, but eventually moles involute and disappear spontaneously. **In the elderly very few, if any, moles are found** – the predominant pigmented skin lesions are **seborrhoeic keratoses** and **solar lentigines** ('liver spots'), both of which increase in number with age.

---

**Helpful tips**

- 90% of moles appear after birth (acquired)
- New moles may appear up to age 30–35 years
- Average mole count 20–30 per adult – fewer in freckled skin
- Moles change slowly – mature then involute – rate varies with site
- Risk of melanoma no greater for moles on palms, soles, genitalia
- Do not worry about moles with diameter of <5 mm
- Sunburn (>3 episodes) correlates with number of moles and risk of melanoma

---

Reasons for removing moles are:
1 Suspicion – is it becoming a melanoma? Experienced clinicians will feel confident about leaving at least 90% of moles *in situ*. Less experienced will excise a higher proportion.
2 Nuisance – repeatedly catching in clothing.
3 Cosmetic – particularly intradermal naevi on the face and neck.

# INFLAMMATORY DISORDERS

## BACTERIAL INFECTIONS

### Boils (furuncles)

These common lesions are due to **staphylococcal** infection of hair follicles. If immunity is impaired (e.g. **diabetes**), infection may extend to adjacent follicles, which can become involved in a necrotizing process and form a carbuncle. Those with recurrent boils are often found to be 'staph. carriers' and swabs should be taken not only from an active lesion, but also from possible carriage sites (the nose, axilla and perineum). It may also be necessary to check for staphylococcal carriage amongst close contacts, e.g. family members. Large lesions need incision and drainage, but most will respond to conservative treatment with an appropriate systemic antibiotic (usually flucloxacillin). Nasal staph. carriage is treated with **mupirocin** nasal ointment and other carriage sites with antiseptic skin cleanser or soap.

### Cellulitis/erysipelas

The terms are interchangeable and describe a painful acute infection of the dermis and subcutis, usually with pyrexia. Erysipelas is sometimes reserved for more superficial infections associated with blistering and classically for those affecting the face. *Streptococcus pyogenes* group A is the most common cause, but *Staphylococcus aureus* is sometimes responsible and there may be a mixed infection. Nowadays, cellulitis is most commonly encountered in the lower limb in association with chronic venous disease, lymphoedema, or simply neglect of foot hygiene. Intravenous benzylpenicillin is needed in the acute phase and appropriate topical therapy for any predisposing skin disease. Recurrent cellulitis may require long-term prophylactic oral penicillin-V or erythromycin.

## VIRAL INFECTIONS

### Warts

Warts (Figure 14.3) are caused by the human papilloma virus (HPV) of which about 65 strains are now recognized. They appear in various guises, depending upon which strain is responsible, e.g. vulgar (hands), plantar (soles of feet), digitate (beard area), filiform (usually face), plane (face and backs of hands), and anogenital. Some of the HPV serotypes responsible for anogenital warts are also the major cause of cervical cancer. **Warts resolve spontaneously** (90% within 2 years) and since they remain confined within the

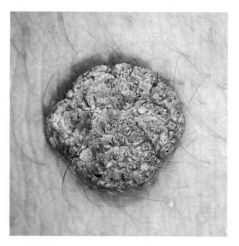

**Figure 14.3** Wart

epidermis, disappear without trace. **Excisional surgery will always leave scarring** and does nothing to stimulate the individual's immune response to the virus. Until a specific anti-HPV chemotherapeutic agent is discovered, treatment will remain both frustrating and unsatisfactory. Strong reassurance for parents that warts resolve spontaneously is probably the best approach for young children; topical therapy with various preparations containing salicylic acid can be of some help and liquid nitrogen cryotherapy is useful for most warts in older children and adults.

The distinction between **plantar warts** and **corns** is important, because the former generally carry a good prognosis, whereas the latter are likely to persist indefinitely. Both can be very painful, but corns are classically situated over weight bearing areas, particularly the metatarsal heads, and represent circumscribed areas of excess keratin caused by persistent pressure and friction. In order to distinguish between the two, it may be necessary to pare away surplus keratin with a scalpel blade. By so doing, considerable relief of pain is achieved and the root of the problem exposed. The corn will be revealed as a virtually endless core of keratin, whereas the papillary architecture of a plantar wart is soon disclosed, often with characteristic little black dots representing thrombosed capillaries.

# NON-INFECTIVE INFLAMMATORY DISORDERS

### Hidradenitis suppurativa

A chronic idiopathic inflammatory disorder of apocrine sweat glands, often confused with 'recurrent boils' in flexural areas (Figure 14.4). Mild examples of hidradenitis suppurativa are relatively common, particularly amongst overweight young women. Early lesions both look and feel like boils and may appear in the axillae, groins and external genitalia in any combination. Less frequently, the breasts themselves may also be affected. More severe disease is characterized by chronic inflammation, purulent discharge and scarring. Microbiological examination of the discharge is unrewarding and treatment is extremely difficult. Excision of all apocrine gland-bearing skin from affected areas is the only definitive solution and can be a practical proposition for axillary disease. Patients with mild disease may respond to conservative therapy:

* Anti-androgens (women only)
* Broad spectrum antibiotics

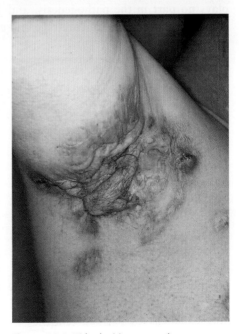

**Figure 14.4** Hidradenitis suppurativa

- Oral retinoids
- Sometimes systemic steroids.

### Stasis (hypostatic; venous) eczema

Eczema is one of several components of the post-thrombotic syndrome. Stasis eczema affects the gaiter area of the lower leg and is usually associated with haemosiderin staining of the skin. There may also be other features of venous insufficiency, particularly oedema and ulceration. Treatment consists of graduated compression bandaging or hosiery combined with an appropriate topical corticosteroid. Patients with stasis eczema may also have allergic contact dermatitis, usually to some ingredient of topically applied medicaments or bandages. Ideally, they should be patch tested in order to discover what can and cannot be used safely on their legs.

### Pyogenic granuloma

Pyogenic granuloma (Figure 14.5) is a rather alarming vascular lesion which grows rapidly following minor trauma (e.g. a bitten lip or prick from a rose thorn). It appears most frequently on the fingers and lips and is essentially a mass of friable granulation tissue, which seems to pop out through the skin and bleeds on contact. Typically, a collar of epidermis is visible around the base. **In spite of the name, infection plays no part in the pathogenesis**, and most can be removed in the outpatient clinic by the technique of curettage and electrocautery.

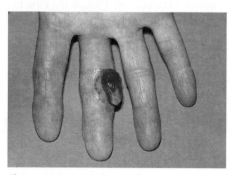

**Figure 14.5** Pyogenic granuloma

> **Note:** An amelanotic nodular malignant melanoma can look very similar to a pyogenic granuloma and must always be considered in the differential diagnosis. If in doubt, the lesion must be fully excised.

### Keloid

Keloids (Figure 14.6) are excess formation of fibrous tissue following trauma. They are thickened scars, looking rather like caterpillars, and have both familial and racial predilections, e.g. Afro-Caribbean. Specific areas of the body are particularly susceptible, notably the **pre-sternal chest, shoulders, and upper back.** Scarring after burns and scalds has a particular tendency to be keloidal. Nodular keloids occur on

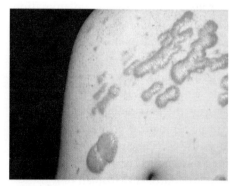

**Figure 14.6** Keloid

the earlobes after ear-piercing. Some unfortunate individuals form keloids spontaneously or after minor acne. Treatment is difficult, but some flattening can be induced by intralesional steroid injections and also by sustaining pressure over the lesions. This is achieved for extensive keloids by wearing special elastic garments, or for more localized scarring with silicone gel dressings. Surgical excision is contraindicated.

### Nodular chondritis

This is a small, excruciatingly painful inflammatory nodule most often encountered on the helix of an ear in middle-aged or elderly men. The degree of discomfort, particularly when lying on the affected side at night, seems surprising for such a subtle lesion which rarely exceeds 5 mm in diameter. The easiest solution is to excise, under local anaesthesia, the nodule together with a sliver of underlying cartilage.

## VASCULAR DISORDERS

### HAEMANGIOMAS

#### Capillary haemangioma (strawberry naevus)

This is a common vascular lesion that appears in early infancy and continues to grow for the first 6–12 months of life (Figure 14.7). Superficial (capillary) and deep (cavernous) components may coexist. The lesions may look alarming but fortunately resolve spontaneously, becoming paler during the second year and involuting completely by 7 years. Parents need continual reassurance. Occasionally, if some vital function is jeopardized, e.g. with periocular or perianal lesions, large doses of systemic steroid can shrink the lesion remarkably if administered during the proliferative phase.

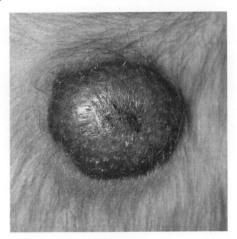

**Figure 14.7** Strawberry naevus

#### Port wine stain (naevus flammeus)

These congenital lesions (Figure 14.8) are, unfortunately, permanent. They are mainly of cosmetic significance, but about 10% of facial port wine stains are associated with the Sturge–Weber syndrome and glaucoma can also occur. Nowadays, there is much interest in the treatment of these lesions with a pulsed dye laser.

#### Cherry angioma (Campbell de Morgan spot)

These are multiple red papules, 1–5 mm in diameter, encountered commonly on the skin of adults from their mid-30s onwards. They tend to be most numerous on the trunk and are of no significance.

### Spider telangiectasis (spider naevus)

These lesions are well known to occur during the terminal stages of liver failure, probably due to an inability to detoxify oestrogens. They are, however, very common in healthy individuals, particularly on the face, the upper trunk and arms. Spider naevi in childhood may resolve spontaneously (parents need reassurance) and the same usually happens to eruptive lesions appearing in pregnancy. If treatment is requested for cosmetic reasons, the central 'feeder' arteriole can be destroyed with a Hyfrecator, or a pulsed dye laser.

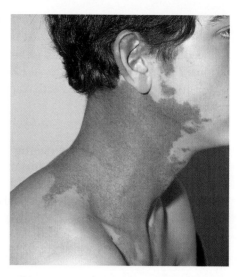

**Figure 14.8** Port wine stain

## NAILS

### Sub-ungual haematoma

Haemorrhage under a nail following minor trauma can be extremely painful (Figure 14.9). The acute problem is solved by piercing the affected nail plate over the haematoma with a red-hot needle, thereby relieving the pressure. An untreated sub-ungual haematoma may be mistaken for a sub-ungual malignant melanoma, because it can be extremely difficult to distinguish between altered blood and melanin under a nail. If in doubt, removing the nail allows accurate assessment.

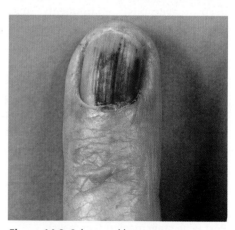

**Figure 14.9** Sub-ungual haematoma

### Paronychia

This is a painful swelling of the nailfold, which in the acute form is caused usually by *Staphylococcus aureus*. Organisms enter through a small break in the skin, which may be intentional (nail biting) or accidental, and sometimes there is no preceding injury. The condition may resolve spontaneously or require oral antibiotics. Persistent lesions with pus require incision and drainage. People whose hands are persistently exposed to water, diabetics and those with cold hands, e.g.

Raynaud's phenomenon, may suffer from chronic paronychia. *Candida albicans* is frequently implicated in the inflammatory process, but other bacteria may play a part, e.g. *Pseudomonas*. Treatment is conservative and consists of keeping the hands as dry as possible, together with topical, or systemic anticandidal and/or antibacterial measures.

### Ingrowing toenail

This is a common, painful condition, multifactorial in its aetiology and most frequently seen in young adults (Figure 14.10). The big toes are most often affected and the main cause seems to be persistent compression from poorly fitting footwear. There may also be a congenital malalignment of the nail plate, and cutting the toenails in a convex manner, rather than straight across may contribute.

The simple inflammatory stage may be treated conservatively, but surgical intervention is often needed. This may vary from simple curettage of excessive granulation tissue forming over the affected nailfold; wedge resection of part of the nail plate; or total ablation of the nail apparatus in particularly difficult cases (**Zadek's procedure**).

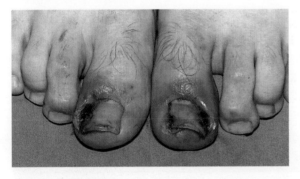

**Figure 14.10** Ingrowing toenails

### Onychogryphosis

This term implies gross thickening of the nail plate and most commonly involves the big toenails. It is encountered usually in the elderly who find routine nail care difficult. The condition is largely attributable to local trauma and continued pressure and friction from footwear. Conservative treatment is undertaken by a chiropodist, who trims and pares the affected nails. If the condition is particularly troublesome, a Zadek's procedure may be necessary. Thickened nails are also seen with fungal infection (tinea unguium) and psoriasis.

### Sub-ungual exostosis

This is a painful bony outgrowth arising from the terminal phalanx, usually in the great toe, which pushes up the free edge of the overlying nail plate. The diagnosis is confirmed by x-ray (Figure 14.11). Treatment consists of excising the excess bone.

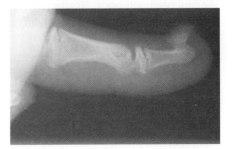

**Figure 14.11** X-ray of sub-ungual exostosis

### Myxoid cyst

This is a common lesion associated with osteoarthritis involving the terminal interphalangeal joint of the affected digit, usually a finger (Figure 14.12). The cyst arises because of degenerative change in connective tissue associated with the extensor mechanism of the joint and may be situated at any point between it and the posterior nailfold. If pierced, the cyst will exude clear gelatinous material, which can be easily expressed. Excision can be undertaken, but dissection may be awkward and difficult to justify. Conservative management by repeatedly evacuating the contents when the cyst refills may be all that is required.

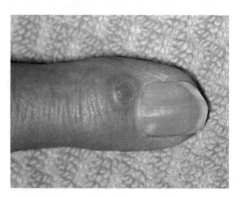

**Figure 14.12** Myxoid cyst

### Glomus tumour

This tumour is an uncommon but acutely painful lesion, particularly situated under a nail. The tumour is unimpressive and presents as a small sub-ungual area of bluish discoloration. The degree of pain seems totally out of proportion to the clinical signs and may be triggered by changes in temperature. Treatment is by surgical removal.

## NEOPLASMS

### BENIGN TUMOURS

#### Skin cysts

The umbrella term **sebaceous cyst** is used for all benign skin cysts containing cheesy or oily material. In fact, because sebum is an oily liquid, the only true sebaceous cyst is relatively rare, sometimes appearing in large numbers in the inherited condition **steatocystoma multiplex**. The usual cysts encountered are extremely common:

- **Pilar (trichilemmal) cyst** – inherited as an autosomal dominant trait and often referred to as a 'wen'. These lesions are generally multiple, occur on the scalp (Figure 14.13) and are only troublesome if large.
- **Epidermoid cyst** – the most common cyst derived from the pilo-sebaceous unit. At first

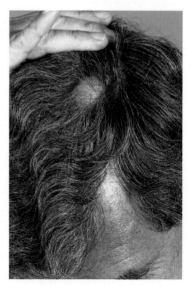

**Figure 14.13** Pilar cyst on scalp

glance, it resembles a pilar cyst, but close inspection reveals **a punctum** near its summit (Figure 14.14). Unlike pilar cysts, epidermoid cysts are prone to episodes of inflammation and are filled with cheesy, white material with a rancid odour. This material is altered keratin, not sebum. Epidermoid cysts are encountered mainly on the face, neck, upper trunk, behind the ears, and on the scrotum.

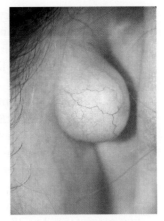

- **Implantation dermoid** – caused when a fragment of skin is driven deep to the dermis by injury (thorn-prick) or operation, and the fragment continues to grow and desquamate. Common on the hand and fingers.

**Figure 14.14** Epidermoid cyst

Troublesome cysts are removed by enucleation. Pilar cysts on the scalp can be persuaded to pop out very easily through a small incision, but epidermoid cysts sometimes require more careful dissection, particularly if they have been inflamed.

## BENIGN PIGMENTED LESIONS

The most important benign pigmented lesion – the melanocytic naevus – has already been considered. Others are listed below and in Table 14.1:

- **Freckle and lentigo** – both are small, uniformly pigmented and flat (macular), the lentigo being the darker of the two. The freckle is characterized by increased activity from a normal number of melanocytes in the basal epidermal layer, whereas in a lentigo, the number of basal melanocytes is dramatically increased. Most lentigines are due to chronic solar damage and are seen on the faces and backs of the hands of the ageing white population ('liver spots').
- **Seborrhoeic keratosis** – also called seborrhoeic wart or senile keratosis. An extremely common pigmented skin lesion which causes problems of diagnosis and management. Typically they seem stuck onto the skin, have a greasy feel and warty appearance. Seborrhoeic keratoses appear on ageing skin and most are situated on the trunk. Numbers vary from one to many hundreds and their size ranges from a millimetre to several centimetres. The degree of pigmentation is variable. Once recognized they are easily differentiated from melanomas. Treatment if required (many people simply wish to be reassured) is liquid nitrogen cryotherapy, or curettage. Surgical excision is only necessary if there is diagnostic doubt.
- **Skin tags** – often appear in large numbers around the neck and in the axillae and groins of obese individuals. They are small, soft protrusions, which may be variably pigmented and, if required, can easily be destroyed using a Hyfrecator without anaesthesia.

- Benign fibrous histiocytoma – a common, firm, dermal nodule (Figure 14.15) which is often pigmented and feels rather like a button within the skin. If compressed between finger and thumb, the lesion puckers in a characteristic fashion (the dimple sign). Most are encountered on the lower legs of women and some are thought to arise as a fibrotic reaction to insect bites and so, not surprisingly, may be multiple. Size varies from 2 to 20 mm and they

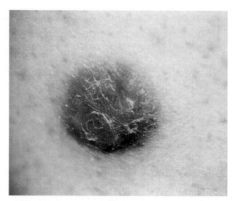

**Figure 14.15** Benign fibrous histiocytoma

are usually asymptomatic. Treatment is not often necessary but lesions may be excised for reasons of nuisance, size or diagnostic uncertainty. The major differential diagnosis for larger examples is nodular malignant melanoma.

## LESIONS WITH MALIGNANT POTENTIAL

Damage to the skin from solar and some artificial sources of ultraviolet radiation has become a major problem for white skinned people. UV photo-damage is cumulative and responsible for most age-related skin changes (e.g. wrinkling) and the bulk of skin cancer. Those with fair, freckled skins are most at risk. By avoiding sunbathing, wearing sensible clothing and applying high protection sunscreens, the risk of skin cancer can probably be reduced by 80% and the skin will remain wrinkle free until advanced middle age.

### Solar keratosis

Such lesions (Figure 14.16) indicate a significant degree of chronic photodamage and are precursors of squamous carcinoma. The risk of this has been estimated at about 1 per 1000 solar keratoses per year. They are small, usually multiple, hyperkeratotic plaques, and sometimes either pink or slightly pigmented. Most are seen on the bald scalp and ears of men and on the faces and backs of the hands of

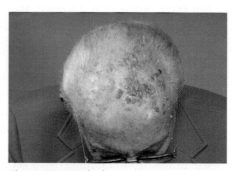

**Figure 14.16** Solar keratosis

both sexes. If few in number, the best treatment is liquid nitrogen cryotherapy. However, for more diffuse lesions, topical 5-fluorouracil cream can be very helpful.

### Bowen's disease

This is true **squamous carcinoma *in situ*** and is mainly due to chronic photodamage. An individual plaque of Bowen's disease (Figure 14.17) resembles a small lesion of psoriasis, being well demarcated, erythematous and scaly. Lesions are encountered mainly on the lower legs of elderly ladies, where they are frequently multiple and associated with solar keratoses. Progression from in-situ to invasive squamous carcinoma is not inevitable; many plaques of Bowen's disease remain unchanged. When considering treatment, the nature of the lesion, its site and the patient's age, must all be taken into account and a conservative approach with topical 5-fluorouracil cream is often better than surgical intervention or cryotherapy.

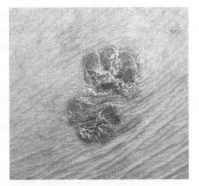

**Figure 14.17** Bowen's disease

### Keratoacanthoma

An impressive lesion, keratoacanthoma (Figure 14.18) is one of the most rapidly growing and also one of the few self-healing tumours found anywhere. It is usually seen on sun-damaged skin, particularly the head and neck and backs of hands. Typically there is a period of rapid growth over 2–3 months, followed by a period of stability for about the same period and finally shrinkage and involution over a slightly

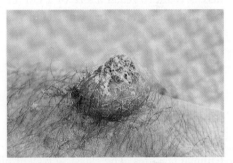

**Figure 14.18** Keratoacanthoma

longer period to leave a pitted scar. The size attained by such lesions varies from half to several centimetres. Histologically, there is often difficulty in differentiating them from invasive squamous carcinoma. The majority of keratoacanthomata behave in a benign manner but **a few ultimately transform into high grade squamous carcinoma and metastasize.** Whilst it is acceptable to adopt a conservative approach in elderly patients with typical lesions, most should be removed surgically.

### Cutaneous horn

This is a purely descriptive term for a keratinizing lesion arising from a solar keratosis, keratoacanthoma, or well-differentiated squamous carcinoma. In view of the latter, such lesions ought to be removed surgically.

## MALIGNANT TUMOURS

Skin cancers are almost exclusively confined to individuals with white skin. The three most common forms of skin cancer are:

1 Basal cell carcinoma
2 Squamous carcinoma
3 Malignant melanoma.

They occur in this order of frequency, but their threat to life is exactly the reverse. Incidence statistics for skin cancer in the United Kingdom grossly underestimate the problem, but **basal cell carcinoma far outnumbers any other malignant disease**. The incidence of all three is rising because of the ageing population and changing habits of sun exposure over the last few decades. There is an inexorable 6% annual increase in the incidence of malignant melanoma.

### Basal cell carcinoma (rodent ulcer; BCC)

**Aetiology** Although the most common human malignancy, it is only locally destructive and very rarely metastasizes (Figure 14.19). The tumour arises from malignant degeneration of basal epidermal cells. It grows very slowly and can take 5 years to reach a size of 1 cm (cf. keratoacanthoma). Fair skinned individuals over the age of 40 are most frequently affected in **sun-exposed areas of the head and neck.** Cumulative UV photo-damage is the most important predisposing factor, but other external carcinogens such as ionizing radiation and inorganic arsenic may be responsible.

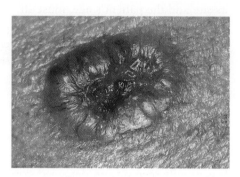

**Figure 14.19** Basal cell carcinoma

**Clinical features** The classical rodent ulcer may vary in size from 2 or 3 mm to a couple of centimetres, and has a rolled, pearly, telangiectatic border surrounding the central, often crusted ulcer. If neglected, the tumour will grow and erode local structures (hence 'rodent') such as the orbit and nose. Fortunately, these tumours do not metastasize.

**Management** Complete surgical excision is the treatment of choice, which for large lesions may involve reconstructive plastic surgery. Other modalities can be used for selected lesions, e.g. curettage and electrocautery, cryotherapy and radiotherapy.

### Squamous cell carcinoma (SCC)

**Aetiology** Most SCCs arise on sun-damaged skin, sometimes in pre-existing solar keratoses or Bowen's disease. Although outnumbered by BCCs in a ratio of 3:1, SCC (Figure 14.20) is a more important tumour because of its **potential to metastasize.** The rate of metastasis varies from 0.5 to 30%, being greatest for tumours on the lip, ear, external genitalia and mucous membranes. SCCs may also appear in old burn scars, areas of radiation injury, chronic ulcers (**Marjolin's ulcer**), sinuses associated with osteomyelitis and in the skin of immunocompromised individuals. In view of this risk, it is essential to give advice about sun protection to all patients on immunosuppressive therapy. Human papilloma virus (the cause of warts) plays an important aetiological role in squamous cancers of the cervix and external genitalia.

**Clinical features** These are very variable but classically an SCC presents as an ulcer with everted margins. However, thickened warty plaques and nodules are not uncommon. There is frequently a scab covering at least part of the tumour, which must be removed before any reasonable diagnosis can be attempted. The regional lymph nodes may be involved.

**Management** Complete surgical excision including involved nodes is the preferred option, but good results can be achieved with radiotherapy, particularly for lesions on the head and neck. There is also a place for 'on the spot'

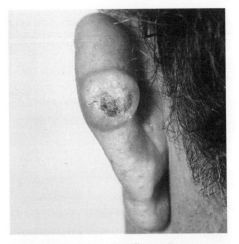

Figure 14.20 Squamous cell carcinoma

curettage and electrocautery for well differentiated SCCs arising in solar keratoses in elderly patients, since these show little tendency to metastasize.

### Malignant melanoma

This is the least frequently encountered, but most feared skin cancer (Figure 14.21). It is exceptionally rare in childhood, when the odd case arises in giant congenital naevi, but after puberty it can affect all age groups. In the United Kingdom, its incidence is rising at about 6% per annum amongst the white population and in 1992 was responsible for 1065 deaths in England alone. In the same year, about 80 000 new cases were diagnosed in the USA, but the highest incidence in the world is found amongst the white population of Australia.

The following clinicopathological types are recognized:
- Superficial spreading melanoma (60%)
- Nodular melanoma (20%)
- Lentigo maligna melanoma (15%)
- Acral lentiginous mucosal melanoma (5%).

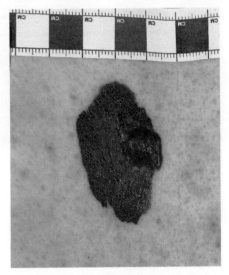

Figure 14.21 Malignant melanoma

**Aetiology** It is not known what predisposes to most examples of nodular melanoma (the most aggressive variant) or the acral variant (the only one likely to affect coloured races). Lentigo maligna melanoma arises in chronically sun-damaged skin, usually where there has been a **pre-existing in-situ melanoma (lentigo maligna, Hutchinson's melanotic freckle** – Figure 14.22). These lesions occur mainly on the face in elderly people and will not be discussed further.

**Superficial spreading melanoma** is the most common, important and possibly preventable subtype for which the major risk factors in order of significance are:

- Number of banal naevi (ordinary moles)
- More than three clinically atypical naevi
- Freckles/solar lentigines
- 'Red' hair.

The number of acquired banal naevi in young adults correlates with the amount of sun exposure, particularly episodes of sunburn in early life. An individual with 50 banal naevi has a lifetime risk approximately 15–20 times above average for melanoma, whereas a person with 'red' hair, typically with freckles and blue eyes, has an approximate fourfold lifetime risk.

**A clinically 'atypical' naevus has the following features:**

- More than 5 mm diameter plus one of – irregular edge, variegated pigment, inflammation throughout.

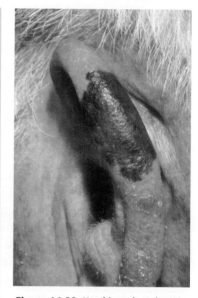

**Figure 14.22** Hutchinson's melanotic freckle (lentigo maligna)

**Diagnosis** When considering the possibility of a malignant melanoma arising in a pre-existing mole, either the British 'seven point checklist' (Table 14.2) or the American 'ABCD' mnemonic can be used.

| ABCD |
|---|
| Asymmetry |
| Border irregularity |
| Colour variation |
| Diameter > 6 mm |

**Table 14.2** Seven point check list

| Major signs | Minor signs |
|---|---|
| Change in size | Inflammation |
| Change in shape | Crusting or bleeding |
| Change in colour | Itch |
| | Diameter >7 mm |

The diagram (Figure 14.23) illustrates the rate of change which might suggest the development of melanoma. Note that these tumours do not appear in a few days – a mole which enlarges over such a short period usually does so because it has been traumatized, e.g. caught in a 'zip', or become infected.

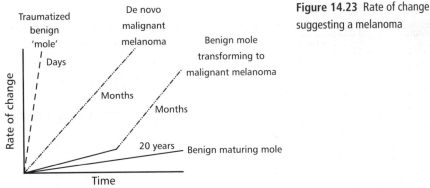

**Figure 14.23** Rate of change suggesting a melanoma

**Prognosis** The most important factor influencing prognosis is tumour thickness, as originally described by Breslow (Figure 14.24). Good prognosis tumours are <1 mm thick and carry a 5-year survival of 95–98%, whereas at the other end of the scale, tumours with a thickness of >3.5 mm carry a 5-year survival of only 40%. Death occurs due to metastatic disease.

**Management** If malignant melanoma is suspected, the patient should see a specialist (dermatologist or appropriate surgeon). If the suspicion is confirmed, the lesion can be excised under local anaesthetic, either at the first visit or very soon after, with 1–2 mm clearance laterally and minimal clearance in depth. On receipt of a positive histopathological diagnosis, the patient should be seen again as soon as possible to plan definitive excision. On this occasion, excision should be undertaken down to fascia, but there is controversy concerning lateral clearance – most

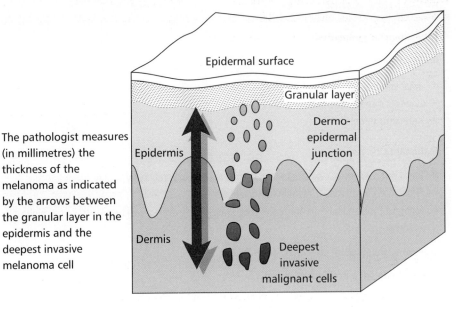

**Figure 14.24** Breslow malignant melanoma thickness measurement

agree that for a thin melanoma (<1 mm Breslow thickness), 1 cm clearance is adequate. Many surgeons will then extend excision margins by 1 cm for each extra millimetre thickness, up to a maximum of 3 cm clearance. It may well be that even for thick tumours, there is nothing to be gained by taking more than 1 cm margins, a dilemma which can hopefully be resolved in the near future.

Patients require careful follow-up, but unfortunately metastatic disease is radio-resistant and very poorly responsive to chemotherapy. Hopefully, effective immunotherapy may soon be available.

## CRIB BOX – SKIN AND APPENDAGES

### Moles

- 90% are acquired; mature then involute; rare/absent in elderly
- Learn to differentiate between moles and other pigmented lesions
- Remove for suspicion/nuisance/cosmetic

### Haemangiomas

- Strawberry naevus (capillary and cavernous)
- Port wine stain
- Campbell de Morgan spot; spider naevus

### Skin cysts

- Sebaceous
- Pilar
- Epidermoid
- Implantation dermoid

### UV damage is cumulative

Pre-malignant:

- Solar keratosis
- Bowen's disease (squamous carcinoma *in situ*)
- Keratoacanthoma

### Malignant skin lesions

- Basal cell carcinoma – most common human malignancy; relatively benign
- Squamous carcinoma – potential for metastasis
- Malignant melanoma – rising by 6% year; almost exclusively in whites; Australia has highest incidence

### Learn the 'seven point checklist' and ABCD

Prognosis related to **Breslow** thickness

Management is surgical

# chapter 15

# ENDOCRINE GLANDS

Endocrine glands mediate changes by means of hormones discharged directly into the bloodstream to affect their target organs; i.e. the pituitary, thyroid, parathyroids, adrenal glands and pancreas. Other tissues also manufacture hormones, in particular the **APUD** (**A**mine **P**recursor **U**ptake and **D**ecarboxylation) cells arising from the neural crest, many of which are associated with the GI tract and secrete hormones such as gastrin and glucagon. Calcitonin is secreted by the C cells which are found mainly in the thyroid.

## THE THYROID GLAND

### Anatomy
• The thyroid gland (Figure 15.1) consists of a lateral lobe on either side of the trachea and larynx joined by the isthmus in front of the second, third and fourth tracheal rings.

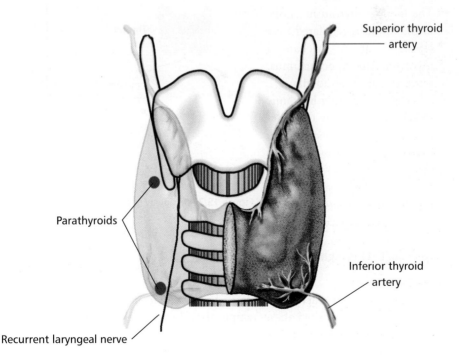

**Figure 15.1** Anatomy of thyroid gland

- The **parathyroid glands** and **recurrent laryngeal nerves** lie between the medial surface of each lobe and the trachea.
- The acini comprise a single layer of cuboidal cells with a rich capillary network and contain the colloid that holds the thyroid hormones in storage. Some 20–30 acini form a **lobule** which is the basic unit of the functioning thyroid gland.
- At any one time some lobules will be resting in involution and others will be active with cellular proliferation and a reduction in the amount of colloid.

## Physiology (Figure 15.2)

- Iodine from water and food becomes attached to the amino acid tyrosine which complex enzyme systems convert into **thyroxine (tetraiodothyronine, T4) and tri-iodothyronine (T3)**.
- 99.95% of T3 and T4 in the blood is bound to plasma proteins. Only unbound **'free'** T3 and T4 have metabolic effects. T3 is the most active. T4 is converted to T3 in peripheral tissues.
- The level of thyroid hormone in the blood is regulated by a classic feedback mechanism involving the hypothalamus, pituitary and thyroid gland.
- **Thyroid stimulating hormone (TSH)** is secreted by the anterior pituitary in response to thyrotrophin releasing hormone (TRH) from the hypothalamus. TRH secretion is inhibited by T3 and T4.
- Thus **in thyrotoxicosis TSH is low** whereas **in hypothyroidism TSH is high**.

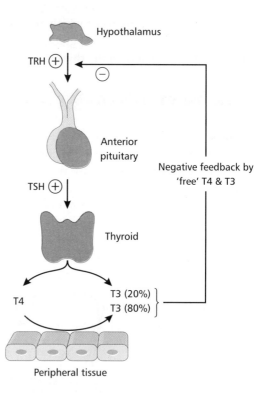

Figure 15.2 Physiology of thyroid gland

## Clinical examination

- **History** – most patients are female and present with a goitre or solitary lump. Patients should be asked about symptoms of hyper- or hypothyroidism, family history, pressure symptoms.
- **Observation** – the thyroid gland and lumps within **move on swallowing**. Does the patient look toxic or myxoedemic? Eye signs, tremor, atrial fibrillation?

- **Palpation** – gently feel the gland from **behind** the patient, using fingertips (Figure 15.3). Is the goitre smooth, nodular, hard and tender? Decide whether lumps are solitary or part of a multinodular goitre. Retrosternal extension can be felt when the patient swallows (have a glass of water ready).
- **Listen** – for bruits over a vascular toxic gland.

### Tests of thyroid function

- **TSH and T4** – are the mainstay investigations and give a satisfactory indication of thyroid status in 90% of patients. However, they are not reliable in patients who are taking thyroxine when the clinical picture is more important. T4 may also be raised in patients with any acute illness, suggesting an erroneous diagnosis of thyrotoxicosis. **Free T3 is raised only in thyrotoxicosis** and can therefore be used as a confirmatory test under these conditions.

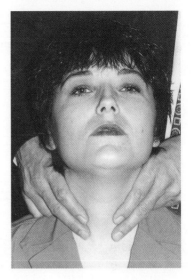

**Figure 15.3** Palpating the thyroid gland

- **Thyroid antibodies** – enables the diagnosis of Hashimoto's disease, differentiating it from anaplastic carcinoma and lymphoma.
- **Thyroglobulin** – marker to detect residual or recurrent follicular carcinoma.
- **Ultrasound scanning** – to confirm a solitary nodule or whether a thyroid nodule is in fact part of a multinodular goitre. It also differentiates cystic from solid nodules.
- **Isotope scanning** – Technetium ($^{99}$Tc) scanning demonstrates whether a nodule is functioning ('hot') or not ('cold'). A cold nodule that is solid on ultrasound may be malignant. Previously, scanning used radioactive iodine ($^{131}$I) but this is now reserved for treatment.
- **X-rays** – of the thoracic inlet will confirm tracheal deviation or narrowing. CT or MRI determines the extent of the malignancy.
- **Fine needle aspiration cytology** (**FNAC**) – particularly in the diagnosis of carcinoma.

**Table 15.1** Incidence of thyroid disease

| Thyroid disorders | Thyroid carcinoma |
|---|---|
| Non-malignant: | Relative incidence |
|    50 cases per 100 000 population per |   Papillary 70% |
|    annum with a female to male ratio of 6:1 |   Follicular 20% |
| |   Anaplastic <5% |
| Malignant: |   Medullary 5% |
|    Female – 2.25 per 100 000 per annum |   (Lymphoma) <2% |
|    Male – 1 per 100 000 per annum | |

## GOITRE

The word goitre describes any enlargement of the thyroid gland, but usually refers to:

1 **Non-toxic goitre** → simple
→ multinodular

2 **Toxic goitre** → diffuse (Graves' disease)
→ multinodular
→ toxic nodule

3 **Neoplastic** → benign
→ malignant

4 **Thyroiditis** → viral
→ Hashimoto's
→ Riedel's.

In females, enlargement of the gland at puberty, during pregnancy and at other times of increased physiological stress is common – **physiological goitre.**

### Non-toxic simple goitre

Simple goitre is much more common in women than men because of higher metabolic demands. An inability to produce sufficient T3 and T4 results in **thyroid hyperplasia driven by increased TSH from the anterior pituitary.**

**Causes**  Simple goitre is caused by:
- **Iodine deficiency** – goitre is **endemic** in mountainous areas, e.g. Alps, Pyrenees, Himalayas and Andes. Lack of iodine in soil and water gives a daily intake insufficient for normal hormone production by the thyroid gland. Patients are either euthyroid or hypothyroid, depending on the degree of insufficiency. Endemic goitre in the UK was formerly called 'Derbyshire neck'.
- **Inborn errors of iodine metabolism** – genetic deficiency of the enzymes (dyshormogenesis) necessary for the conversion of mono- and di-iodotyrosine to T3 and T4. There is often a family history of goitre with **sporadic** clusters. The absence of thyroid hormone in the fetus results in a **cretin.** Familial goitre with nerve deafness is recognized as **Pendred's syndrome.**

**Treatment**  Adequate intake of iodine prevents simple endemic goitre and in many countries table salt is iodized for this purpose. Sporadic goitre is treated with thyroxine. **Left untreated, simple goitres will eventually become nodular under the constant stimulation of TSH.**

### Non-toxic multinodular/colloid goitre

This is the most common goitre of middle age and older (Figure 15.4). Most are asymptomatic apart from cosmesis. Large goitres cause **pressure symptoms** on:
- **Trachea** – may be displaced to one side so that breathing is difficult in certain positions, especially at night. Narrowing by pressure from each side until it produces a slit shaped **scabbard trachea.** Haemorrhage into a thyroid nodule may cause urgent dyspnoea.

- Oesophagus – dysphagia rarely.
- **Superior mediastinal veins** – engorgement of neck veins and facial cyanosis due to mediastinal extension.

**Treatment** Multinodular goitre diagnosed before it becomes large enough to produce pressure symptoms is treated with thyroxine; a small dose suppresses TSH and prevents further thyroid enlargement.

**Pressure symptoms or retrosternal enlargement demand surgery** – subtotal thyroidectomy is performed and the patient then requires replacement thyroxine for life.

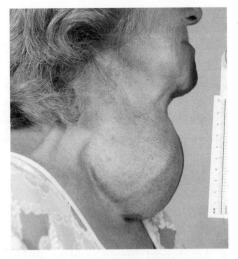

**Figure 15.4** Multinode goitre

### Toxic goitre: primary thyrotoxicosis (Graves' disease)

Parry, a physician of Bath, first described hyperthyroidism in 1786. In 1935 Robert Graves of Dublin rediscovered it.

Primary thyrotoxicosis (Figure 15.5) occurs in **young** people, arises in what was a previously normal thyroid gland and its **effects are mainly metabolic**. It is an **autoimmune disease** with the development of thyroid stimulating antibodies (TsAb) that bind to TSH receptors on the thyroid membrane.

**Pathology** The gland is uniformly enlarged to two or three times normal, and is smooth, not nodular. It is

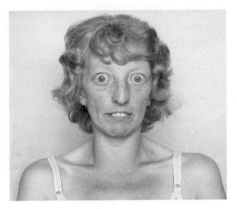

**Figure 15.5** Graves' disease

extremely vascular. Cells lining the acini are taller than normal and the acini contain scant colloid. Lymphocytes are found throughout the gland and there may be collections of lymphoid tissue arranged as in lymph nodes.

### Symptoms and signs:

- **Metabolic** – hyperactivity, tremor, sweating of palms; loss of weight despite increased appetite; dislike of hot weather.
- **Cardiac** – tachycardia, even during sleep; apex beat thrusting; increased blood flow may produce apical systolic murmur.
- **Thyroid** – typically the thyroid is only moderately enlarged, smooth and with an **audible bruit**.
- **Exophthalmos** – increased prominence of the eyes due to **lymphocytic infiltra-**

tion and increased fat in the posterior part of the orbit is common and occasionally the first sign of the disease. Caused by **exophthalmos producing substance** from the anterior pituitary gland. The eyes stare and both upper and lower lids retract so that white sclera is visible above and below the pupil; poor co-ordination of eye and lid movement causes 'lid lag'. In severe exophthalmos the eye muscles become progressively paralysed, resulting in **exophthalmic ophthalmoplegia** and corneal ulceration.

**Investigations** The T4 and T3 will be markedly elevated and TSH suppressed.

**Treatment**

> There are three methods of treating hyperthyroidism: antithyroid drugs, radio-iodine and surgery.

- **Antithyroid drugs** – carbimazole has the lowest incidence of toxic side-effects. It acts by inhibiting the biosynthesis of thyroid hormones. After 1–2 years the drug is stopped and remission will have occurred in about 50% of cases. All antithyroid drugs tend to increase the size of the thyroid gland; it is therefore advisable to give a small dose of thyroxine at the same time to suppress pituitary secretion of TSH. **Carbimazole may cause agranulocytosis and patients must be warned to report sore throats and other symptoms.** Propranolol (beta-blocker) will control the symptoms of hyperthyroidism within 48 hours.
- **Radio-iodine therapy** – oral radio-iodine $^{131}$I **is the treatment of choice** in virtually all adult patients. There is an appreciable incidence of hypothyroidism that may not be manifest until many years after the treatment – easily corrected with oral thyroxine.
- **Surgery** – subtotal thyroidectomy is restricted to those patients with large unsightly goitres or pressure symptoms, where there is a contraindication to irradiation, such as pregnancy, and in those patients who elect to have surgery rather than irradiation. The hyperthyroidism must first be controlled with carbimazole and/or propranolol.

---

**Specific complications of thyroidectomy**

**Bleeding** – a surgical emergency which threatens the patient's airway. Patients are returned **immediately** to theatre for intubation and re-exploration to control the haemorrhage.

**Tetany** – due to damage or inadvertent removal of parathyroid glands. The serum calcium should be determined after the operation.

**Hoarseness** – may result from **damage to the recurrent or external laryngeal nerves.** The vocal cords should be inspected before surgery and afterwards if there is any doubt about damage to the nerves.

**Hypothyroidism** – occurs in about 30% of cases but is readily corrected by giving thyroxine.

**Thyroid crisis or storm** – precipitated by surgery to an unprepared toxic gland and rarely by procedures of any kind in an undiagnosed toxic individual. Characterized by hyperpyrexia, tachycardia, restlessness, with delirium, collapse and death in severe cases. Treatment consists of cold sponging, oxygen, resuscitation with intravenous fluids and propranolol to control the toxicity.

### Toxic multinodular goitre (secondary thyrotoxicosis)
- Secondary thyrotoxicosis is an uncommon condition where the enlarged gland produces excessive thyroxine **autonomously.**
- **It arises in multinodular goitres in middle age and presents with cardiac problems such as atrial fibrillation.**
- The metabolic effects are much less marked than in the younger patients with primary thyrotoxicosis.

**IMPORTANT LESSON**
Appreciate the differences between primary (Graves') and secondary thyrotoxicosis. The first is young people (generally); autoimmune in a previously normal gland; mainly metabolic effects and eye signs. The second is older people; multinodular goitre; cardiac effects and, rarely, eye signs.

**Pathology** The gland shows multiple areas of involution and hyperplasia interspersed with fibrosis. Hyperplasia is often seen in the tissue between the nodules; rarely there is a single large area of hyperplasia present. It is not possible to diagnose toxicity with certainty from the histological appearance.

**Symptoms and signs** Patients with toxic multinodular goitre present a different clinical picture from the younger patients with Graves' disease. **The disease primarily affects the cardiovascular system** and is of insidious onset. Patients present with congestive heart failure, swollen ankles, atrial fibrillation, dyspnoea, tiredness and restlessness. Eye changes are rare. There is usually weight loss. The levels of T4 and T3 are raised and TSH suppressed.

**Treatment** Any of the three methods outlined for Graves' disease can be used but:
- Remission after 2 years of treatment with antithyroid drugs is uncommon
- Response to radio-iodine is less certain
- The nodularity may be causing pressure symptoms
- There is a slight risk of malignant change.

Therefore **surgery is the treatment of choice.** Prior to operation the patient is rendered euthyroid with antithyroid drugs and propranolol. Other medical problems are also treated, such as cardiac failure, atrial fibrillation, etc. The treatment of thyrotoxicosis is shown in Table 15.2.

**Table 15.2** Treatment of thyrotoxicosis

| Antithyroid drugs | Thyroidectomy | Radioactive iodine |
|---|---|---|
| Children and young patients | Long-term medical supervision not available or not desirable | Adults. Not in pregnancy |
| Mild hyperthyroidism | Bulky nodular glands with pressure symptoms | Diffuse rather than nodular glandular enlargement |
| Ancillary to other forms of treatment, especially as preoperative preparation | Toxic multinodular goitre Toxic adenoma | Hyperthyroidism recurring after thyroidectomy because of risk to parathyroids and recurrent nerves at reoperation |

## THE SOLITARY NODULE

Diagnosis of an apparently solitary thyroid nodule is a common clinical problem. Clinically it may be the only nodule large enough to be palpable in what is really a multinodular goitre. Solitary nodules always raise the suspicion of neoplasia – either a benign adenoma or a malignant adenocarcinoma.

**Investigations** These aim to answer the following questions:
- Is the lump truly solitary?
- Is it solid or cystic?
- Is it benign or malignant?

**Ultrasound scan** This differentiates cystic or colloid nodules from solid lesions and indicates whether it is a true solitary nodule or part of a multinodular goitre. **Isotope scan** This demonstrates normal or excess uptake, or whether there is no uptake, i.e. a 'cold' nodule; 10–20% of 'cold' nodules will prove to be malignant. **FNAC** aims to differentiate benign from malignant prior to definitive surgery.

**Treatment** Treatment of a solitary nodule depends in part on the result of investigations. In practice most lumps are excised even if they are benign adenomas or colloid nodules. The differential diagnosis of goitre is shown in Table 15.3.

**Table 15.3** Differential diagnosis of goitre

| Toxic goitre | Malignancy | Acute thyroiditis | Hashimoto's disease |
|---|---|---|---|
| Distinguish from non-toxic goitre with anxiety state – by thyroid function tests | Suspected if: rapid enlargement; feels hard; palpable nodes; hoarse voice; solitary nodule, especially if solid on ultrasound scan and 'cold' on isotope scan | Pain radiating to the ears; gland enlarged and tender | Moderate enlargement but firm + antibodies ↑ |

## THYROID NEOPLASMS

These frequently present as solitary nodules and may be:
- Benign (adenoma)
- Malignant – carcinoma (papillary; follicular; anaplastic; medullary); lymphoma.

### Thyroid adenoma

These usually demonstrate a normal or decreased radioisotope uptake. Difficulty in FNAC interpretation and the patient's anxiety about the lump make surgery the usual treatment option. **Occasionally a patient presents with a solitary nodule and thyrotoxicosis – a toxic adenoma.** Radioisotope uptake will indicate a 'hot' nodule with complete suppression of the normal thyroid tissue and is diagnostic. Treatment can be either radioactive iodine or surgery.

### Thyroid carcinoma

- Carcinoma arising from the true thyroxine-producing cells in the gland is either **differentiated** (papillary or follicular pattern) or **undifferentiated** (anaplastic) (Table 15.4).
- **Medullary** carcinoma in the thyroid gland is in fact derived from the parafollicular or C cells from the neural crest which migrate forward in the fetus.
- **Lymphoma**, although not carcinoma, is seen in the thyroid gland.

### Papillary carcinoma

This occurs typically **under the age of 40,** and accounts for almost all cases seen in childhood and adolescence. A small, hard, non-encapsulated, slow growing nodule occurs in one lobe of the thyroid, but careful microscopical examination of the gland will often show the tumour to be multicentric. **Spread is via the lymphatics** to nodes:
- Above the isthmus of the gland
- In the groove between the oesophagus and trachea

**Table 15.4** Thyroid carcinoma

|  | Papillary | Follicular | Anaplastic |
|---|---|---|---|
| Age | Young | Middle | Old |
| Spread | Nodes (lateral aberrant thyroid) | Blood → Skeleton → Lungs | Direct |
| $^{131}$I uptake | No | Yes | No |
| Treatment | Lobectomy/total thyroidectomy plus nodes Thyroxine to suppress TSH | Total thyroidectomy $^{131}$I for metastases Thyroxine to suppress TSH | Surgery for diagnosis and decompression Rarely responds to DXT |
| Prognosis | Good – 92% 5-year survival | Fair – 75% 5-year survival | Bad – 0% 5-year survival |

- In the thymus
- Along both jugular chains.

**Pathology** Histologically, the metastases resemble thyroid tissue, with papillary processes and varying amounts of colloid. **'Former lateral aberrant'** thyroids are metastases of differentiated thyroid carcinoma to lymph nodes in the neck.

**Symptoms and signs** A solitary firm nodule in the thyroid gland of a young patient should raise a suspicion of carcinoma. When enlarged lymph nodes are palpable, the diagnosis is almost certain. Uncommonly, spread may occur via the bloodstream to the lungs and bones.

**Tests** If the primary tumour is impalpable the diagnosis is made by excising a lymph node for histology or by FNAC. In a palpable solitary thyroid nodule, FNAC may confirm the diagnosis and allow definitive treatment to be planned.

**Treatment Total thyroidectomy** is the ideal treatment for papillary carcinoma if the diagnosis has been confirmed prior to surgery, since the disease may be multi-centric. If it is difficult to achieve, removal should be as complete as possible followed by an ablative dose of $^{131}$I. One or more parathyroids must be preserved and both recurrent laryngeal nerves if possible. All visible and palpable lymph nodes are excised.

Frequently the correct diagnosis is only made by the pathologist when examining sections of the lesion; **therefore total lobectomy is recommended for all solitary nodules,** as it is in these that carcinomas are usually discovered. Following operation, full replacement therapy with thyroxine is needed for the rest of the patient's life. **It is extremely important that the dose of thyroxine is sufficient to suppress TSH** below physiological norms to diminish the stimulus to further growth of any cancer cells that remain in the neck or elsewhere (Figure 15.6).

During follow-up any suspicious node found on palpation is excised.

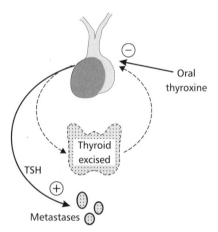

**Figure 15.6** Suppression of metastases using oral thyroxine

The prognosis in young patients is good and the disease is compatible with long life. Adverse prognostic factors are a large primary tumour, i.e. >2 cm in diameter, lymph node spread and age over 40 years. The disease is more aggressive in males than females.

### Follicular carcinoma

Typically, this type of tumour occurs in the middle years of life.

**Pathology** The carcinoma reproduces in varying degree the follicular pattern of the thyroid, and the better differentiated it is, the better chance there is of eradicating the disease. **Spread is more often by the bloodstream rather than by the lymphatics** and therefore metastases are found in the lungs and skeleton. **The classical metastatic tumour in the head of a humerus is usually from a thyroid primary.**

**Tests** More than half of these patients have noticed a nodule for years which latterly has grown more quickly. A third present with symptoms of metastasis to lung or bones (pathological fracture). Chest x-ray, bone scan and FNAC or biopsy of a metastasis are needed.

**Treatment Total thyroidectomy** is done first in order to remove the primary tumour and all normal functioning thyroid tissue or all the tumour is removed and the rest of the gland destroyed with $^{131}$I. Full thyroxine replacement therapy is needed. Metastases are treated with radio-iodine if differentiated enough to absorb it. When metastases do not take up radio-iodine, they are treated by conventional radiotherapy.

### Undifferentiated carcinoma
Undifferentiated or anaplastic carcinoma of the thyroid usually occurs in the elderly, and is more common in women than men.

**Pathology** There are undifferentiated sheets of irregular or spindle shaped cells.

**Symptoms and signs** There is rapid painless growth of the thyroid gland, which may already be enlarged due to multinodular goitre. Hoarseness occurs early due to laryngeal nerve invasion, and compression of the trachea leads to dyspnoea and stridor. Dysphagia due to involvement of the oesophagus occurs later.

**Tests** It is essential to differentiate anaplastic carcinoma from **thyroiditis** and **lymphoma** which are clinically similar – thyroid antibody tests and biopsy are required. Radiography of the neck will show the extent of the tumour as well as tracheal compression or displacement.

**Treatment** The treatment of undifferentiated thyroid carcinoma is radiotherapy. Airway obstruction requires tracheostomy. Thyroxine is given since the gland is rapidly destroyed. The prognosis is poor with an expectation of life rarely more than 3 months.

### Medullary carcinoma
This is a slow growing tumour of the **parafollicular** or **C cells**. The tumour spreads to lymph nodes and the mediastinum and is often calcified. A rare familial type is associated with phaeochromocytomas (MEN-2) and with mucosal neuromas (MEN-2b), (MEN, multiple endocrine neoplasia). It is therefore important to check the patient for other endocrine problems and the patient's family should be investigated.

**Symptoms and signs** Growth is slow with lymph node and mediastinal involvement. After a latent period of many years, the tumour may show a spurt of growth and metastasize. The presence of this tumour is accompanied by high levels of **calcitonin** in the blood and this is a useful way of monitoring the patient for recurrence after treatment.

**Treatment** Surgical excision is the treatment of choice, because it is unaffected by radio-iodine and radiotherapy. The 5-year survival rate is 70%.

### Lymphoma
A lymphoma may develop within the thyroid gland as in many other organs that are rich in lymphoid tissue. It has a similar variable prognosis but frequently responds well to radiotherapy or chemotherapy and long survival times are not uncommon. It is because it is eminently treatable that it is important to establish a tissue diagnosis and differentiate it from anaplastic carcinoma.

## THYROIDITIS

### Acute thyroiditis: de Quervain's thyroiditis
This is due to a viral infection and presents with acute pain and tenderness of the thyroid gland. The **pain classically radiates to the ears** and is a diagnostic feature. There is general malaise and fever. The thyroid gland is moderately enlarged, firm and tender. Because of the cellular destruction, there is release of large amounts of thyroid hormones into the bloodstream and **frank thyrotoxicosis is common**. There will be elevation of T3 and T4 as well as suppression of TSH and the **ESR is high**. In all but mild cases it will be necessary to treat the thyrotoxicosis with antithyroid drugs, and steroids will usually shorten the course of the disease. Full recovery is the norm but occasionally the gland is destroyed and hypothyroidism results.

### Hashimoto's disease: chronic lymphocytic thyroiditis
First described by a Japanese surgeon in 1912. The thyroid gland is only moderately enlarged and the histological changes are characteristic. The cells lining the follicles become plump and eosinophilic with granular cytoplasm, and are known as **Hürthle cells**. There is infiltration with lymphocytes, and the parenchyma of the gland is progressively replaced by lymphoid tissue and varying amounts of fibrosis. **This is an autoimmune disease with antithyroid and thyroglobulin antibodies.** The cause is unknown.

**Symptoms and signs** This disease occurs most commonly in women, usually between the ages of 30 and 50. The thyroid gland is moderately enlarged, non-painful, feels rubbery with well defined borders, and is often remarkably mobile. Initially there may be mild signs of hyperthyroidism, followed inevitably by increasing hypothyroidism, which in untreated patients progresses to myxoedema.

**Tests** The diagnosis is made on clinical suspicion confirmed by positive thyroid antibody titres. FNAC provides histological proof of the condition.

**Treatment** The patient requires full thyroid replacement therapy for the rest of her/his life.

### Riedel's thyroiditis
This condition was described by Riedel in 1896 as ligneous or woody thyroiditis. It is exceedingly rare, occurring twice as commonly in women as men in the 30–60-year age group.

**Symptoms and signs** The onset is insidious, with the gland becoming stony hard and bound to all the surrounding structures by fibrosis. There may be little evidence of hypothyroidism, but dyspnoea, dysphagia and hoarseness become progressively worse. Association with mediastinal fibrosis, sclerosing cholangitis and retroperitoneal fibrosis is described. Both clinically and at operation **it is indistinguishable from anaplastic carcinoma;** biopsy for pathological examination is essential.

**Treatment** As in Hashimoto's thyroiditis the thyroid gland is destroyed and hormone replacement is required.

**Table 15.5** Differential diagnosis – goitre

| Non-toxic | Toxic | Malignant | Other |
|---|---|---|---|
| SIMPLE | DIFFUSE | ADENOCARCINOMA | AUTOIMMUNE |
| Physiological endemic | Graves' disease | (Differentiated) | Hashimoto's disease |
| sporadic (IEM) | (primary) | papillary follicular | Riedel's thyroiditis |
| MULTINODULAR | MULTINODULAR | ANAPLASTIC | INFLAMMATORY |
| Usually euthyroid but | (secondary | (undifferentiated) | Acute viral thyroiditis |
| may be: | thyrotoxicosis) | | |
|   hypo- | | | |
|   hyper- | | | |
| SOLITARY NODULE | SOLITARY NODULE | MEDULLARY | |
| | Toxic adenoma | LYMPHOMA | |

## HYPOTHYROIDISM

Hypothyroidism, or in its extreme form, **myxoedema** (Figure 15.7), is not a surgically treated condition; but it so often complicates other diseases that the surgeon should always keep it in mind. **It is often overlooked.**

Hypothyroidsim produces general sluggishness of mind and body. Weight is increased and typical fatty pads appear above the clavicles. In severe cases patients become difficult to manage, paranoid and hate the cold.

**Treatment** Treatment is achieved with simple hormone replacement – to prevent untoward cardiac effects the initial dose of thyroxine is low, slowly increasing over a period of 2–3 months to a maintenance dose of around 0.2 mg.

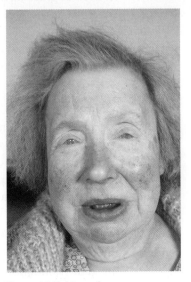

**Figure 15.7** Myxoedema

# THE ADRENAL GLANDS

## Anatomy
The adrenal glands are crescentic in shape and overlie the upper poles of the kidneys. Each gland comprises a cortex surrounding a medulla; they have separate endocrine functions.

## THE ADRENAL CORTEX

The adrenal cortex, comprising the golden coloured outer layer of the adrenal, secretes a large number of hormones that are grouped in three main categories:

1 **Glucocorticoids** – of which cortisol (hydrocortisone) is the most important, regulate carbohydrate metabolism and help the tissues to deal with stress (including surgery) and infection.
2 **Mineralocorticoids** – of which the chief is aldosterone, control transport of sodium across cell membranes and the excretion of potassium by the kidney.
3 **Androgens** – secreted by the adrenal cortex as well as by the testes.

> The production of the glucocorticoids is controlled by adrenocorticotrophin (ACTH) from the anterior pituitary by a feedback mechanism, in which a reduction in the level of corticoids stimulates the pituitary to secrete more ACTH. Therapeutic administration of corticosteroids (e.g. prednisolone) will suppress ACTH and eventually lead to atrophy of the adrenal cortices. **This is important to the surgeon because if major surgery is needed, it is essential to supplement the steroid dose, since the patient cannot produce the additional adrenal secretion required.**

## Pathology
Increased secretion of glucocorticoids, mineralocorticoids and androgens may be due to:
- Pituitary tumour
- Hyperplasia of both adrenal cortices
- One or more cortical adenomas
- Rarely, a carcinoma.

## Cushing's syndrome
This is due to excessive secretion of glucocorticoids:
- Usually caused by an ACTH-secreting **microadenoma of the anterior pituitary,** resulting in **hyperplasia of both adrenal cortices.** The tumour is rarely large enough to expand the sella turcica and be seen in radiographs of the skull.
- **Rarely, an adenoma or carcinoma arising in the cortex of one adrenal.**
- Sometimes bilateral adrenal hyperplasia is caused by **ectopic ACTH from a non-pituitary tumour** (e.g. lung, pancreas).

## Symptoms and signs
- Women are more commonly affected than men, most commonly in the age group 20–40.

- The onset is gradual, with obesity, hirsutism, amenorrhoea (or impotence), muscle weakness, backache, pathological fractures and symptoms due to hypertensive heart disease and mental depression (Figure 15.8).
- The face is moon shaped and purplish, the face and hair are greasy with acne, purple striae develop in the skin over the flanks.
- **'Cushingoid' features are seen regularly in patients receiving large doses of therapeutic steroids for various disorders.**

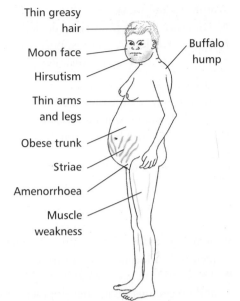

Thin greasy hair — Moon face — Hirsutism — Thin arms and legs — Obese trunk — Striae — Amenorrhoea — Muscle weakness — Buffalo hump

**Figure 15.8** Cushing's syndrome

### Tests

- Hyperglycaemia and glycosuria are common.
- The urine contains increased amounts of 17-hydroxycorticosteroids but a high 24-hour urinary free cortisol is more specific.
- **Plasma cortisol is persistently raised and will not suppress with dexamethasone.**
- Plasma ACTH is raised with a pituitary tumour or ectopic ACTH production, but low (i.e. suppressed) with an adrenal adenoma.
- A CT or MRI scan reveals bilateral adrenal hyperplasia, or a solitary adrenal adenoma.
- Pituitary scanning may show an adenoma but they are often very small.
- Ectopic ACTH production from tumours outside the pituitary needs consideration (chest x-ray).
- It is important to differentiate those patients who merely have hypertension, obesity and glycosuria from the true Cushing's syndrome.

### Treatment

- Hypertension, heart failure, hyperglycaemia and hypokalaemia need attention.
- Synthesis of adrenal steroids can be blocked with metyrapone or aminoglutethamide but surgery is usually preferred.
- Pituitary adenomas are removed surgically via a trans-sphenoidal route or occasionally ablated by inserting radioactive yttrium.
- Bilateral adrenalectomy with subsequent hormone replacement is used for otherwise untreatable ectopic ACTH production or pituitary recurrence.
- An adrenal adenoma is excised by unilateral adrenalectomy.

### Conn's syndrome

This is primary hyperaldosteronism due to a **solitary cortical adenoma** of golden yellow colour.

Symptoms and signs
- These are due to potassium depletion, sodium retention and hypertension.
- Muscle weakness, cramps, polyuria and headache are common.
- **The condition may be mistaken for renal failure associated with hypertension.**

Treatment
- Preliminary treatment is medical, i.e. control of hypertension and correction of hypokalaemia – spironolactone; amiloride; potassium supplements.
- This is followed by excision of the adenoma.

### Adrenogenital syndrome
This is caused by excess secretion of cortical androgens.

**Congenital** An inborn defect in adrenal cortisol synthesis results in ACTH-driven hyperplasia which in turn causes excess androgen secretion.
- Signs and symptoms are due to deficiency of cortisol and/or aldosterone coupled with androgenic virilization.
- The condition presents at birth or early childhood with virilism in the female and precocious sexual development in the male.
- Growth is rapid at first, but early epiphyseal fusion occurs.
- A female child at birth may have clitoral hypertrophy and fused labia (pseudohermaphrodite).

**Acquired** This is usually an adrenal cortical tumour which is benign or malignant. In adults it may be associated with bilateral adrenal hyperplasia, e.g. Cushing's.

Treatment
- Corticosteroid replacement therapy suppresses ACTH and androgen secretion. Tumours are excised.

## THE ADRENAL MEDULLA

The adrenal medulla is composed of two kinds of cells, one nervous in type, the other endocrine. The latter stain brown with chromic acid (phaeochromocytes). **The phaeochromocytes may form adenomas which secrete adrenaline and noradrenaline. The nerve cells may produce benign ganglioneuromas or highly malignant neuroblastomas.**

### Phaeochromocytoma
The chromaffin cells of the adrenal medulla secrete adrenaline and noradrenaline; tumours of these cells produce **hypertension**, which is typically paroxysmal, but may be continuous.

Symptoms and signs
- There are attacks of sudden increase in blood pressure, with blinding headache, anxiety, personality changes and convulsions.
- The patient goes pale in an attack, sweats and may suffer from dyspnoea and anginal pain.

## Tests
- CT/MRI scanning and radioactive metaiodobenzylguanidine ($^{131}$I MIBG) scanning have superseded intravenous pyelography and aortography as tumour localization procedures.
- Pressure over the loin may start an attack of hypertension.
- The urine is assayed for **vanillyl mandelic acid** (VMA) and catecholamines.
- An injection of 5 mg phentolamine will reduce the blood pressure.

## Treatment
- Preliminary treatment for 1 or 2 weeks is directed at minimizing the hypertension by giving the alpha-adrenergic blocking agent, phenoxybenzamine, and the beta-blocker propranolol.
- The tumour with the adrenal gland is excised with great care, as handling releases noradrenaline and causes hypertension.

# THE PARATHYROIDS

## HYPERPARATHYROIDISM

### Primary
**This is not a rare disease and occurs in 1 in 700 of the population.** It is probably often overlooked. Excess parathyroid hormone (PTH) leads to a raised blood level of calcium and excess urinary excretion of calcium. It is **usually due to an adenoma** occurring in one of the parathyroid glands, occasionally there are two such tumours, and in about 5% of patients there is hyperplasia of all four glands. Carcinoma of the parathyroids is rare.

### Secondary
Secondary hyperparathyroidism clinically resembles the primary disease but all four parathyroids are hyperplastic. The commonest cause is severe renal damage, hence it usually complicates renal failure. Malabsorption in the gut is another cause.

### Tertiary
This is usually due to the chronic calcium loss of renal failure or steatorrhoea. All four parathyroids become hyperplastic and eventually adenomatous. The **adenomas become autonomous** and continue to secrete excess PTH, even if the cause of calcium loss is removed, e.g. by kidney transplant in renal failure.

**Symptoms and signs** Biochemical screening discovers many patients with asymptomatic hypercalcaemia. Many of these apparently fit individuals have a small parathyroid adenoma which should

| Differential diagnosis of hypercalcaemia |
| --- |
| • Bone metastases |
| • Hyperparathyroidism |
| • Multiple myeloma |
| • Sarcoidosis |
| • Renal disease |
| • Thyrotoxicosis |
| • Vitamin D overdose |

be removed because of the risk of insidious renal damage and the accompanying complications. These fall into four groups: bone disease, urinary tract disease, hypercalcaemic changes and peptic ulcer and pancreatitis. Hyperparathyroidism is a disease of **bones, stones, psychological moans, and abdominal groans:**

- **Bone disease** – the reason why some patients with hyperparathyroidism develop bone disease and some do not is unknown. **The basic change is subperiosteal resorption and is best seen in x-rays of the middle phalanges.** Von Recklinghausen's disease or osteitis fibrosa cystica (Figure 15.9) is a generalized decalcification of the skeleton with cyst formation and the presence of tumour-like masses of osteoclasts. Vertebrae may collapse and a patient loses height, this being accentuated by the bowing of the femora. Bone pain, especially backache, is common. Pathological fractures may occur.

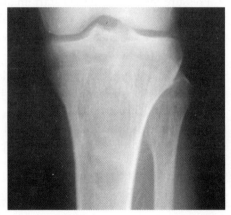

**Figure 15.9** Osteitis fibrosa cystica in the tibia

- **Urinary tract disease** – urinary calculi are common. The stones are often bilateral and recur after removal. Calcification of the renal tubules may be demonstrated by radiography – nephrocalcinosis.
- **Hypercalcaemia** – this leads to hypotonia of the muscles and generalized weakness. Deposition of calcium occurs in many tissues and in the eye produces a band of keratitis adjacent to the limbus. The electrocardiogram shows shortening of the Q-T interval. Depression and **psychological problems** occur.
- **Chronic peptic ulcer and acute pancreatitis** – these may also be presenting features of hyperparathyroidism and should lead to a search for the other endocrine abnormalities of the MEN syndrome.

Tests
- **Calcium** – levels vary from day to day and tests must be repeated more than once. The patient should be fasting and tourniquets should not be used when obtaining blood.
- **Phosphate** – typically lowered.
- **Parathormone (PTH)** – assays now give accurate estimations of PTH levels. Therefore any patient with a high serum calcium and raised PTH is suffering from primary hyperparathyroidism. All other causes of raised serum calcium suppress parathormone.
- **Radiography** – may show subperiosteal erosion (phalanges); loss of lamina dura around the teeth; bone cysts; renal calculi and nephrocalcinosis.

- **Isotope subtraction scan** – Radiothallium ($^{201}$Th) is taken up by both the thyroid and parathyroid glands, $^{99}$Tc only by the thyroid. Computerized subtraction of these images (Figure 15.10) reveals an adenoma as a 'hot' spot.
- **Venous sampling** – PTH estimation at different levels in the jugular vein has largely been superseded by the subtraction scan.

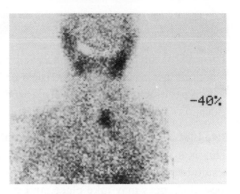

**Figure 15.10** Isotope subtraction scan showing adenoma of left lower parathyroid

Treatment

- Removal of the parathyroid gland containing the adenoma, or subtotal parathyroidectomy if all the glands are involved by hyperplasia.
- In the latter patients the possibility of a MEN syndrome also involving pituitary, pancreas and adrenal cortex should be suspected.
- The first operative attempt to find the parathyroid tumour is the most important one, and the search may have to include the thymus and upper mediastinum, where parathyroids may also occur.
- In severe hyperparathyroidism there is **usually post-operative tetany** due to 'rebound' hypocalcaemia. Immediate treatment is by intravenous calcium gluconate and subsequently effervescent calcium by mouth.
- Bone takes time to replenish calcium stores. Renal damage is usually permanent.

**Table 15.6** Multiple endocrine neoplasia

| MEN-1 | MEN-2A | MEN-2B |
|---|---|---|
| Parathyroid | Medullary carcinoma of the thyroid | Medullary carcinoma of the thyroid |
| Pituitary | Parathyroid hyperplasia | Phaeochromocytomas |
| Pancreatic islet hyperplasia neoplasia | Bilateral phaeochromocytoma | Multiple mucosal neuromas lips and tongue throughout the gastrointestinal tract |
| and, rarely, Carcinoid tumours | and, rarely, Cutaneous lichen amyloidosis | |

## THE PANCREAS

The bulk of the pancreas is concerned with its exocrine functions. The endocrine functions are performed by the islets of Langerhans, which contain a number of cell types including beta-cells (producing insulin), alpha-cells (producing glucagon) and others of the APUD type.

### Beta islet cell tumour (insulinoma; nesidioblastoma)

This is a rare tumour of beta-cells which produces hyperinsulinism, and as a result, hypoglycaemia. Because it may go undiagnosed for many years, permanent mental changes may take place, and patients with this disease have been discovered in mental institutions.

**Symptoms and signs**  There are three, the 'triad of Whipple':

1 **Fasting** causes measurable hypoglycaemia. In severe cases this starts within a few hours of eating but can take a day or more.
2 **Hypoglycaemic attack** – often begins with a recognizable aura followed by giddiness, apprehension, fear, aggression, disorientation, fitting, coma. Hypoglycaemia is associated with adrenaline release and a fight/flight reaction; thus there is accompanying sweating, cardiovascular changes and sometimes incontinence.
3 **Sugar** in any form during an attack brings it to an end. Intravenous glucose is the most dramatic way of doing this.

**Tests**  All patients who have epileptiform attacks should have a blood sugar estimation, since a level under 2 mmol/l is strongly suggestive of an insulinoma and demands further investigation. Serum insulin levels are raised inappropriately. CT/MRI or selective angiography may demonstrate the position of the tumour or tumours; 80% are due to a single adenoma.

**Treatment**  The pancreas is explored through a transverse abdominal incision and the tumour excised. If no tumour is discovered, subtotal pancreatectomy is performed in the hope of removing either a tumour or a sufficient number of hyperplastic islets (MEN-1).

### Zollinger–Ellison syndrome

This is a rare non-beta-cell tumour which secretes gastrin (**gastrinoma**), found usually in the pancreatic head and presents with peptic ulceration (see Chapter 27).

## THE PITUITARY

Tumours of the pituitary produce symptoms in two different ways:

1 **Raised intracranial pressure** produces vomiting, headache and poor vision. Local pressure on the optic chiasma leads to reduction of the visual fields (bitemporal hemianopia) and eventual blindness.

2   **Hypersecretion of hormones** leads to endocrine changes.

### Pituitary tumours

There are three types of tumour arising from different types of cell in the **anterior lobe of the pituitary: chromophobe, eosinophil and basophil.**

- **Chromophobe adenoma** – is the commonest, and grows to a large size, producing most of its changes by pressure on the surrounding structures and an increase in the general pressure inside the skull. Atrophy of the remainder of the pituitary produces hypopituitarism. Some present when they are still small as the cause of amenorrhoea, infertility in women and impotence in men, due to excess **prolactin** secretion (**prolactinoma**).
- **Eosinophil adenoma** – secretes growth hormone; it is rare, and in childhood leads to gigantism and in an adult to acromegaly.
- **Basophil adenoma** – is also rare and frequently very small, but it may produce large quantities of ACTH and Cushing's syndrome.

**Treatment**   The treatment of tumours of the pituitary is usually surgical excision; microsurgery may permit removal of individual secreting tumours.

## THE THYMUS

The thymus gland is composed of fatty tissue, with many thymocytes, lymphocytes and some lymphoid tissue. It is relatively large at birth and until puberty, but becomes smaller in adults and is atrophic in the elderly. In the young it produces immunologically competent lymphocytes. It is occasionally enlarged in adults in hyperthyroidism and myasthenia gravis.

### Myasthenia gravis

Myasthenia gravis is a disease in which there is progressive weakness of the skeletal muscles, which may end in respiratory paralysis and death. The disease often progresses very slowly over many years, and is usually controlled by giving neostigmine in a gradually increasing dosage.

**Treatment**   Thymectomy is used for myasthenia with somewhat unpredictable results, although young patients with disease of recent onset do best.

## CRIB BOX – ENDOCRINE GLANDS

**Goitre** – non-toxic; toxic; neoplastic; thyroiditis. Also physiological

### Thyrotoxicosis

- Primary (Graves' disease) – autoimmune; eye signs; young people
- Secondary (multinodular goitre) – older people; no eye signs; cardiac presentation

**Solitary nodule** – is it solitary?; solid or cystic; benign or malignant

### Thyroid cancer

- Papillary – under 40; good prognosis; nodal spread
- Follicular – over 40; intermediate prognosis; haematogenous spread
- Anaplastic – elderly; poor prognosis; locally very invasive

Remember medullary and lymphoma

### Adrenals

- Cortex – cortisol (Cushing's); aldosterone (Conn's); androgens (adrenogenital syndrome)
- Medulla – adrenaline and noradrenaline (phaeochromocytoma); malignant neuroblastomas

### Hyperparathyroidism

- Primary, secondary and tertiary
- Disease of bones, stones, psychological moans and abdominal groans

### REMEMBER THE DIFFERENTIAL DIAGNOSES OF HYPERCALCAEMIA.

**Pancreas** – insulinoma (triad of Whipple); Zollinger–Ellison syndrome

### Pituitary adenomas

- Chromophobe – pressure only; panhypopituitarism; prolactinoma
- Eosinophil – acromegaly; gigantism
- Basophil – Cushing's

# chapter 16

# FACE AND NECK

Surgery is required for many face and neck conditions. In adults, infection and malignant disease predominate, whereas in the young, congenital lesions are more prevalent. The regional anatomy is complex – superficial lesions such as epidermoid cysts are common but pathology in deeper structures often presents a diagnostic challenge.

## HISTORY

### Pain
- Pain is usually due to **infection**, e.g. parotitis or lymphadenitis secondary to intra-oral sepsis.
- Pain on eating suggests salivary gland obstruction and may be accompanied by swelling of the affected gland.
- Painless swelling indicates tumour.
- Cystic swellings are usually intermittent.

## EXAMINATION

### Observation
- A lump in the neck, **which moves on swallowing**, is either in the **thyroid** gland or attached to the pretracheal fascia, e.g. lymph nodes.
- A midline swelling which moves upwards when the **tongue is protruded** is a **thyroglossal cyst**.
- Lymph nodes closely associated with the carotid artery will often transmit visible pulsation.

- With all swellings in the neck it is important to inspect the mouth, oro- and nasopharynx since otherwise even gross tumours in these areas may be overlooked.

- Some systemic diseases such as Cushing's, thyrotoxicosis and myxoedema have typical facial signs.

### Palpation
- Palpation of the neck should be performed with the examiner standing behind the patient who is usually on a low backed stool.
- The anterior and posterior triangles of the neck are examined systematically, particular attention being paid to fixity and consistency of any mass.

- A retrosternal goitre can be felt to move up into the neck when the patient swallows.
- Salivary glands of the floor of the mouth or cheek need to be examined by bimanual palpation.
- Cysts can usually be transilluminated.

- **It is especially important to examine areas drained by lymph nodes in the neck** – malignant tumours within the testes, abdomen, chest, breast and oropharynx may all present with involved neck glands.

## Percussion
- Percussion of the upper chest, sternum and clavicles may elicit dullness with a retrosternal goitre or apical lung tumour.

## Auscultation
- Bruits may be heard in association with cervical ribs, thyrotoxicosis and carotid disease.

# LESIONS IN ADULTS

## SWELLINGS IN THE NECK

The **majority of swellings in the neck are due to lymph nodes** which may be involved with infection or malignant disease. Bacterial infection is common, most often related to dental sepsis and is painful. Conversely, **lymphatic malignancy usually causes painless enlargement**. Carcinoma of the lip, tongue, mouth or salivary glands spreads to the submental, submandibular and jugular lymph nodes. Supraclavicular nodes may indicate spread from carcinoma of the breast and especially on the left side may be a late presentation of abdominal malignancy. Hodgkin's disease, non-Hodgkin's lymphoma and chronic lymphatic leukaemia can present with firm, rubbery, discrete neck nodes. **Neck glands which are clinically malignant should not be excised before the oropharynx, nasopharynx, hypopharynx and larynx have been thoroughly examined for a primary tumour.** Fine needle aspiration cytology avoids the need for excision biopsy in most cases.

### Specific infections
- **Actinomycosis** is a rare infection in the neck but occasionally follows dental extractions. Diagnosis is made by examination of pus for 'sulphur granules' and mycelial masses are seen on microscopy.
- **Ludwig's angina** is cellulitis in the submandibular, submental and sublingual spaces limited by the deep cervical fascia. Oedema spreads backwards and downwards to involve the larynx, leading to respiratory obstruction. Management is by decompression of the deep cervical fascia in the submandibular/submental region and large doses of antibiotics. Endotracheal intubation and ventilation may be required.

- **Tuberculous** glands are encountered world wide and may suppurate to produce a cold abscess.

### Pharyngeal pouch

This is a pulsion diverticulum of the mucous membrane between the fibres of the inferior constrictor and cricopharyngeus muscles of the pharynx and is more common on the left side of the neck. It causes dysphagia and contents may be regurgitated to produce inhalation pneumonia. It is diagnosed on barium swallow or endoscopy (see Chapter 26).

### Thyroglossal cyst

A thyroglossal cyst (Figure 16.1) may occur anywhere along the thyroglossal tract from the foramen caecum of the tongue to the thyroid isthmus. Presentation is usually with a smooth **midline swelling** commonly in the subhyoid region which **moves up when the tongue is protruded.** Since they are prone to infection, thyroglossal cysts should be excised together with the thyroglossal tract up towards the foramen caecum, including the mid-portion of the hyoid bone.

### Carotid body tumour (chemodectoma)

This is a rare tumour of chromaffin tissue arising between the internal and external carotid arteries (Figure 16.2). The tumour is very slow growing, ovoid in shape and is usually benign. Excision is difficult and is sometimes impossible without arterial reconstruction.

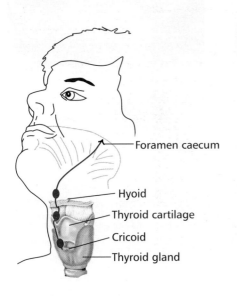

Foramen caecum

Hyoid

Thyroid cartilage

Cricoid

Thyroid gland

**Figure 16.1** Thyroglossal cyst

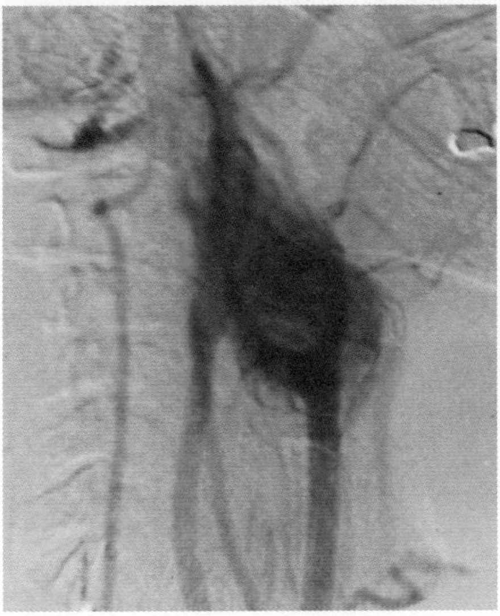

**Figure 16.2** Subtraction angiogram of carotid body tumour (note splaying of internal and external carotid arteries)

## THE SALIVARY GLANDS

Diseases affecting the salivary glands are **infection, calculi, cysts, tumour, and autoimmune disease.**

### Parotid gland

- Parotitis or infection of the gland is most often due to the mumps virus. Recurrent parotitis gives a classical appearance of globular sialectasis on sialography – the Epstein–Barr virus has been postulated as the infective organism. Management is usually with systemic antibiotics to limit damage due to secondary infection.
- Bacterial infection can occur in patients who become dehydrated, e.g. postoperatively – reduced salivary flow allows infection to ascend from the mouth into the gland, occasionally causing an abscess which requires drainage.
- Calculi are uncommon in the parotid duct but present as pain and swelling of the gland after meals. Diagnosis is made by sialography as parotid stones tend not to be radio-opaque.

- **Benign tumours – Ninety per cent of parotid tumours are pleomorphic adenomas**, presenting with a superficial mobile mass near the angle of the jaw (Figure 16.3). These benign tumours consist of epithelial cells in a matrix of mucoid myxomatous or chondroid tissue. They are slow growing and are surrounded by a pseudo-capsule. Treatment is by excision of the mass – **superficial parotidectomy with preservation of the branches of the facial nerve.** Occasionally total parotidectomy, again with preservation of the facial nerves, is required. Soft swellings of the parotid gland may sometimes be due to other benign conditions such as adenolymphoma or parotid cysts.

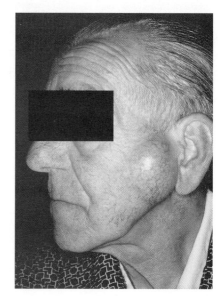

**Figure 16.3** Parotid tumour

- **Malignant tumours** – Carcinoma of the parotid gland is a serious disease, difficult to eradicate and prone to local spread – fixation to masseter muscle and **facial palsy** are indications of late presentation. Squamous, adenocystic and adenocarcinoma are all seen. Metastatic spread is to the cervical lymph nodes of the neck and late to the lungs and liver. Treatment is by total parotidectomy with sacrifice of the facial nerve (which can be reconstructed with nerve grafts) and may cure the disease in the early stages. Block dissection of the neck glands may be necessary (see page 215). High voltage radiation can be used post-operatively or occasionally as the first line treatment in advanced local disease but the majority are relatively radio-resistant.

## Submandibular gland

- **Stones are common** in the duct of the submandibular gland (Figure 16.4) and cause pain and swelling in the submandibular triangle at meal times.

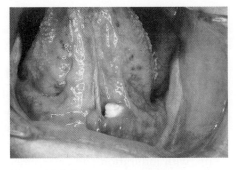

**Figure 16.4** Submandibular calculus

- Intraductal calculi located in the accessible part of the submandibular duct can be removed through an incision into the duct in the floor of the mouth.
- Multiple calculi are not uncommon and can be confirmed on sialography.
- Excision of the submandibular gland is required if the calculi causing obstruction are lying within the substance of the gland.
- Benign and malignant tumours of the submandibular gland are rare and are treated by excision of the whole gland.

## Mikulicz–Sjögren's disease

- This is a rare condition in which some or all of the salivary glands are enlarged and lose their power of secretion so that the patient complains of dry eyes and a dry mouth. It is due to an autoimmune process similar to that of Hashimoto's thyroiditis.

## LIPS, TONGUE AND MOUTH

### Carcinoma of the lip

- Any chronic thickening of the lower lip should raise suspicion of carcinoma.
- It is more common in elderly men, the main cause being **solar radiation damage**.
- The tumour is invariably **squamous cell carcinoma** presenting as a thickened, firm warty growth or ulcer (Figure 16.5).
- Spread is **local** and via the **lymphatics** to the submental and submandibular nodes.
- If the growth is untreated, death may follow fungation of secondary deposits in the neck; haemorrhage from ulcerated vessels occasionally occurring.

**Treatment** The primary tumour can be treated either surgically or with radiotherapy; part of the mandible sometimes needs to be resected and

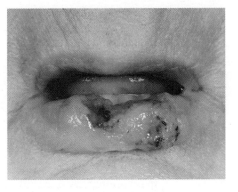

**Figure 16.5** Carcinoma of the lip

reconstructed. A block dissection of the neck is required if and when the lymph nodes become involved (see page 215).

### Ulcers of the tongue
- **Aphthous ulcers** are small, superficial and probably viral. They occur on the tip and lateral border of the tongue and on the inside of the lips, are extremely uncomfortable and usually heal within a week.
- **Syphilis of the tongue** is now extremely rare in Britain but may occur in any of the three stages of the disease. The primary sore is an indolent ulcer near the tip, with induration and enlargement of the submental nodes. The secondary stage produces superficial fissures and ulcers on the sides and back of the tongue (snail track ulcers). The tertiary stage may produce a diffuse gumma with a large painless swelling breaking down to form a typical indolent ulcer in the middle of the dorsum of the tongue.
- **Tuberculous ulcers** are extremely rare in Britain and occur at the tip of the tongue secondary to bacilli coughed up in open disease.

### Leukoplakia
This term is no longer used by facio-maxillary surgeons but is included here because it continues to be heard in other circles.

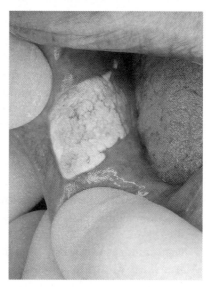

- It literally means white plaques and describes a condition characterized by pale areas of hyperkeratosis overlying hyperplastic or dysplastic squamous epithelium anywhere in the mouth (Figure 16.6).
- It is associated with smoking, intra-oral irritation from irregular teeth, spirits and syphilis.
- The term is misleading since hyperplasia can also appear as **red patches** (**erythroplakia**) and any shade in between. Its importance is that, rarely, it undergoes malignant transformation.
- Once diagnosed, dysplastic areas can be destroyed by diathermy, laser or excision.

**Figure 16.6** White patch (leukoplakia)

### Carcinoma of the tongue and mouth
This is more common in men than women, usually over the age of 50. Predisposing factors are classically, smoking, sepsis, spirits, spices and syphilis; candidal infection is also implicated. **Most tumours are squamous carcinoma and are often multifocal.**

### Signs and symptoms
- Tumour may present as a papilliferous growth but more commonly as an indurated fissure or ulcer on the lateral border of the tongue (Figure 16.7).

- With advanced disease the tongue becomes fixed, impeding speech and swallowing.
- Pain may be a prominent feature with radiation to the ears.
- Later there is involvement of the submental, submandibular and deep cervical lymph nodes.

**Treatment** Following histological confirmation of the disease, if the primary lesion is small and accessible it is widely excised with diathermy and an appropriate reconstruction carried out. Alternatively, implantation or external beam radiotherapy can be used for the primary tumour.

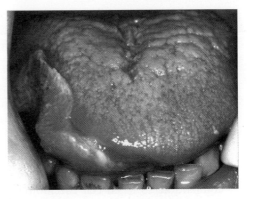

**Figure 16.7** Carcinoma of the tongue

**Radical block dissection is performed for metastatic neck nodes** – this involves removing the sternomastoid muscle, the internal jugular vein, the spinal accessory nerve together with cervical fascia, lymph nodes of the anterior and posterior triangles of the neck and the submandibular salivary gland. When the lymph nodes are involved on both sides of the neck, it is usual to perform a modified block dissection (leaving the internal jugular vein intact) on the less affected side.

## THE JAWS

- **Tooth infection** occurs as a result of dental caries or periodontal disease. Regular oral hygiene and preventative dentistry will avert most infections. When they do occur, radiography of the teeth and jaws is useful in aiding diagnosis. Infected dental cysts may require removal of the offending tooth but can often be treated with apical root surgery.
- **Acute osteomyelitis** of the jaws is rare and almost always due to *Staphylococcus*. In the infant it is associated with spread of infection from the maxillary antrum. In the mandible it is invariably due to blood-borne infection from a primary septic focus elsewhere, or complicates an open fracture.
- **Chronic osteomyelitis** associated with long-standing dental infection is more common.

### Cysts and odontogenic tumours of the jaws

- **Radicular cysts** (Figure 16.8) account for 60% of radiolucent swellings within the jaw. They are usually found around the apices of old infected roots. Treatment is by removal of the tooth or marsupialization.
- **Odontogenic keratocysts** account for 5–10% of all cysts. Following excision there is a very high rate of recurrence due to a thin friable capsule. They can become very large and cause considerable surgical problems.

- **Follicular (dentigerous) cysts** arise from unerupted teeth and produce cystic swellings associated with the crown of the tooth. Treatment is removal of the tooth and its associated cyst.

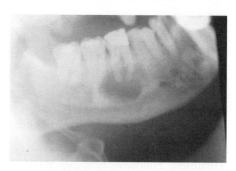

**Figure 16.8** Radicular cyst

- **Ameloblastoma** accounts for 1% of all oral tumours. They are slow growing, locally invasive tumours of odontogenic epithelium and are comparable to basal cell carcinoma of skin. Most patients present between the third and sixth decade and 80% of ameloblastomas occur as uni- or multilocular cystic swellings in the mandible, usually at the angle. Treatment is *en bloc* resection of the involved bone with a margin of healthy bone and reconstruction with a vascularized graft.

### Malignant disease

Primary malignancy (e.g. osteosarcoma) is rare in the jaws. Malignancy is usually due to direct spread from surrounding tissues, most commonly:

- **Carcinoma of the maxillary antrum** (Figure 16.9) invades the upper jaw, producing pain in the face, bloody nasal discharge and diplopia if the orbit is involved. Clinical and radiological examination including CT and MRI scanning reveals the extent of the disease. **It is usually a squamous cell carcinoma although adenocarcinoma and adenocystic carcinoma are encountered.** Treatment is radiotherapy and/or surgery. A reconstruction of the jaw can be carried out by importing the patient's own tissue in the form of a free flap or by replacing the tissue with a prosthesis.

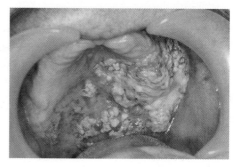

**Figure 16.9** Carcinoma of maxilla

- **Sarcomas** are very malignant and extremely rare. Prognosis is extremely poor but radiotherapy and chemotherapy may be useful as palliation.

### NOSE

#### Epistaxis (nosebleed)

- Occurs at any age and may be due to trauma, foreign body, sepsis, hypertension and bleeding disorders – many have no apparent cause.
- The commonest bleeding point is on the septum near the anterior nares in **Little's area** and usually responds to cautery with silver nitrate although the nose may sometimes need to be packed or tamponaded with a balloon.

- Very rarely, it may be necessary to tie off the ethmoidal, external carotid or maxillary arteries.
- Nasal infection causing epistaxis needs to be treated by antibiotics and occasionally a blood transfusion is necessary.
- The underlying cause for the bleed should always be sought and if possible eradicated.

### Rhinitis

Acute nasal infection is extremely common (common cold). It is aggravated by allergies such as hayfever and chronic allergy leads to hypertrophy of the lining mucosa with polyp formation which in turn leads to reduction in aeration of the nasal sinuses with further polyp production. Treatment is medical in the first instance with decongestants and local steroids.

Chronic disease is treated by removal of the polyps and opening up the airways into the sinuses.

### Nasal obstruction

Apart from obstruction caused by rhinitis and associated polyps, nasal obstruction also occurs due to congenital or acquired (trauma) deviation of the nasal septum. The obstruction is treated either by repositioning the septum correctly (**septoplasty**) or by removing that part of the septal cartilage causing the obstruction from beneath its mucous covering, **submucous resection** (SMR).

## LARYNX

- Tumours of the larynx are best classified as:
  - Supraglottic (including epiglottis)
  - Glottic (vocal cords)
  - Subglottic (cricothyroid region).
- There is usually **hoarseness, the patient is often a smoker** and in time develops dysphagia.
- Fibreoptic nasal endoscopy is used to make the diagnosis and obtain adequate biopsies.
- **Ninety per cent are squamous carcinomas.**
- CT and MRI determine the extent of both the primary lesion and metastatic spread to neck glands.
- Most small laryngeal carcinomas are treated initially with radiotherapy.
- **Recurrent laryngeal tumours require laryngectomy and a permanent tracheostomy.** Post-operatively the patient has to be taught to speak by swallowing and belching air from the oesophagus.

## LESIONS IN THE YOUNG

## NECK

### Tonsils and adenoids

These are part of **Waldeyer's ring** and guard the upper respiratory and digestive tract against ingested pathogens. The tonsil is composed of lymphoid tissue and is particularly liable to infection. Acute tonsillitis is accompanied by a raised temperature, difficulty in swallowing and general malaise. Draining lymph nodes which lie near the angle of the jaw may be enlarged and tender on palpation. The tonsils themselves are bright red and often shows spots of exudate in their crypts. Treatment of the acute infection is with antibiotics.

Occasionally the acute infection progresses to a **peritonsillar abscess (quinsy)** behind the upper pole of the tonsil and causes great difficulty in swallowing. Clinically there is acute pain, severe swelling and toxicity. **The patient often feels that he is choking** due to the accompanying oedema. Treatment is by incision, care being taken not to allow the patient to aspirate the pus which may flood the trachea and later cause a lung abscess. Quinsy is one of the few indications for tonsillectomy but this should be deferred for at least 6 weeks until the acute symptoms have subsided.

### Chronic tonsillitis

This is a rather ill-defined condition that consists of large infected tonsils which frequently undergo attacks of inflammation. The indications for tonsillectomy are repeated attacks of **tonsillitis, quinsy and tonsillar tumour.**

### The adenoids

These consist of a pad of vascular lymphoid tissue on the posterior wall of the nasopharynx surrounding the opening of the Eustachian tube. Swelling can obstruct normal aeration of the middle ear to produce infection and glue ear. Management is removal of the adenoids (usually with tonsillectomy) and re-aeration of the middle ear by a grommet.

### Branchial cyst and fistula

Branchial cysts and fistulae are derived from the embryological **second branchial cleft** which is normally obliterated to leave the tonsillar fossa in life. Remnants of the cleft will produce a cyst, fistula or sinus.

- **A branchial cyst** (Figure 16.10) appears deep to the **upper third** of the sternomastoid muscle and presents as an oval cystic swelling. It often is first noticed when it becomes enlarged following a respiratory tract infection. Enlargement may occur at any age and it can be difficult to distinguish from cervical adenitis. There is a small incidence of cysts developing epidermoid carcinoma. Treatment is by excision as recurrent infection can lead to the formation of a sinus or fistula.

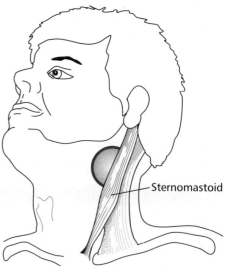

Sternomastoid

**Figure 16.10** Branchial cyst

- **A branchial fistula** (Figure 16.11) presents as a small skin opening at the **lower anterior border** of the sternomastoid which discharges viscous fluid. They are usually present from birth, may be bilateral, and track from the skin to the tonsillar fossa between the carotid arteries, or end blindly as a sinus. The condition is often familial and associated with pre-auricular sinuses. The fistula is excised through small step-ladder incisions in the neck.

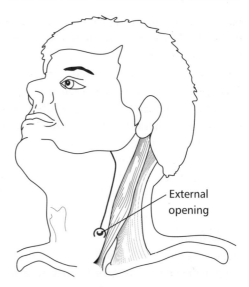

External opening

**Figure 16.11** Branchial fistula

### Dermoids

Dermoids in the face and neck occur as cystic swellings lined by squamous epithelium containing keratin. They occur at lines of junction between developmental blocks of tissue (i.e. **inclusion** dermoids). The commonest are:

- **Periorbital dermoid** (Figure 16.12) – occurs at the upper border of the eye just beneath the extremity of the eyebrow and there is often an underlying pit in the skull. Occasionally a defect in it communicates with an extradural dermoid. Very rarely it communicates with the meninges. Treatment is by excision mainly for cosmetic reasons but also because they tend to enlarge if left.
- **Submental dermoid** – occurs beneath the chin in the midline in or superficial to the mylohyoid raphe. The differential diagnosis includes thyroglossal cyst and lymph node.
- **Sublingual dermoid** – occurs in the midline, beneath the tongue and projects into the floor of the mouth. Differential diagnosis is from a ranula which lies slightly more lateral and is associated with the sublingual gland. Unlike the ranula it does not transilluminate.

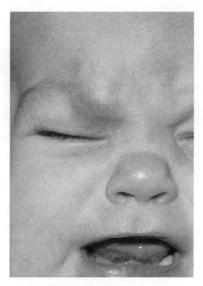

**Figure 16.12** Periorbital dermoid

### Sternomastoid tumour (wry-neck)

This is a solid oval swelling in the lower third of the sternocleidomastoid muscle, usually diagnosed in the second or third week of life. Because it is in the muscle the mass can **only be moved laterally** and not in the line of the muscle fibres. It is presumed to be due to trauma to the muscle or its blood supply. If untreated, fibrous contraction ensues with eventual torticollis. Initial management is under the supervision of the physiotherapist who manipulates the neck to stretch the affected muscle. Treatment can usually be discontinued after a year but occasionally fibrous contraction of the muscle and cervical fascia requires surgical correction by tenotomy or excision.

### Cystic hygroma

This is a form of multilocular lymphangioma presenting as a **brilliantly transilluminable** swelling in the lateral or posterior aspect of the neck in a newborn baby (Figure 16.13). Complete excision is extremely difficult and is indeed not often possible.

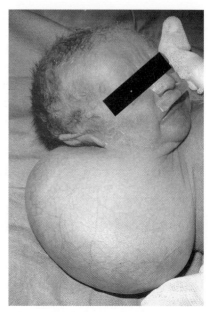

**Figure 16.13** Cystic hygroma

## CERVICAL RIB

- This is a fairly common deformity (0.5%) which consists of an additional rib, usually bilateral, arising from the transverse process of the seventh, or occasionally the sixth cervical vertebra.
- It may be cartilaginous or bony. Sometimes the end continues as a fibrous band attached to the first rib.
- **Symptoms occur due to upward traction on the subclavian artery or lower branches of the brachial plexus.**
- Interference with the arterial supply can be shown by abolition of the radial pulse when the arm is flexed backwards.
- Pressure on the lower branches of the brachial plexus (**C8, T1**) may result in pain and **wasting of the small muscles of the hand.**
- Plain x-ray will show the rib if it is bony.
- Although congenital, symptoms tend to occur in adulthood and treatment is excision of the rib.

## LIPS, TONGUE AND MOUTH

### Cleft lip

**Embryology** The frontonasal process develops into the forehead, nose and filtrum of the upper lip. From each side the two maxillary processes grow inwards to produce the cheeks and the more lateral parts of the upper lip on each side. The paired mandibular processes unite in the midline to form the chin and lower lip.

- Cleft lip – failure of fusion of the frontonasal processes with one of the maxillary processes will give rise to a unilateral cleft lip (Figure 16.14) which is a little more common on the right and more common in males. The incidence is 2–3 per thousand.
- The commonest complication of a cleft lip is a cleft palate. With cleft lip alone the infant is still able to suck and thrive.

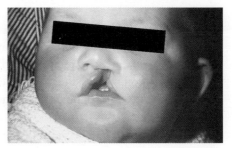

**Figure 16.14** Cleft lip

## Treatment

- Is undertaken around the age of 3 months and classically when the child is 10 lb (4.5 kg), 10 weeks and has a haemoglobin of 10 g/dl.
- Repair of the lip is performed as a functional repair, i.e. the muscles of the lip are repaired in such a manner that muscle activity enhances the normal growth of the face.
- Bilateral clefts of the lip are more difficult to repair.

### Cleft palate

**Embryology** The palate is formed by horizontal processes of the maxilla on each side anteriorly and the palatine bones behind uniting from the front backwards with the cartilage and bone of the nasal septum from above. The uvula and soft palate fuse last.

- Cleft palate – is a serious disability, preventing the baby from suckling properly. To a large extent this can be resolved by using a broad teat on the feeding bottle and by the use of a feeding plate to cover the defect.

## Treatment

- Is a hazard in the neonatal period but palatal repair should be carried out before formal babbling occurs as then there is less problem with normal speech development.
- Mucoperiosteal incisions are made close to the midline and layered repairs involving the nasal mucosa, muscle and oral mucosa of the uvula and soft palate and two-layer closure of the hard palate are carried out. Occasionally a pharyngoplasty may be required at a later date if nasal speech persists.

### Tongue tie

In tongue tie the frenulum beneath the tongue is unduly short, preventing the tongue tip from protruding as far as the lower lip. Tongue tie may be familial and is often blamed for delay in a child learning to speak but is rarely, if ever, the cause for this. Correction is easily carried out in the very young without anaesthesia by cutting the frenum with scissors. Care should be taken to avoid the blood vessels lying lateral to the frenum. In the older child the operation can be uneventfully carried out under local anaesthesia.

### Ranula

A ranula is a translucent cystic swelling which arises on one side of the underside of the tongue and is a mucous retention cyst from the sublingual salivary gland. Definitive treatment is by removal of the cyst and its associated sublingual salivary gland although occasionally marsupialization, that is unroofing of the cyst, may defer the need for definitive treatment.

## THE EAR

Absence of the pinna is very rare and associated with deafness. The **most common abnormality is an accessory auricle** – a small tag of skin enclosing a rod of cartilage situated anterior to the ear. They are often multiple and treatment is by excision.

### Pre-auricular sinus

This is a blind pit situated just anterior to the external auditory meatus. The opening is surrounded by scaly skin and there may be an associated mass of cartilage. The pit frequently becomes infected and never heals. Treatment is excision but as they occasionally extend into deeper tissues care should be taken to prevent **damage to the facial nerve**.

## FACIAL TRAUMA

There is often severe swelling of the face following trauma (Figure 16.15). This can be due to haematoma from lacerations, or bleeding from fractures in the underlying bony skeleton. In addition, the swelling can be increased due to surgical emphysema with air escaping from the nasal sinuses into the lax tissues of the face, especially around the orbits and lower jaw. The nasal bones are most commonly fractured.

**Figure 16.15** Facial trauma

### Middle third fractures of the face

Middle third fractures of the face can occur at three levels, classified as Le Fort I, II and III (Figure 16.16).

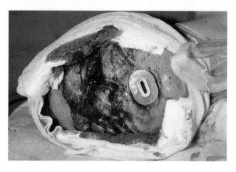

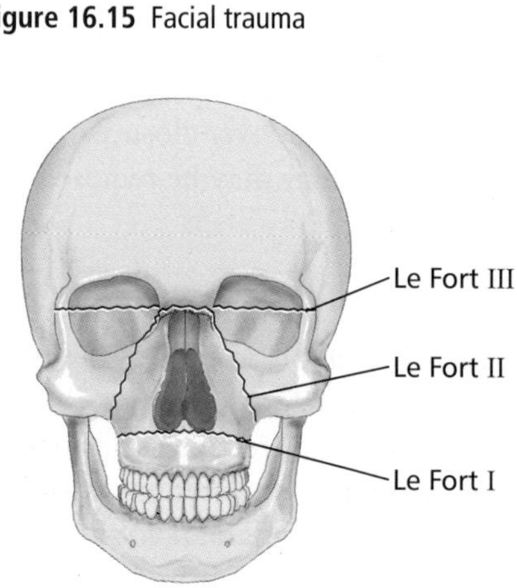

Le Fort III

Le Fort II

Le Fort I

**Figure 16.16** Le Fort's fractures

- **The Le Fort I** is low level and occurs above the palate separating the upper jaw from the rest of the face.
- **The Le Fort II** is pyramidal shaped passing through the lateral wall of the antrum through the anterior orbital rim, across the medial wall of the orbit often involving the cribriform plate and then down again through the opposite medial wall of the orbit, infra-orbital rim and lateral wall of the antrum. Middle third fractures are associated often with a **compromise of the upper airway** as the maxilla moves backwards and downwards, the airway being further compromised by teeth fragments, dentures and blood.
- The high level fracture (**Le Fort III**) occurs at the frontozygomatic suture laterally and the cribriform plate medially.

Any of these fractures can occur bilaterally or unilaterally, singly or in combination with each other. In addition, there may well be a fracture of the zygomatic complex and also the nasal bones.

### Mandibular fractures

Mandibular fractures (Figure 16.17) tend to be much more painful than middle third fractures of the face. This is due to displacement which is caused not only by the initial injury but also by pull from the muscles of mastication around the fracture sites. Within the lower jaw there are sites of potential weakness; these include the condylar neck, the angle of the mandible where there is often an unerupted wisdom tooth and the parasymphyseal region where the long root of the lower canine tooth reduces the amount of bone in this area.

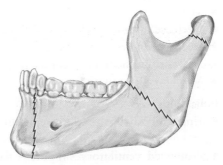

**Figure 16.17** Mandibular fractures

Unlike bone, teeth do not remodel and consequently it is **essential that the occlusion is restored as perfectly as possible** when reduction and fixation of the jaw fracture is carried out.

**Treatment of facial fractures** Fixation of facial fractures can be achieved either directly or indirectly. Direct fixation is achieved with mini plates following repositioning of the displaced bones. Indirect fixation of jaw fractures is achieved by using the teeth of one jaw as a splint against which the teeth of the fractured jaw are placed and wired.

Due to the excellent vasculature in the head and neck osteomyelitis is a rare complication of fractures of the facial skeleton. However, haemorrhage and infection associated with facial fractures can often involve other structures such as the globe of the eye.

## TRACHEOSTOMY

A tracheostomy is a temporary or permanent fistula fashioned between the skin and trachea at the level of the third or fourth cartilaginous rings, through which it is possible to breathe – usually a tracheostomy tube is inserted to maintain patency (Figure 16.18). The most obvious indication **is to relieve upper airway obstruction, or following laryngectomy, but tracheostomy is also used for long-term mechanical ventilation or when control of the airway is needed** (e.g. extensive facio-maxillary surgery; neurological disorders). When the need for a tracheostomy has passed, the fistula will heal spontaneously once the tracheostomy tube is removed. Some benefits of tracheostomy are listed:

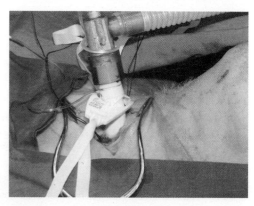

**Figure 16.18** Tracheostomy

- Temporary or permanent relief of upper airway obstruction
- Decrease in dead-space of 30–50%
- Decrease in airway resistance
- Access to bronchial tree for sucking out secretions
- Mechanical ventilation possible whilst eating and drinking normally.

### Indications

- **Upper airway obstruction** – epiglottitis; Ludwig's angina; tumours of the head and neck; facio-maxillary trauma; foreign body
- **Prolonged ventilatory support** – flail chest injury; neuromuscular disorders associated with respiratory muscle paralysis (e.g. Guillain–Barré syndrome); poliomyelitis; acute respiratory distress syndrome
- **Tracheobronchial toilet** – during prolonged recovery from any of the above when on-going nasotracheal or orotracheal intubation is not tolerated.

Tracheostomy is usually undertaken when the less invasive procedure of endotracheal intubation is impossible (laryngectomy), or likely to be prolonged (e.g. in the ITU situation when a patient needs mechanical ventilation over a period of many weeks).

Endotracheal intubation gains rapid access to the upper respiratory tract and is part of the preparation for elective or urgent tracheostomy. Emergency tracheostomy without such preparation is very seldom necessary. In such a situation the operation of **cricothyroidotomy** is easier and safer.

### Cricothyroidotomy

In complete upper airway obstruction when the patient is in imminent danger of death by asphyxiation and endotracheal intubation via mouth or nose is not possible, the easiest access to the trachea is via the cricothyroid membrane. This membrane is easily identified immediately below the thyroid cartilage where it is practically subcutaneous with no vascular structure or thyroid tissue overlying it.

**Procedure** In the unconscious patient no local anaesthetic is required even if it is available (the indications for this procedure seldom arise within the hospital environment). The patient is positioned supine with the neck extended over a towel, rolled up jacket or shoe.

A vertical incision is made through the skin over the cricothyroid membrane and the edges of this wound retracted by the index finger and thumb of one hand either side of the wound. The cricothyroid membrane is then incised transversely to enter the lumen of the trachea. If a small endotracheal tube is available it is inserted. If the operation is being performed in the high street (for example) the barrel of a ball-point pen is a useful substitute.

Once the acute emergency life-threatening situation has been relieved, the patient is transferred to hospital for further treatment such as removal of the impacted boiled sweet from the larynx or formal tracheotomy.

## CRIB BOX – FACE AND NECK

- Face and neck lesions – often **congenital in the young; acquired in the adult**
- **Neck swelling in the adult** – most often lymph nodes (infective or malignant)
- **Other adult swellings** – pharyngeal pouch, thyroglossal cyst, carotid body tumour
- **Parotid tumours** – pleomorphic adenoma, adenolymphoma, carcinoma
- **Carcinoma of lip** – elderly, sun damage, squamous Ca
- **Ca tongue and mouth** – squamous, treat by excision or radiotherapy, radical block dissection for involved neck nodes
- **Ca maxilla** – usually squamous, treat by excision and/or radiotherapy with reconstruction
- **Epistaxis** - Little's area, ? underlying pathology
- **Childhood swellings** – branchial cyst/fistula, cystic hygroma, inclusion dermoids, sternocleidomastoid tumour, cervical rib
- **Cleft lip** – 2–3/1000, repair at 10 weeks; 10 lb; Hb 10
- **Facial trauma** – Le Fort I, II & III
- **Tracheostomy** – learn the indications; learn cricothyroidotomy, you may need it!

# chapter 17

# THE BREAST

Benign breast disease is very common and breast cancer affects 1 in 12 women in developed Western countries. Any breast symptom is likely to be perceived as breast cancer by the patient and causes anxiety and psychological morbidity. **Prompt investigation and diagnosis in a fully equipped 'one-stop' diagnostic breast clinic is the most efficient and kindly way of managing these patients.**

## ANATOMY

The adult female breast (Figure 17.1) is a modified apocrine gland composed of compound tubular glands draining into approximately seven lactiferous sinuses which lie just deep to the nipple. The nipple is surrounded by the areola in which the tubercles of Montgomery (large sebaceous glands) are embedded. The ligaments of Cooper are strands of dense connective tissue radiating from the nipple

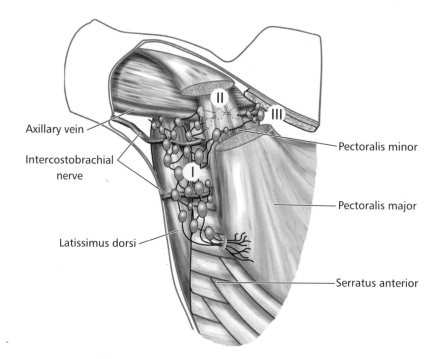

**Figure 17.1** The lymphatic drainage of the breast

and the dermis of the breast to the fascia covering pectoralis major. The glandular parenchyma of the breast lies between these ligaments and is composed of **ducts** and the terminal **lobuloalveolar** units surrounded by fine connective tissue. After the menopause this fine connective tissue is replaced by fat and the glandular parenchyma involutes although a few normal glands may persist into old age.

## HISTORY

- **Lump in the breast** – this requires careful assessment and a decision must be made whether it is benign or malignant. Tender lumps which vary in size with the menstrual cycle are likely to be benign. An **insidious increase in size** unrelated to the cycle may be **a fibroadenoma or a cancer**. Sudden appearance of a lump may be a cyst or a cancer.
- **Discharge from the nipple** – note whether the discharge is from a single duct or from multiple ducts. Note the colour, volume and presence of **blood** in the discharge and whether it stains the clothes.
- **Pain in the breast** – may be cyclical or unrelated to the menstrual cycle. Note the severity of the pain and association of a lump or discharge from the nipple.
- **Risk factors for breast cancer** – note the family history, age at first full term pregnancy, number of children, age at menarche and menopause, oral contraceptive and hormone replacement therapy.

## EXAMINATION AND INVESTIGATIONS

### Inspection
- Inspect the breasts with the patient sitting on the edge of the couch (Figure 17.2a).
- Look for lumps, distortion, asymmetry, skin tethering, fixation, ulceration and nipple retraction.

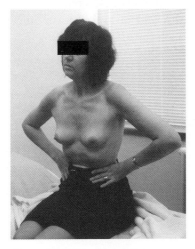 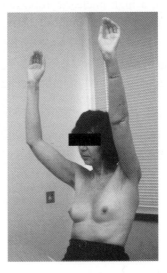

**Figure 17.2** Breast inspection

- Then ask the patient to raise her arms and look for the same abnormalities and again with the hands pressed into the hips (Figure 17.2b).
- These manoeuvres are designed to tense the ligaments of Cooper and cause the appearance of a skin dimple or eccentric retraction of the nipple in the case of breast cancer.

## Palpation

- The breasts are palpated bimanually in the sitting position.
- The axillae and supraclavicular fossae are examined for lymph nodes – noting if they are fixed or mobile.
- The examination is completed with the patient semi-reclined, using the flat of the hand in each quadrant and in the retroareolar area (Figure 17.3).

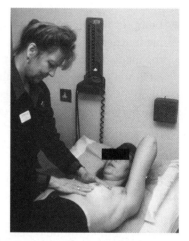

## Fine needle aspiration cytology (FNAC)

If a lump is found, then a 21G needle on a 10 ml syringe is introduced into the lump and aspiration attempted. A cyst will disappear on aspiration. The fluid is discarded unless it is blood-stained; in this case the patient may have an intracystic cancer and the fluid should be sent for cytology. If the lump is solid then it may

**Figure 17.3** Breast palpation

be a cancer, fibroadenoma, fat necrosis or benign lumpiness. The aspirate is smeared onto a slide, air dried or fixed with alcohol, and sent for cytological examination.

## Cytology

The characteristics of **malignancy** are nuclear and cellular **pleomorphism**, obvious **nucleoli**, a **high nuclear:cytoplasmic ratio** and loss of adherence between cells. Cytology cannot distinguish between in-situ and invasive breast cancer. Core biopsy (e.g. Trucut needle) is necessary in such cases.

## Mammography

- Craniocaudal and oblique mediolateral views are taken of each breast (Figure 17.4).
- **10–16% of breast cancers do not show on mammography.**
- The characteristic picture of malignancy is a stellate mass with asymmetry and clustered microcalcification (Figure 17.5).

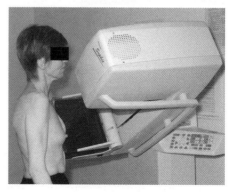

**Figure 17.4** Mammography

### Ultrasound

Ultrasound is used as an adjunct to mammography to improve diagnostic accuracy or as the first line investigation in patients younger than 35 with a discrete lump.

### MRI

MRI may be useful in deciding on responses to drug treatment and for the detection of ductal carcinoma *in situ*.

### Hook-wire localization

Non-palpable suspicious mammographic lesions (typically a small area of microcalcification) can be biopsied or excised by inserting a hooked guidewire into the lesion during mammography (Figure 17.6). The surgeon then excises the wire and surrounding tissue for histology.

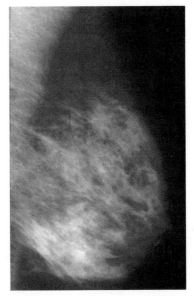

**Figure 17.5** Mammogram

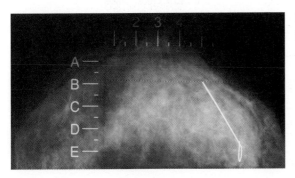

**Figure 17.6** Hook-wire mammogram

## PATHOLOGY

The most common clinical and pathological problems are listed in Table 17.1.

## BENIGN DISEASES

### LUMPINESS OF THE BREAST

This is the commonest condition presenting to general practitioners and the breast clinic. It usually presents as focal **asymmetrical lumpiness in the upper outer quadrant** of the breast which may or may not be tender. It may be difficult to discriminate between lumpiness and a true discrete lump. Lumpiness in the week prior to the menses is common. Pregnancy may present as tender lumpiness. If the lumpi-

**Table 17.1** Common clinical and pathological problems of the breast

|  | Problem |
| --- | --- |
| Whole breast | Gynaecomastia |
|  | Accessory nipple/breast |
|  | Aplasia/hypoplasia of the breast |
| Nipple and areola | Eczema |
|  | Papilloma of the nipple |
|  | Paget's disease of the nipple |
| Lactiferous sinuses and major ducts | Duct ectasia |
|  | Periductal mastitis |
|  | Intraduct papilloma |
| Terminal lobuloalveolar units & small ducts | Pyogenic abscess |
|  | Benign cystic disease |
|  | Epithelial hyperplasia ± atypia |
|  | Ductal carcinoma *in situ* |
|  | Lobular carcinoma *in situ* |
|  | Invasive breast cancer |
| Terminal units & connective tissue | Fibroadenoma |
|  | Phylloides tumour |
| Terminal units & nerves | Cyclical breast pain |
| Chest wall pain radiating to the breast | Tietze syndrome – non-cyclical pain |
| Connective tissue | Fat necrosis |
|  | Lipoma & adenolipoma |

ness resolves after one or two menstrual cycles then the woman can be reassured and discharged. Persistent focal lumpiness should be investigated. Histology of the breast tissue in these cases may show no abnormality, multiple small cysts, hyperplasia of the ductal epithelium with or without cell atypia, radial scars, diffuse cellular infiltrates, e.g. lymphocytes, and ductal or lobular carcinoma *in situ*. **Synonyms are benign fibrocystic disease, chronic mastitis and mastopathy.**

## GYNAECOMASTIA

This is a general enlargement of the breast in females prior to development of the true breast or in males at any time (Figure 17.7). It may be unilateral or bilateral. The cause is **excessive oestrogen or prolactin stimulation:**

- Increased oestrogen levels occur just after birth and at puberty.
- Increased oestrogen production may occur in germ cell tumours or other ectopic hormone producing tumours, e.g. **testicular and lung cancers.**

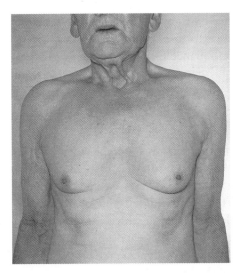

Figure 17.7 Gynaecomastia

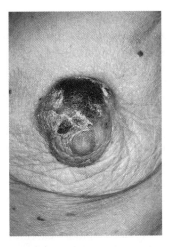

Figure 17.8 Paget's disease of the nipple

- Hyperprolactinaemia occurs with pituitary tumours, thiazides, tricyclics, phenothiazines and cimetidine.
- Lack of oestrogen catabolism occurs in **liver disease,** e.g. alcoholic cirrhosis.
- About 20% of cases are idiopathic and will usually resolve spontaneously.

Surgery is indicated if the condition is painful or results in embarrassment.

### ECZEMA OF THE NIPPLE

This is a contact dermatitis and is treated with steroid cream and avoidance of the allergen. It is important to distinguish this from **Paget's disease of the nipple (Figure 17.8) which is caused by malignant spread of breast cancer.** Biopsy under local anaesthetic may be necessary to make a diagnosis.

### PERIDUCTAL MASTITIS

This is a general term for inflammatory diseases of the major ducts. The cause of this inflammatory disease is unknown. The ducts adjacent to the nipple become dilated (**duct ectasia**) and surrounded by inflammatory cells (**plasma cell mastitis and granulomatous mastitis**). In most cases the only symptom is a bothersome clear, brown, or green nipple discharge from multiple ducts. This can be cured by subareolar excision of the major ducts. A single duct may rupture resulting in a periareolar abscess – if this abscess ruptures through the skin or is incised then a **mammillary fistula** ensues. The fistula does not usually close spontaneously (because of distal duct obstruction and/or disease in the tract) and requires excision.

### PYOGENIC ABSCESS

This is usually due to *Staphylococcus* and **most often occurs during lactation and breast-feeding**. Initially there is a cellulitis presenting as pain and erythema of the overlying skin – antibiotics given at this stage may abort the infection. Numerous micro-abscesses then develop which coalesce to form a multiloculated abscess. The abscess may be aspirated to allow continuance of breast-feeding or incised and drained under general anaesthetic.

## BENIGN CYSTIC DISEASE

This commonly occurs in the **5–10 years prior to the menopause**. It is probably due to sequestration of ductal epithelium from the main system, resulting in isolated segments which continue to produce fluid that results in a cyst. Cysts do not need excision and can be treated by simple aspiration. They are commonly multiple, but are only palpable when the cyst is tense with fluid. Cytological examination of the fluid is only necessary if it is blood-stained in which case it may be a rare intracystic papillary carcinoma. The majority of patients should have mammography and ultrasound after aspiration of the cyst. **Benign cystic disease is the main differential diagnosis for carcinoma of the breast.**

## INTRADUCT PAPILLOMA

This is a benign proliferation of the epithelium of the major ducts. It presents as a straw coloured or **bloody nipple discharge from a single duct** (Figure 17.9). Ductal carcinoma *in situ* is the main differential diagnosis. Occasionally there may be a small palpable lump adjacent to the nipple and often pressure on a certain small segment of the breast or areolar margin will produce a droplet of blood at the nipple. Ultrasound may identify the lesion within the duct which is subsequently excised by microdochectomy.

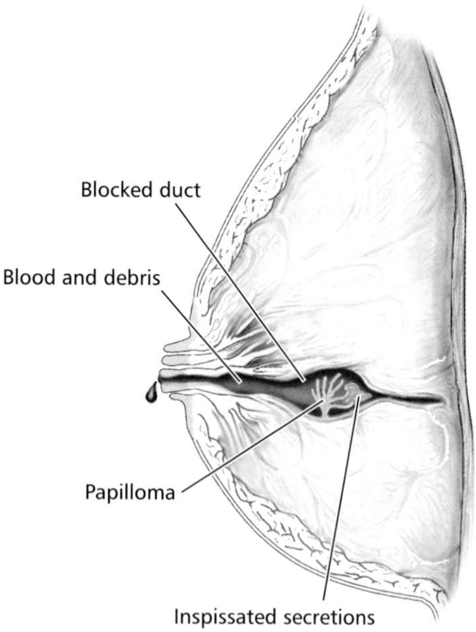

Blocked duct

Blood and debris

Papilloma

Inspissated secretions

**Figure 17.9** Intraduct papilloma

## FIBROADENOMA

This is a benign tumour of the breast commonly presenting between the ages of **15 and 35 years**. The lesion grows from the connective tissue and epithelium of the terminal lobuloalveolar unit. The clinical presentation is typically a young woman with a 2–4 cm smooth, rounded, discrete breast lump which is very mobile when palpated (**a breast mouse**). The diagnosis should be confirmed by ultrasound and aspiration cytology. The patient should be given the choice of excision. Some surgeons avoid excision if the diagnosis can be made reliably. In patients aged 25–40 fibroadenoma is the main differential diagnosis for carcinoma of the breast. **Giant or juvenile fibroadenoma** is a rare massive growth of a fibroadenoma, usually occurring close to the menarche.

## PHYLLOIDES (FERN-LIKE) TUMOUR

This is a rare fibroepithelial tumour of the breast named for its leaf-like microscopical appearance. It is not a sarcoma but is liable to local recurrence if inadequately excised. Mastectomy may be necessary in large tumours of the infiltrating type. The histology may be difficult to differentiate from a true sarcoma of the breast.

## BREAST CANCER

### Incidence
- There are **24 000 new cases** and **14 000 deaths** from breast cancer in England and Wales per year, representing 5% of all deaths in females.
- **One in 12 women will develop breast cancer in their lifetime.**
- Although the cause is unknown, differing incidence rates in various countries suggest behavioural and/or environmental factors are important (e.g. Japan has a low incidence).
- **Male breast cancer is 0.8%** of all breast cancers and is managed in the same way as female breast cancer.

### Clinical signs of breast cancer
Breast cancer may have no clinical signs and be detected only on mammogaphy. Conversely, patients may present at a late stage with a fungating growth ulcerating through the skin and fixed to the chest wall; or with symptoms caused by distant metastases. Local signs in the breast include:
- **Lump** – visible; palpable; indiscrete edges; hard; irregular
- **Skin tethering** – dimpling (Figure 17.10) due to muscle or skin fixity
- **Nipple inversion** (Figure 17.10) or bloody discharge
- **Paget's disease of nipple** – caused by infiltration of malignant cells
- **Deformity** – enlargement; asymmetry of breasts or nipples
- *Peau d'orange* – skin oedema resembling an orange due to lymph blockage
- **Inflammation** – rare; usually lactational; 'mastitis carcinomatosa'
- **Ulceration** (Figure 17.11) – late stage; often elderly recluse
- **Lymph glands** – axillary and/or supraclavicular; mobile or fixed.

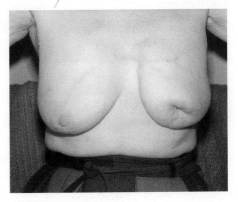

**Figure 17.10** Nipple retraction

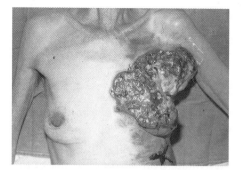

**Figure 17.11** Ulcerating breast

**Risk factors for breast cancer**

**Increasing age** – increased risk

**Genetics**

- BRCA1&2 – 70% develop breast cancer
- Li-Fraumeni (P53) – increased risk

**Family history**

- Post-menopausal 1st degree relative – × (1.8–2.0)
- Premenopausal 1st degree relative – × (4.0–7.0)

**Previous breast cancer** – 0.5–1%/year will develop contralateral BC

**Benign breast disease** – atypical hyperplasia, 20% develop BC in 20 years

**Menstrual history & pregnancy**

- Early menarche <12 – × 1.4
- Late menopause >55 – × 1.4
- First full pregnancy <20 – × 0.5

**Oral contraceptives & HRT** – early use for more than 5 years × 1.4

**Environment**

- High alcohol intake & radiation – increased risk
- Diet effect – uncertain

## The staging of breast cancer

- **Clinical staging** governs decisions concerning the treatment of invasive breast cancer. Clinical staging also provides information on the prognosis. It relies on clinical examination of the patient and simple tests to detect distant metastases (e.g. chest x-ray, haematology, liver function).
- **Pathological staging** after excision of the primary tumour and the axillary lymph nodes is more accurate in predicting prognosis and provides a rational

basis for subsequent treatment after surgery for early breast cancer. For example, if more than four axillary nodes have metastases, aggressive chemotherapy may be indicated.

**The staging (Table 17.2) and TNM (tumour, node, metastasis) (Table 17.3) classifications are used universally to enable accurate recording and communication, and to plan appropriate treatment.**

By convention, **early** breast cancer is defined as **stage 1 or 2**, or up to and including **T2 N1 M0**. The term 'early' is based on the historical precept that breast cancer spreads first to the local lymph glands and thereafter to distant sites. In such circumstances and when technically possible, surgery to excise completely the primary tumour and involved lymph nodes should be curative: experience proves that this is not necessarily correct (see Natural history).

**Table 17.2** Staging classification for breast cancer

| Stage 1 | Early | A cancer of any size confined to the breast |
|---|---|---|
| Stage 2 | Early | Stage 1 + mobile palpable nodes |
| Stage 3 | Locally advanced | Stage 2 ± fixed axillary nodes<br>± skin fixation or to underlying muscle<br>± supraclavicular nodes<br>± fixation to chest wall |
| Stage 4 | Advanced | + distant metastases |

**Table 17.3** TNM classification for breast cancer

| **Primary tumour** | Greatest diameter |
|---|---|
| T0 | None demonstrable |
| T1 | <2 cm |
| T2 | 2–5 cm |
| T3 | >5 cm |
| T4 | Any size + involvement of chest wall and/or skin |
| **Axillary nodes** | |
| N0 | None palpable |
| N1 | Mobile palpable nodes |
| N2 | Fixed nodes |
| N3 | + supraclavicular nodes and/or arm oedema |
| **Distant metastases** | |
| M0 | Undetectable |
| M1 | Distant metastases |

## Natural history

> The present treatment of breast cancer is based on the hypothesis that the primary carcinoma can metastasize at any time to form distant micrometastases which grow and later present as recurrent disease. Metastasis occurs coincidentally to the regional nodes and **the number of involved axillary nodes is a reflection of the likelihood of systemic metastases**. Thus local therapy (surgery, radiotherapy) provides control of the primary tumour, but the patient also requires some form of adjuvant systemic therapy (endocrine and/or cytotoxic chemotherapy) to destroy the putative micrometastases.

## Treatment

The treatment options for breast cancer (as in all cancers) are **surgery, radiotherapy and drugs**, or a combination of all three.

### Ductal carcinoma *in situ*

- When ductal carcinoma has not invaded through the basement membrane of the duct then it is known as ductal carcinoma *in situ* (DCIS).
- This condition is often diagnosed on mammography as an area of microcalcification.
- If the tumour is impalpable then localization biopsy or stereotactic guided needle biopsy is required to distinguish benign and malignant causes of calcification. Mastectomy cures the patient in 96% of cases.
- Local excision and radiotherapy prevents recurrence in 93% at 5 years.
- The correct treatment is uncertain and currently the subject of trials.

### Lobular carcinoma *in situ*

- This is a rare condition.
- About 17% of patients will develop invasive breast cancer 15 years after biopsy.
- The correct treatment is uncertain.

## INVASIVE BREAST CANCER

### Early breast cancer

#### Surgery

- Breast conserving surgery (lumpectomy, Figure 17.12, quadrantectomy) is the treatment of choice for the majority of women presenting with stage 1 and 2 breast cancer.
- Mastectomy (Figure 17.13) is reserved for patients with multiple primary breast cancers, large tumours in relatively small breasts, diffuse microcalcification and factors which indicate a high probability of local recurrence (incomplete excision, extensive intraduct cancer, lymphovascular permeation and age <39).
- **Patients undergoing mastectomy should be offered reconstruction of the breast** by latissimus dorsi flap or transverse rectus abdominis (TRAM) flap.

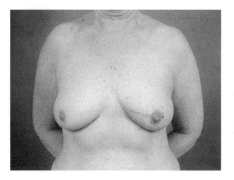

**Figure 17.12** Lumpectomy

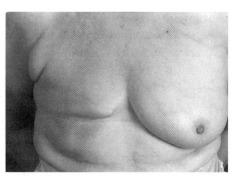

**Figure 17.13** Mastectomy

- The axillary nodes are either sampled or cleared up to the inferior border of the axillary vein (level 1) or beyond (level 2 and 3). This serves to rid the axilla of tumour and provide accurate pathological staging of the axillary nodes.

### Radiotherapy (DXT)

- Radiotherapy to the chest wall after mastectomy or to the breast after breast conserving surgery reduces the risk of local recurrence by 50%.
- It is not thought to affect prognosis.
- A dose of 50–55 Gy of supravoltage therapy is given over a period of 5 weeks (1.8–2 Gy/fraction). Boost doses may be added to the tumour bed at a dose of 10—15 Gy by electron or photon beam or iridium-192 wires.
- About 60% of patients suffer lethargy, skin reactions, nausea and/or sore throat during radiotherapy.
- Lymphoedema of the breast and/or radiation mastitis occurs in about 8% of patients.
- Radiation pneumonitis occurs in 5–10% of cases.

### Adjuvant systemic therapy

- Systemic therapy should be given to the majority of patients with early breast cancer.
- The selection of a specific adjuvant therapy depends on the prognosis for the patient, with regard to both local recurrence and survival.
  - Tamoxifen (20 mg/day for 2 years or more) is an anti-oestrogen which reduces the risk of recurrence by 25% and **improves survival** by 17% in post-menopausal women. It is also effective in premenopausal women. The side-effects include hot flushes and other menopausal symptoms.
  - Cytotoxic chemotherapy produces similar reductions in the risk of recurrence and death in premenopausal women. The side-effects depend on the drugs, but include exhaustion, nausea, vomiting, bone marrow suppression and hair loss. CMF (cyclophosphamide, methotrexate and 5-fluorouracil) given once per month for six cycles is a typical regimen.
  - Ovarian ablation in premenopausal women also reduces the risk of recurrence and death. Ovarian ablation may have adverse effects on bone mineralization, protection against coronary artery disease and libido.

**Prognosis and survival** Pathological staging using the maximum diameter of the tumour, the grade of the tumour and the number of lymph nodes (Figure 17.14) containing metastases provides an estimate of the prognosis. On balance, around 80% of stage 1 and 50% of stage 2 patients are alive at 5 years.

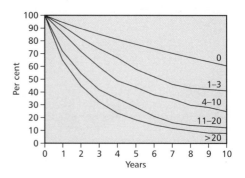

**Figure 17.14** Survival by number of involved nodes

**Elderly women** Women over the age of 70 or who are unfit for surgery may be offered tamoxifen therapy as initial treatment. About 60% will respond and avoid surgery and/or radiotherapy.

**Psychological support and counselling** About 25% of women will have significant depression and anxiety 1 year after treatment for breast cancer. In extreme cases there may be disintegration of relationships with family and friends. Preoperative counselling and support in the post-treatment period is essential in reducing this morbidity.

### Late breast cancer

### Locally advanced breast cancer
- Patients presenting with stage 3 breast cancer are not suitable for primary surgery.
- These cases are treated with cytotoxic chemotherapy and/or endocrine therapy.
- Surgery and/or radiotherapy are reserved for cases that have a good response to this initial treatment, or if the tumour becomes massive, or for bleeding ulceration (toilet mastectomy).

### Metastatic breast cancer
- Patients may present with the symptoms of metastatic disease or develop metastases (stage 4) some time after the treatment of early breast cancer.
- Local recurrence in the residual breast or in the scar of a previous mastectomy or in the regional lymph nodes is often the first sign of systemic metastases.
- Investigations are full blood count, urea and electrolytes, serum calcium, liver ultrasound, chest x-ray and bone scan. MRI scans are useful for the diagnosis of bone metastases.

The majority of patients are treated with systemic therapy and specific symptoms are also treated (Table 17.4).

**Sites of metastatic disease: effects and treatment** These are displayed in Table 17.5.

## Screening for breast cancer

The NHS mammographic breast screening programme for women aged 50–65 began in 1988. Screening gives a potential reduction of 30% in death from breast cancer in women over 50. Benefit for younger women remains uncertain.

**Table 17.4** Systemic therapy for metastatic disease

| | | |
|---|---|---|
| Antimetabolites | 5-Fluorouracil<br>Methotrexate | |
| Alkylating agents | Cyclophosphamide<br>Melphalan | |
| Cytotoxic antibiotics | Adriamycin<br>Mitomycin C | |
| Plant products | Vincristine<br>Vinblastine<br>Taxanes | |
| Endocrine therapy | Drugs<br>  Anti-oestrogens<br>  Aromatase inhibitors<br>  LHRH agonists<br>  Progestins<br>  Tamoxifen<br>  Aminoglutethimide<br>  Zoladex®<br>  Methylprogesterone | Ablative<br>  Oophorectomy by surgery or DXT |

**Table 17.5** Sites, effects and treatment of metastatic disease

| Site | Effects | Treatment |
|---|---|---|
| Bone | Pain<br>Hypercalcaemia<br>Pathological fracture<br>Spinal cord compression | Analgesics + DXT<br>Diuresis/biphosphonates<br>Orthopaedic fixation + DXT<br>Laminectomy + DXT |
| Bone marrow | Anaemia | Transfusion |
| Lungs | Pleural effusion | Intrapleural drainage |
| Pericardium | Effusion | Ultrasound aspiration |
| Liver | Bile duct obstruction<br>Ascites | Biliary stent<br>Diuretics |
| Brain | Focal signs | Corticosteroids + DXT |

**CRIB BOX – THE BREAST**

**Breast disease** – very common; best assessed in dedicated one-stop breast clinics

**Breast lump** – can be diffuse/discrete; benign/malignant; solid/cystic

**History**

- Lump – slow/rapid onset; varies/fixed in size; tender/painless
- Discharge – single/multiple ducts; bloody/other colour
- Pain – cyclical is breast; non-cyclical probably musculoskeletal
- Risk factors for cancer

**Examination**

- Observation – lump; distortion; asymmetry; tethering; nipple retraction
- Palpation – diffuse/discrete lump; mobile/fixed; feel the nodes!

**Investigations** – FNAC; Trucut biopsy; mammography; ultrasound; MRI; hook-wire biopsy

**Breast cancer** – 1 in 12 women

- Remember the risk factors
- Learn the Staging and TNM classifications
- Appreciate the difference between clinical and pathological staging

**Breast cancer treatment** – surgery and/or radiotherapy and/or drugs

- Early – stage 1 and 2, i.e. primary and nodes amenable to surgery
- Late – stage 3, locally advanced; stage 4, metastases. Treat both systemically

# chapter 18

# THORACIC SURGERY

## THE PLEURA

The pleura is a continuous membrane which lines the walls of the thoracic cavity including the rib cage, mediastinum and diaphragm (parietal pleura) and is then reflected at the root of the lung to cover the lung (visceral pleura). The potential space between the parietal and visceral parts of the pleural membrane contains a film of fluid to allow the two layers of pleura to move over each other without friction during respiration.

In abnormal circumstances this potential space becomes a real space when the two layers of pleura become separated by collections of:

- **Air** – pneumothorax
- **Blood** – haemothorax
- **Exudate or Transuclate** – pleural effusion
- **Pus** – empyema thoracis
- **Lymph** – chylothorax.

## PNEUMOTHORAX

A pneumothorax follows the entry of air into the pleural space through a rupture of the lung surface, oesophageal wall or open chest wall injury. Such defects may be either spontaneous or traumatic:

- **Spontaneous** – rupture of congenital lung bullae;
  - rupture of acquired emphysematous bullae.
- **Traumatic** – rib fracture;
  - penetrating injury of chest wall;
  - iatrogenic (pleural aspiration, central venous line insertion, dilatation of oesophageal stricture).

**Tension pneumothorax** (Figure 18.1) is a complication of any pneumothorax when the site of the air leak allows more air to enter the pleural space than can escape. A high positive pressure is thus built up in the pneumothorax, forcing the mediastinum into the opposite side of the chest and compressing the normal and only functioning lung. This situation is an **emergency** requiring **urgent treatment**.

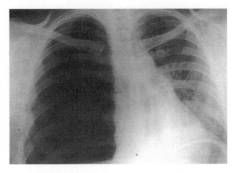

**Figure 18.1** Tension pneumothorax with shift of mediastinum

### Diagnosis of pneumothorax

There may be a history of trauma or emphysematous chest disease. Chest pain and/or dyspnoea are typical presenting symptoms. Dyspnoea at rest is caused by:

- Large pneumothorax
- Degenerative lung disease
- Tension pneumothorax
- Bilateral pneumothoraces
- Absence or non-function of the contralateral lung.

Examination of the affected side reveals a **hyper-resonant percussion note** and greatly **diminished breath sounds. Chest x-ray** shows the collapsed lung with mediastinal shift if there is tension. In **haemopneumothorax** the percussion note will be hyper-resonant above and stony dull beneath the fluid level of blood.

### Treatment of pneumothorax

An uncomplicated pneumothorax which is not making the patient dyspnoeic at rest may be expected to resolve spontaneously and no active treatment is indicated.

- **If the patient is dyspnoeic then active drainage of air from the pleural space is indicated.** This can be done by inserting a fine intravenous cannula into the chest through the second intercostal space in the mid-clavicular line; aspiration using a large syringe and three-way tap will remove intrapleural air and allow the lung to re-expand (Figure 18.2).
- **Persistent leaks require more continuous drainage using an underwater-seal intercostal chest drain.** The ideal site to place an intercostal tube to drain air from the pleural cavity is in the mid-axillary line at the level of the sternal angle. In the axilla this point will be in the 4th or 5th intercostal space (Figure 18.3).

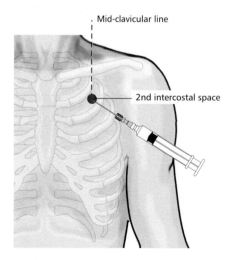

**Figure 18.2** Aspiration of pneumothorax

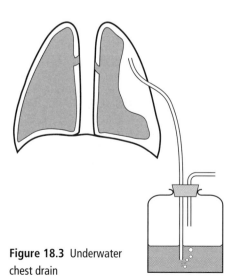

**Figure 18.3** Underwater chest drain

## Complications of pneumothorax

- **Persisting air leak** – if the defect in the lung producing the pneumothorax fails to heal spontaneously after 8–10 days, then further definitive action to close it is indicated. This may be achieved by producing a chemical pleuritis (with talc or tetracycline) and encouraging the parietal and visceral pleurae at the site of leakage to adhere to each other (**pleurodesis**). While the sticking process is taking place the two surfaces must be kept in contact and therefore all air must be continually removed from the pleural space via an intercostal apical drain with suction. If this procedure fails, open thoracotomy will be required to deal with the leak.

- **Recurrent spontaneous pneumothorax** – this is treated as a persisting air leak but if thoracotomy is eventually required, the parietal pleura may be stripped from the inner aspect of the rib cage (**parietal pleurectomy**), producing dense adhesion between the lung surface and chest wall. The pleural space is thus largely obliterated and further pneumothorax is impossible.

- **Chronic pneumothorax** – this is the result of an untreated pneumothorax which has not resolved spontaneously and a fibrous cortex has formed over the surface of the collapsed lung. Once this situation is established, thoracotomy and decortication of the lung is indicated.

- **Surgical emphysema** – occasionally air from a pneumothorax will enter the subcutaneous tissues, gaining access along the track of a fractured rib or a chest drain. The skin swells with subcutaneous emphysema which is felt as a distinctive crackling beneath the fingers. Extensive surgical emphysema can produce an alarming 'Michelin man' appearance. The air is eventually absorbed without special treatment.

> **Complications of pneumothorax**
>
> - Persisting leak
> - Recurrence
> - Chronicity
> - Surgical emphysema

## HAEMOTHORAX

Bleeding into the pleural space may be caused by:

- Chest trauma
- Leaking fusiform or dissecting aneurysm of the thoracic aorta
- Coagulation abnormalities.

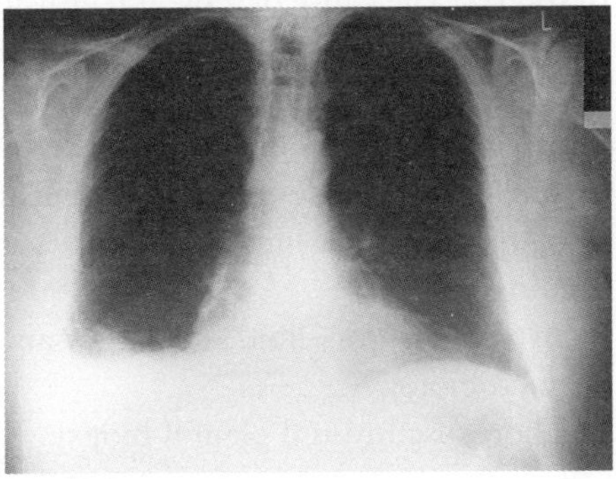

### Diagnosis of haemothorax

A history of trauma or chest pain with shock is usually obvious. Examination reveals:

**Figure 18.4** Erect chest radiograph of a haemothorax, showing blunting of the costophrenic angle

- Diminished movement of chest wall on affected side
- Stony dull percussion note and absent breath sounds
- Erect chest x-ray (Figure 18.4) shows dense opacification on the affected side
- Pleural aspiration produces blood.

### Treatment of haemothorax

Blood in the pleural space may or may not clot as the movements of the lung and chest wall will defibrinate the blood to varying degrees. Whether it clots or not, blood should be removed from the chest as:

- It is a pleural irritant and causes pain
- It impairs the function of the underlying lung
- It may form a fibrinous and later fibrous cortex over the lung, restricting its function.

Blood (or other fluid) in the pleural space will gravitate to the lowest part of the chest; in a patient nursed supine in bed this will be in the gutter formed by the posterior angle of the ribs. Blood can be removed by aspiration using a syringe and cannula inserted into this area. In practice the point of insertion is in the posterior axillary line at the level of the nipple.

Should the haemothorax recur, then it must be assumed that bleeding is continuing and an intercostal tube drain should be inserted. This should be at the same site as for aspiration. Continuous blood loss via the drain is an indication for exploratory thoracotomy.

## PLEURAL EFFUSION

The accumulation of fluid within the pleural space may be associated with:

- **Heart failure** or hypoproteinaemic diseases such as the **nephrotic syndrome** or **cirrhosis** of the liver when the fluid is a **transudate** and low in protein.
- **Pleural inflammation, pulmonary infarction** and primary or secondary **malignant tumour** when the fluid is an **exudate** and rich in protein.

### Diagnosis of pleural effusion

The clinical signs are as in haemothorax. Large effusions (Figure 18.5) will cause dyspnoea. The cause of a pleural effusion should be established. If it is not clearly associated with another condition such as heart failure or a hypoproteinaemic state, it becomes of paramount importance to determine whether the effusion is due to **inflammatory** or **neoplastic** disease. The clinical history and physical examination may provide the answer, but if not, then further investigations are required:

- Aspiration for fluid cytology and microbiology
- Thoracoscopy and pleural biopsy.

**Thoracoscopy** is performed with full operating theatre facilities under general anaesthesia and tracheal intubation. A cannula is introduced via an intercostal space into the fluid-filled part of the pleural space and the effusion withdrawn by suction. Air is

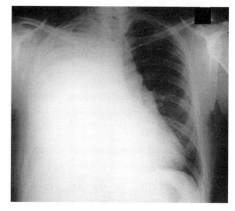

**Figure 18.5** Chest x-ray of effusion

allowed to enter the pleural space through the cannula to replace the effusion. An illuminating telescope with biopsy forceps is passed through the cannula into what is now a pneumothorax and the pleural surfaces inspected. Suspicious areas are then biopsied under direct vision. The lung is then re-inflated by positive pressure via the endotracheal tube and the cannula withdrawn.

---

**IMPORTANT LESSON**
It is only safe to completely remove a large effusion in one procedure if the lung can be re-inflated immediately by positive pressure ventilation. Under any other circumstances complete aspiration will result in a sudden shift of the mediastinum as the lung will not immediately re-expand spontaneously to fill the space previously filled by the effusion. This shift may induce sudden circulatory collapse.

---

### Management of pleural effusion

Effusions due to heart failure, inflammatory or hypoproteinaemic disease will not recur after successful treatment of the cause. Aspiration, if required to relieve dyspnoea, should be performed as for haemothorax.

Persistent effusions due to malignant pleural tumours present a difficult problem. Some secondary tumour deposits may be controlled by systemic endocrine or chemotherapy but mostly they cannot. The dyspnoea produced by a large malignant effusion may be palliated by aspiration in the early stage as the lung will re-expand and ventilate with the movements of the chest wall and diaphragm.

As the disease progresses, however, the two layers of pleura become so thickened by tumour and fibrosis that neither can the lung re-expand nor the chest wall and diaphragm move to ventilate it. When this stage is reached the actual presence of the effusion is irrelevant and its removal makes no difference to the dyspnoea.

## EMPYEMA THORACIS

An empyema is a collection of pus in the pleural space and is the result of an effusion which has become infected by bacteria from an underlying pulmonary infection. The pus becomes localized by a fibrinous and later fibrous cortex and is thus sequestrated from the rest of the pleural space. As most patients in the process of developing an empyema are nursed in or choose to adopt a semi-sitting up position, the effusion gravitates to the **posterior and lowest part of the pleural space** and so that is where the empyema localizes.

### Diagnosis of empyema

The clinical history is of a respiratory infection which persists despite appropriate antibiotic treatment. The clinical signs are of a pyrexial patient with a pleural effusion. Investigations include a chest x-ray, ultrasound scan and microscopy and culture of the pleural aspirate.

### Treatment of empyema

- Systemic antibiotic therapy and repeated aspiration of the infected effusion may be successful in eradicating the infection and minimalizing the effusion to extinction. If such conservative measures fail, **a chronic pyothorax or empyema is established.**
- When this stage is reached the empyema space must be drained continuously at its lowest point found by ultrasonography. An intercostal tube drain keeps the space empty until the overlying lung re-expands to obliterate the empyema.
- If this treatment fails after 2 weeks and an infected space persists, then long-term drainage of the empyema becomes necessary. This is accomplished by resecting a section of rib over the lowest point of the space, placing a catheter into the space and draining it into a stoma bag stuck to the patient's chest. There is no need to connect the catheter to an underwater-seal drainage bottle as the empyema space does not communicate with the rest of the pleural space. Resection of the portion of rib facilitates easy replacement of the tube, should it become dislodged. The tube remains in place until the space is obliterated as shown by x-ray contrast studies obtained via the catheter.
- Should the space still fail to close, the only alternative to continued tube drainage is **decortication of the lung**. This entails a thoracotomy at which the empyema wall is peeled off the lung, chest wall and diaphragm, thus allowing the lung to expand into and close the space.

## CHEST INJURIES

Chest injuries are usefully classified as either **blunt** (including deceleration) or **penetrating**. Any chest trauma is likely to compromise breathing and may be associated with injury to the lungs, heart, great vessels or abdominal viscera. In the initial assessment of a patient who has sustained an injury to the chest it is of primary importance to establish:

- Whether or not **spontaneous respiration** can be maintained
- The degree of **hypotension and/or hypovolaemia** and its cause
- The presence of **other injuries.**

### BLUNT TRAUMA

#### Rib fracture

Fracture of one or several ribs of only one side will only interfere with respiration due to the pain of the fracture. The diagnosis is suspected if crepitus is felt at the site of pain and confirmed by x-ray.

Treatment is aimed at **relieving pain until the fracture unites.**

Complications of rib fracture  A simple rib fracture may be complicated by injury to an adjacent structure either above or below the diaphragm. A displaced fracture of any but the twelfth rib is certain to breach the parietal pleura.

*Haemothorax* This may ensue from bleeding from the fracture site or torn intercostal vessels. The x-ray appearance will depend on whether the film was taken with the patient supine or erect (Figures 18.6, 18.7). It is easy to forget that the film is of a horizontal patient when looking at a vertical film on a viewing box.

*Pneumothorax* A sharp fractured bone end often lacerates the adjacent lung to produce a pneumothorax or haemopneumothorax. If blood (fluid) and air (gas) are present in the pleural space, then a fluid level will be seen at the fluid/gas interface on the postero-anterior x-ray of the vertical patient (Figure 18.8) or the lateral film of the horizontal patient.

*Visceral injury* Fractures of the lower four ribs may be associated with injuries to the upper abdominal viscera, i.e. spleen, liver and kidneys.

*Flail segment* This occurs when a section of the rib cage becomes detached from the wall of the thorax and moves paradoxically in respiration. This 'flail' segment will be produced by:

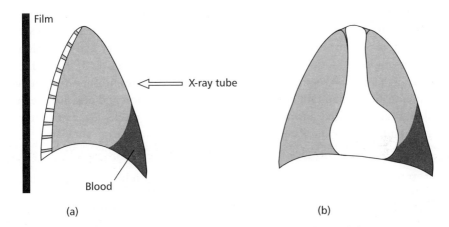

**Figure 18.6** (a) and (b) The appearance of a haemothorax on x-ray taken with the patient erect

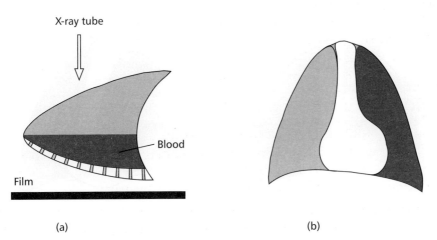

**Figure 18.7** (a) and (b) The appearance of a haemothorax on x-ray taken with the patient horizontal

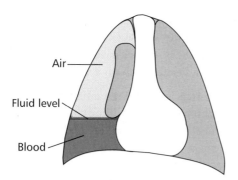

**Figure 18.8** X-ray appearance of haemopneumothorax taken with patient vertical

- Double fractures of a number of adjacent ribs of one hemithorax – this injury is produced by a lateral blow and is often associated with a fracture in the shoulder;
- Multiple bilateral fractures of ribs in the anterior chest wall. As the anterior ends of the ribs and costal cartilages do not show well on x-ray, a radiological diagnosis may not be possible and so the diagnosis is a clinical one.

A flail segment moves inwards with inspiration (paradoxical movement). This reduces the tidal volume and may compromise respiration to a certain extent. Respiration is compromised to a much greater degree by **injury and contusion of the underlying lung,** and impaired breathing due to pain (**Figures 18.9, 18.10**).

Treatment of a flail segment depends on the degree of respiratory dysfunction. **If a patient cannot maintain normal blood gases, intubation and positive pressure ventilation are required and may need to continue for weeks, i.e. until the ribs heal, the flail segment stabilizes, and the lung injury resolves.**

### Deceleration trauma

Blunt trauma associated with rapid deceleration produces two recognized injuries:

**1. Transection of the thoracic aorta** (see also Chapter 19). This occurs just distal to the left subclavian artery and the patient will only reach the hospital if the

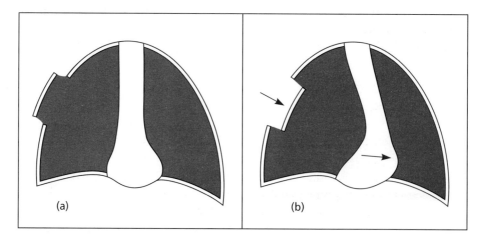

**Figure 18.9** Lateral flail segment: (a) expiration; (b) inspiration

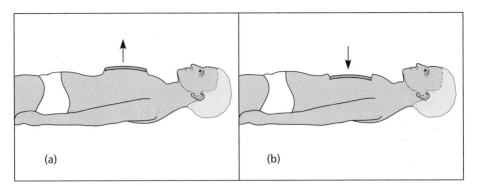

**Figure 18.10** Anterior flail segment: (a) expiration; (b) inspiration

transection is incomplete. The diagnosis is suggested in the hypotensive patient who complains of pain in the region of the upper thoracic spine and whose chest x-ray shows a widened mediastinum. Confirmation of the diagnosis is by a CT or MRI scan. Treatment consists of resuscitation and surgical repair.

2. **Avulsion of a main bronchus.** As the thorax decelerates suddenly to a stop, the lung and its hilum may continue in the direction of travel for a short distance, thus avulsing the mobile main bronchus from the relatively fixed trachea. Such an injury may produces haemoptysis, pneumothorax, or mediastinal surgical emphysema, or all of these. The diagnosis when suspected is confirmed by bronchoscopy. Treatment is by thoracotomy and re-anastomosis of the bronchus.

## PENETRATING TRAUMA

This is usually the result of a knife or firearm attack. Any of the complications associated with blunt trauma above and below the diaphragm can follow a penetrating injury but usually without rib fracture. **Injury to the heart is much more common in penetrating trauma.**

A stab or bullet wound to the heart can produce:

- Cardiac tamponade (Figure 18.11)
- Intracardiac shunts.

### Cardiac tamponade

The lacerations in the pericardium and heart by the knife or missile are usually not large. Blood escapes from the heart under high pressure and too fast to escape through the small pericardial laceration. This shed blood is therefore retained within the pericardium and as the pericardium is unable to expand acutely, the accumulating blood compresses the heart. The main effect of this tamponade is to inhibit diastolic filling of the heart from the vena cavae.

The patient with cardiac tamponade will thus have **a high venous pressure with distended neck veins, hypotension and poor cardiac output.**

Deep inspiration will exaggerate these signs (Figure 18.11b) – when the central tendon of the diaphragm descends, it pulls the base of the pericardium with it, thereby elongating the distended pericardial sac and increasing the tamponade effect.

**Treatment of cardiac tamponade**
Traumatic tamponade is an acute surgical emergency. Needle aspiration of pericardial blood is not helpful as the shed blood soon clots and it is important to arrest the haemorrhage from the heart laceration. Surgical repair is required via midline sternotomy or thoracotomy.

### Intracardiac shunts

Such complications are rare but a penetrating injury passing through the anterior chest wall, the right ventricle, interventricular septum and into the left ventricle will produce a left-to-right shunt. The effects of this shunting of blood from the left to the right ventricle will depend on the size of the septal injury and volume of blood flowing through it. If significant, the lungs will become flooded and the patient dyspnoeic. Positive pressure ventilation of the lungs may relieve the acute emergency but open heart surgery with cardiopulmonary bypass facilities will be required to repair the injury.

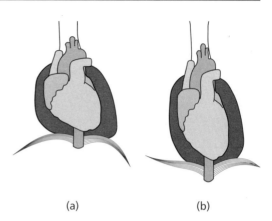

(a)                                      (b)

**Figure 18.11** (a) Cardiac tamponade. (b) The effect of deep inspiration

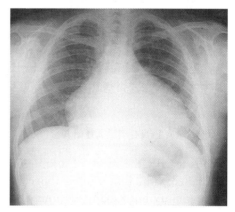

**Figure 18.12** Pericardial effusion

## LUNG TUMOURS

Tumours of the lung may be **benign** or **malignant** and a malignant tumour may be **primary** or **secondary**.

Secondary (i.e. metastatic) lung tumours are the most common.

## BENIGN TUMOURS

Such tumours may arise in the lung **parenchyma** or the bronchial **mucosa**. Benign **parenchymal** tumours are **hamartomas** (an abnormal arrangement of normal tissue):

- Chondroma
- Haemangioma
- Lymphangioma
- Fibroma
- Lipoma.

Benign bronchial **mucosal** tumours are **adenomas**, the most common of which is the **carcinoid** tumour.

Other bronchial adenomas are muco-epidermoid and spindle cell variants.

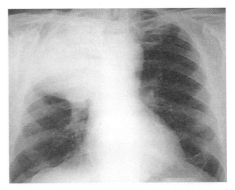

**Figure 18.13** Right upper lobar pneumonia

- **Presentation** – usually haemoptysis with lobar pneumonia (Figure 18.13) due to bronchial obstruction.
- **Diagnosis** – chest x-ray, MRI, and bronchoscopy with biopsy.
- **Treatment** – in patients suitable for major surgery, treatment is by thoracotomy and resection of the tumour. If the tumour is small and localized, local excision of the tumour and bronchus with repair or re-anastomosis of the remaining bronchus with preservation of lung tissue will suffice. If the tumour is locally extensive or malignant, lobectomy or even pneumonectomy will be required.

### Carcinoid tumour

Although usually benign, a small percentage become malignant and metastasize. Patients with liver metastases secreting 5-HT may develop attacks of skin flushing, diarrhoea and bronchospasm, the so-called 'carcinoid syndrome'. Venous blood containing high concentrations of 5-HT draining into the right side of the heart via the vena cavae provoke an endothelial fibrosis in the right atrium and ventricle and eventually pulmonary and tricuspid valve stenosis.

## MALIGNANT TUMOURS

### Primary bronchial carcinoma

This is the greatest single cause of death from malignant disease in England and Wales with around 34 000 deaths per year. The incidence is higher in men and smoking is the most common predisposing factor (Figure 18.14).

Bronchial carcinomas are divided into **two groups: small cell and non-small-cell tumours**. The second group is subdivided into squamous, adeno- and undifferentiated carcinomas. The incidence of these cell type groups is:

- Small cell carcinoma, 20%
- Non-small-cell carcinoma – squamous carcinoma, 40%; adenocarcinoma, 20%; undifferentiated carcinoma, 20%.

**Presenting symptoms** depend on the stage the disease has reached at the time of presentation.

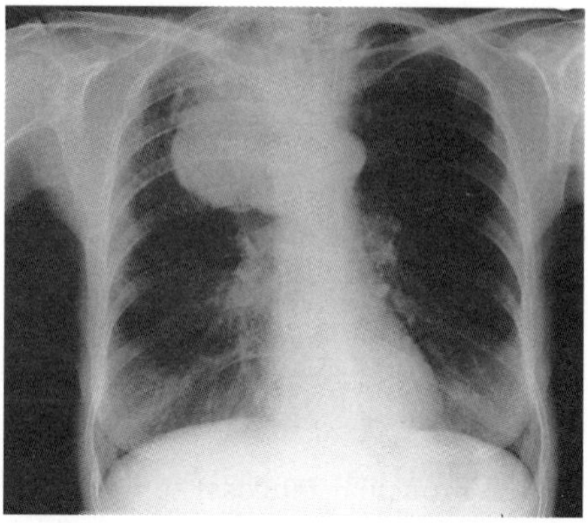

**Stage 1. Local disease** Symptoms are due to the effects of the tumour within the lumen of a bronchus:

- **Cough**
- **Haemoptysis**
- **Dyspnoea on exertion**
- **Recurrent respiratory tract infection**
- **Unresolving pneumonia** – an obstructed bronchus will lead to collapse or consolidation and loss of function with or without infection of that lung, lobe or segment distal to the obstruction, resulting in:

**Figure 18.14** Primary bronchial carcinoma

**Symptoms of primary carcinoma of lung are caused by:**

- Local disease
- Invasive disease
- Metastatic disease
- Systemic effects

**Stage 2. Invasive disease** Symptoms are due to direct invasion by the tumour of other structures within the thorax:

- **Chest wall pain** – peripheral tumour invading chest wall
- **Pleural effusion** – pleural trans-coelomic spread
- **Obstructive dysphagia** – tumour of left main bronchus or involved subcarinal lymph nodes invading the oesophagus
- **Hoarse voice and bovine (cow) cough** – invasion of recurrent laryngeal branch of left vagus nerve under the aortic arch
- **Pain in shoulder and arm with Horner's syndrome** – invasion of the neck of the first rib, stellate ganglion and T1 nerve root by a tumour at the apex of an upper lobe (**Pancoast tumour**)
- **Palpitations and heart failure** – invasion of the pericardium, inducing ectopic ventricular beats and a pericardial effusion with cardiac tamponade
- **Superior vena caval obstruction** – tumours of the right lung may invade and occlude the SVC. Obstructed venous return from the upper limbs, head and neck produces cyanosis, engorgement and distended neck veins.

**Stage 3. Metastatic disease** Symptoms are due to metastases – haematogenous and/or lymphatic spread to distant sites – commonly **bone, brain, liver and lymph nodes**. Secondary tumour at these sites may present as:

- Bone – skeletal pain; pathological fractures

- Brain – headache; late onset epilepsy; stroke; personality changes
- Liver – right hypochondral mass; jaundice
- Lymph nodes – almost invariably the first nodes to enlarge by tumour spread beyond the thorax are those of the right deep cervical group. Palpable as a right supraclavicular mass.

**A tumour at any stage can present with systemic effects:**
- **Hypertrophic pulmonary osteoarthropathy** – painful inflammation of peripheral joints with clubbing of the fingernails
- **Inappropriate hormone secretion** – e.g. ADH
- **Dermatomyositis** – skin rash and wasting and weakness of proximal limb muscles.

**Investigations** After taking a full clinical history and conducting a physical examination, a diagnosis of bronchial carcinoma may be confirmed by:
- PA chest x-ray
- Sputum cytology
- Bronchoscopy and biopsy
- X-ray guided needle biopsy of peripheral tumours.

## Treatment
- **Curative** treatment of bronchial carcinoma is surgical resection of the tumour by pneumonectomy (removal of an entire lung) or lobectomy (removal of one lobe of a lung), whichever is appropriate. This is only feasible if:

1  The tumour type is of the non-small-cell variety.
2  The tumour is confined to the lung and has not invaded other intrathoracic structures or metastasized to distant sites.
3  The patient will tolerate the loss of lung function with pneumonectomy or lobectomy.
4  The patient's general medical state will tolerate the trauma of the major surgery involved.

> Thus only about 20% of patients with lung cancer are deemed suitable for operation. Of these, 25% survive 5 years, those without lymph node involvement having the better prognosis.

- **Palliative** treatment is aimed at relieving painful or distressing symptoms and hopefully prolonging survival time. Small-cell tumours are treated by combined chemotherapy and radiotherapy. Distressing conditions such as painful bone metastases, obstructive dysphagia and SVC obstruction are relieved by local radiotherapy.

### Secondary bronchial carcinoma
The lungs are frequently the site of secondary deposits from malignancy throughout the body, particularly **breast, kidney, bone, melanoma**. The chest x-ray appearance (Figure 18.15) is often single or multiple rounded opacities (cannonball metastases). Treatment is that for the primary malignancy.

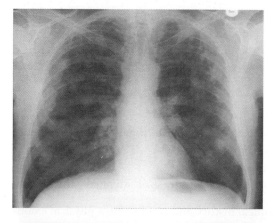

**Figure 18.15** Multiple lung metastases

## MEDIASTINAL MASSES

The mediastinum is that space within the thorax situated between the two pleural cavities, bounded above by the thoracic inlet and below by the diaphragm (Figure 18.16). For descriptive purposes it is divided into a superior and inferior compartment by a line drawn from the sternal angle to the lower border of the body of the 4th thoracic vertebra. The inferior compartment is subdivided into anterior, middle and posterior parts. The anterior mediastinum is the part between the body of the sternum and the pericardium, the posterior mediastinum the part between the pericardium and the vertebral column, leaving the pericardium as the middle mediastinum.

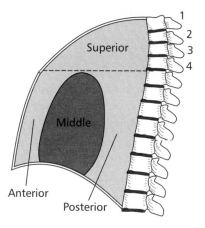

**Figure 18.16** Side view of chest – cross-section to show mediastinum

Various mediastinal masses occur more commonly in each of the compartments.

### Occurrence of mediastinal masses

**Superior mediastinum**
- Thymoma and thymic cyst
- Malignant lymphoma
- Thyroid and parathyroid masses

| **Anterior mediastinum** | **Middle mediastinum** | **Posterior mediastinum** |
|---|---|---|
| • Thymoma and thymic cysts | • Lymphoma | • Neurogenic tumours |
| • Germ cell tumours | • Pericardial cysts | • Gastroenteric cysts |
| • Thyroid and parathyroid masses | (Figure 18.17) | (Hiatus hernia) |
| • Malignant lymphoma | | |
| • Lymphangioma | | |

## Thymomas

Thymomas are tumours arising in the thymic epithelial cells of Hassall's corpuscles. They may be benign or malignant and the malignant ones vary in degree of aggression. The benign and less malignant tumours are often associated with myasthenia gravis.

## Germ cell tumours

These tumours resemble their counterparts in the ovary and testis. They occur in young adults and may be benign or malignant; 75% are benign and cystic and may be termed cystic teratomas.

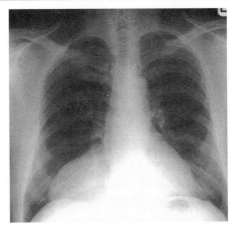

**Figure 18.17** A pleuropericardial cyst

## Malignant lymphoma

These are either Hodgkin's or non-Hodgkin's lymphomas. Not all lymph node masses developing in the mediastinum are lymphomas but may be metastatic disease from a primary tumour elsewhere in the body. Inflammatory tuberculous lymph node masses also occur.

## Neurogenic tumours

These tumours, which arise almost exclusively in the posterior mediastinum, develop from either the sympathetic or peripheral nervous system. Those developed from the sympathetic chain occur in children below the age of 10 and are:
- Ganglioneuroma – good prognosis
- Ganglioneuroblastoma – intermediate prognosis
- Neuroblastoma – poor prognosis.

Tumours of peripheral nerves of the mediastinum, usually an intercostal nerve, are benign and arise in adults.

## Paragangliomas

Such tumours can arise in any part of the paraganglionic system from the base of the skull to the pelvis. Ninety per cent of such tumours are phaeochromocytomas in suprarenal glands but the equivalent tumour arising in the aortopulmonary chemoreceptors does not usually produce catecholamines and hypertension. Extra-adrenal tumours have an incidence of malignancy of up to 50%.

## Thyroid and parathyroid masses

Retrosternal thyroid swellings (goitres) are almost always an extension of a goitre developed from a normally situated thyroid gland in the neck and not from ectopic thyroid tissue in the mediastinum. As the goitre enlarges it passes through the thoracic inlet into the superior and then the anterior mediastinum. As the thoracic inlet is a rigid ring of bone, progressive enlargement of the goitre compresses other structures within this ring, notably the trachea. As this structure is compressed from side to side a so-called **scabbard** trachea is formed and stridor becomes audible. At this stage the patient is in imminent danger of suffocation. Parathyroid tumours in the anterior mediastinum do not present as mediastinal masses but by the effects of parathormone hypersecretion.

## CRIB BOX – THORACIC SURGERY

### Pneumothorax

- **Spontaneous** (rupture of congenital or acquired bullae)
- **Traumatic** (rib fracture; penetrating wounds; iatrogenic)
- **Presentation** – pain, dyspnoea, hyper-resonant percussion and absent breath sounds
- **Treatment** – only if dyspnoeic – needle aspiration; chest drain; pleurodesis; pleurectomy

### Haemothorax

- Trauma; aneurysm; coagulation problems
- **Signs** – diminished movement of chest wall on affected side; stony dull percussion note and absent breath sounds; dense opacification on CXR; pleural aspiration produces blood
- **Treatment** – blood should be removed; aspiration or chest drain

### Pleural effusion

- **Transudate** – heart failure; hypoproteinaemia
- **Exudate** – infection; inflammation; infarction; **malignancy**. Most important to differentiate between malignancy and the other causes – aspirate for cytology; thoracoscopy
- **Treat** underlying condition and/or drain the effusion for dyspnoea

### Empyema

- A walled off **abscess** usually at the lowest part of the pleural space
- **Treat** by drainage (aspiration or tube); decortication if this fails

### Chest trauma

- **Blunt** (inc. deceleration) and **penetrating**
- Understand flail chest and cardiac tamponade

### Lung tumours

- Benign – parenchymal (hamartomas) or mucosal (adenomas)
- Malignant – primary and secondary (very common)

### Primary bronchial carcinoma

- The most common malignancy – **34 000** deaths per year
- Strongly associated with smoking
- Small cell carcinoma 20%
- Non-small-cell carcinoma – squamous carcinoma 40%; adenocarcinoma 20%; undifferentiated carcinoma 20%
- Symptoms produced by **local, invasive and metastatic disease**, and **systemic effects** (remember these)
- **Treatment is curative or palliative**
- **Surgery for non-small-cell only**

# chapter 19

# CARDIAC SURGERY

## CORONARY ARTERY DISEASE

The myocardium derives its oxygen and nutrients from blood supplied by the coronary arteries (Figure 19.1).

Atherosclerotic ischaemic heart disease is the most common cause of death in the UK.

- In more than 70% of cases two or three coronary arteries are affected.
- The disease usually involves the **proximal** portions of the coronary arteries.
- Gradual narrowing causes increasingly limiting **angina**.
- Plaque rupture or haemorrhage with thrombosis can cause sudden occlusion (Figure 19.2), leading to unstable angina or **myocardial infarction**.
- A healed transmural infarct may become **aneurysmal**.
- Occasionally a septal infarct leads to the development of a ventricular septal defect which carries a high mortality and always requires surgical closure.
- Sometimes infarction leads to free wall rupture, which is usually fatal.

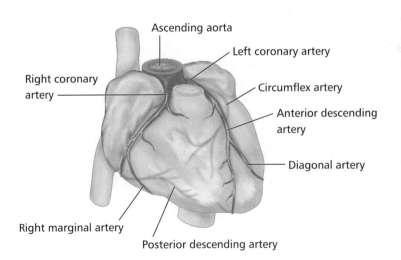

**Figure 19.1** Anatomy of coronary vessels

Surgical treatment of this disease involves treatment of:

1 Coronary insufficiency
2 The sequelae of myocardial infarction.

## CORONARY INSUFFICIENCY

Improving coronary blood flow in stable or unstable angina can be achieved by:

1 Percutaneous transluminal coronary angioplasty (PTCA) ± stent
2 Coronary artery bypass graft (CABG).

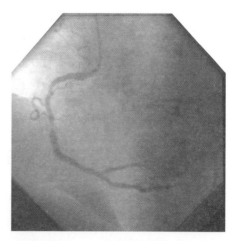

**Figure 19.2** Coronary angiogram showing stenosis

It is estimated that 1000 interventions are necessary per million population in the UK and that 400 will be suitable for PTCA ± stent and 600 for coronary bypass surgery.

### PTCA

- Uses a guided balloon placed across the stenosis in a coronary artery and inflated under great pressure. The atherosclerotic plaque is compressed, leaving a larger lumen for blood flow. Unfortunately, 30–40% restenose within 6 months.
- This problem is overcome to a certain extent by deploying **wire stents** that minimize the chances of restenosis (down to 10–15%).

For multiple vessel disease and certain types of single vessel disease, **coronary bypass surgery is the best option.**

### CABG

This procedure uses an autologous conduit to bypass the coronary stenosis.
- Long saphenous vein is harvested from the leg.
- A median sternotomy is performed and the pericardium opened. A large cannula is placed in the right atrium for venous drainage into a reservoir.
- The blood is oxygenated in a disposable membrane oxygenator and returned to the body via a cannula placed in the ascending aorta. The oxygenator takes over the function of the lungs whilst a pump circulates the blood from the atrium to the aorta and takes on the function of the heart – **cardiopulmonary bypass.**
- The heart is either fibrillated or arrested by clamping the aortic root and instilling a $K^+$-rich solution – **cardioplegia.**
- The coronary artery is opened for a length of 6–8 mm distal to the stenosis. The vein is reversed and anastomosed to the coronary using a 7/0 Prolene suture. All the necessary anastomoses are performed with lengths of vein.

- The aortic clamp is removed and the heart usually starts to beat spontaneously. The vein grafts are then all anastomosed to the ascending aorta. Blood from the aorta now goes through the vein grafts into the coronary arteries distal to the stenoses.
- Ventilation of the lungs is recommenced and cardiopulmonary bypass is discontinued. The atrial and aortic cannulae are removed and the chest closed.

CABG has been one of the most comprehensively studied surgical procedures in history. In the UK alone, nearly 30 000 such operations are performed every year with a mortality of 2–3%.

### Results
The saphenous vein undergoes fibrointimal hyperplasia and atherosclerotic changes, resulting in a **patency rate of 50% at 8–10 years**. Use of the internal thoracic (mammary) arteries as a conduit to the left anterior descending artery of the heart has resulted in better event-free survival. Arterial conduits (e.g. radial artery, inferior epigastric and right gastroepiploic artery) are increasingly used as they offer better long term patency.

Patients help by controlling their risk factors, e.g. smoking, diabetes, hypertension, hyperlipidaemia. Regular aspirin (75–150 mg) improves graft patency.

## SEQUELAE OF MYOCARDIAL INFARCTION

### Left ventricular aneurysm
Improved treatment of myocardial infarction has led to a decrease in this complication.
- Total occlusion of the left anterior descending artery and poorly developed collateral flow may cause a left ventricular aneurysm. The non-aneurysmal portion of the ventricle can dilate and lead to failure.
- The presence of thrombus and episodes of life-threatening ventricular arrhythmias necessitate an operation. Under cardiopulmonary bypass the aneurysm is excised, leaving a 1 cm rim of fibrous tissue for suturing with Teflon strips or by a circular patch so as to remodel the ventricular cavity. A 5-year survival of 65% is better than non-surgical management.

### Post-infarction ventricular septal defect
Complete obstruction of an artery with poor collaterals leads to ventricular septal infarction and rupture.
- Only 50% survive 1 week and 30% survive 2 weeks after the event.
- The development of a pansystolic murmur at the left sternal edge is suspicious.
- Renal function has to be monitored closely. Although a delay of 2–4 weeks will offer better tissue for suturing a patch for closure, it is rarely possible to wait that long. Early surgical closure with a Dacron patch offers the best chance of survival.

## MITRAL VALVE DISEASE

The mitral valve is essentially a bicuspid valve.

### MITRAL STENOSIS

This is almost always due to **rheumatic heart disease** (Figure 19.3).

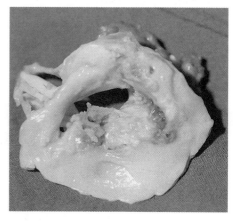

**Figure 19.3** Rheumatic mitral stenosis

- The chordae tendinae are variably involved with fusion, shortening and thickening. The mitral valve looks funnel shaped and the left atrium is enlarged and thickened. The left ventricle is usually normal.
- Typically, rheumatic fever in childhood or early teens is followed by clinical signs of stenosis by the age of 20 years and symptoms start in the 30s.
- Patients with moderate stenosis are often asymptomatic but can develop pulmonary oedema suddenly with severe exertion.
- Those with severe stenosis have easy fatiguability, dyspnoea on exertion, orthopnoea and paroxysmal nocturnal dyspnoea. It takes another 10 years to progress to a state of total disability.
- The average age of death in patients not surgically treated is between 40 and 50 years.
- Atrial fibrillation, systemic embolization from auricular thrombus and pulmonary haemorrhage are all troublesome complications.

### Diagnosis
- Auscultation
- Chest x-ray showing left atrial enlargement and pulmonary hypertension
- Doppler echo identifies severity of stenosis, valve area and gradient
- Coronary angiography in patients over 40 years to identify coronary artery disease.

### Treatment
- Digoxin – for atrial fibrillation
- Warfarin – to prevent emboli.

If valve cusps appear pliable on echo and without calcification, a **balloon mitral valvuloplasty** can be performed. This is particularly useful during pregnancy. It is used frequently in poorer countries as it is a very economical procedure.

**Surgical closed mitral valvotomy** can be performed through a left anterior thoracotomy. A finger is introduced through the left auricle to assess the mitral valve and split open the fused commissures. This procedure would sometimes lead to unintentional tears in the leaflets and gross mitral regurgitation, necessitating valve replacement.

As cardiopulmonary bypass has become a safe procedure, **mitral commissurotomy** is increasingly performed under direct vision. This allows a more accurate procedure with minimal mitral incompetence and can be converted to valve replacement if necessary.

## MITRAL INCOMPETENCE

### Causes
- Rheumatic valve disease
- Mitral valve prolapse
- Idiopathic chordal rupture
- Infective endocarditis
- Ischaemic papillary muscle dysfunction or rupture.

### Rheumatic mitral incompetence
- Annular dilatation is the prime cause and can improve with remission of the acute process.
- Progressive worsening with annular dilatation is invariably seen.
- Untreated, the 5-year survival is 46–80%.

### Mitral valve prolapse
- This is common.
- The abnormal strain placed on the chordae may lead to elongation and rupture, causing increased incompetence.
- Symptoms mimicking thyrotoxicosis, hyperadrenergic state and hypoglycaemia may be seen.

### Infective endocarditis
- Abnormal valves may become infected, leading to vegetations (Figure 19.4) causing destruction of cusps and chordae.
- When the aortic valve is infected and incompetent, 'jet lesions' may infect the mitral valve, producing perforation and incompetence.

### Ischaemic papillary muscle
- Myocardial ischaemia can cause papillary muscle dysfunction, leading to mitral regurgitation. Infarction of papillary muscle can rupture the tip and lead to flail chordae and cusp, causing gross acute mitral incompetence.

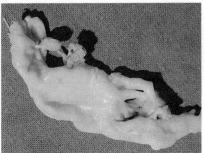

### Treatment
- Mitral valve repair under cardiopulmonary bypass is established as the best treatment for chordal rupture and floppy valves.
- If the valve cannot be repaired, it is replaced with a mechanical prosthesis.

**Figure 19.4** Vegetations on mitral valves

# AORTIC VALVE DISEASE

Disease of this valve leads to:

1 Stenosis of its orifice and pressure loading of the left ventricle
2 Incompetence and volume loading of the left ventricle.

Pathology is best discussed under the headings of stenosis and incompetence.

## AORTIC STENOSIS

The aetiology of aortic stenosis in adults is:
- Calcific aortic stenosis in a congenitally abnormal valve, 61%
- Rheumatic, 13%
- Atherosclerotic, 24%
- Other, 2%.

### Clinical features and diagnosis
Although some patients may be discovered by the chance finding of a murmur, the majority are symptomatic:
- Two-thirds of patients will have angina
- Half will have dyspnoea
- Half will have syncope.

- A third will have the **classic triad of effort dyspnoea, angina and syncope.**

- **Physical examination** reveals a small volume arterial pulse with a slow upstroke and an aortic ejection murmur.
- Chest x-ray shows left ventricular hypertrophy and calcification in the aortic valve.

### Treatment
- In patients with surgically untreated severe aortic stenosis, the average survival after the onset of angina or syncope is 3 years.
- Twenty per cent of deaths will be **sudden** and the rest from left ventricular failure.
- **The only treatment for aortic stenosis is aortic valve replacement.** The mortality of this procedure is 3% and there is a 1–2% incidence of cerebrovascular accident.

## AORTIC INCOMPETENCE

This has a widely varied aetiology:
- Rheumatic, 45%
- Medionecrosis, 18%
- Congenital bicuspid, 13%
- Bacterial endocarditis, 13%.

## Clinical features and diagnosis

- There is a prolonged asymptomatic phase.
- A third of patients will have dyspnoea or paroxysmal nocturnal dyspnoea.
- Twenty per cent will have angina.
- The pulse is collapsing due to the wide pulse pressure.
- The regurgitant jet may cause fluttering of the anterior mitral leaflet leading to a mid-diastolic murmur (**Austin Flint** murmur).
- Echocardiography with colour flow Doppler establishes the diagnosis.

## Treatment

- **Mild or moderate aortic incompetence** has little effect on activity and life expectancy.
- **Severe incompetence** affects the structure and function of the left ventricle and hence the symptoms and prognosis. In this group 80% will be alive at 5 years and only 10% by 8 years.

Asymptomatic patients are kept under observation. If the left ventricular systolic and diastolic dimensions reach significant proportions, aortic valve replacement is carried out.

The diseased valve is replaced with a mechanical prosthesis in the younger age group and bioprosthesis (porcine aortic valve, bovine pericardial valve) in those over 60 years of age. The ascending aorta is replaced if aneurysmal.

> Patients who develop acute severe aortic regurgitation due to bacterial endocarditis need urgent surgical intervention to prevent death.

# DISEASES OF THE THORACIC AORTA

## ANEURYSMS

- Typically seen in men over 50 years.
- Approximately half are atherosclerotic or degenerative type.
- The rest are secondary to chronic aortic dissection with persisting false channel, ectasia and or aortitis (rare).
- The ascending aorta is involved in 45%, the arch in 10% and descending aorta in 35%.

## Clinical features and diagnosis

Many are asymptomatic and discovered on routine chest x-ray (Figure 19.5a).

- Symptoms when present are of **sudden onset** due to extension of the aneurysm.
- Ascending aneurysms give precordial pain radiating to the neck and descending ones produce back pain.
- Compression of various structures can give a variety of symptoms including **superior vena caval obstruction, hoarseness due to stretching of the recurrent laryngeal nerve and wheezing due to airway compression.**

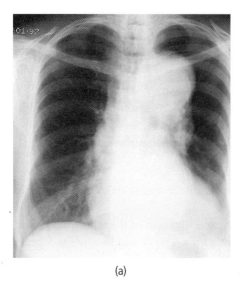

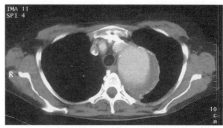

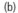

(b)

**Figure 19.5** (a) X-ray of thoracic aneurysm.
(b) CT of thoracic aneurysm

(a)

- A CT scan (Figure 19.5b) with contrast or MRI is the best method of evaluating the aneurysm.

### Treatment
The natural history of all aneurysms is gradual enlargement and eventual rupture.
- 5-year survival of surgically untreated aneurysms is less than 20%.
- Descending thoracic aneurysms can be treated by suturing an inlay Dacron tube graft.
- Ascending and arch aneurysms can only be treated on cardiopulmonary bypass. Arch aneurysm repair needs incorporation of the origins of the head and neck vessels to the side of the tube graft.

The hospital mortality of ascending aortic aneurysm surgery is less than 10% but that of the descending aortic aneurysm is 15–17% and of the arch >40%!

## ACUTE AORTIC DISSECTION

This condition occurs when blood enters an intimal tear and by force of pressure dissects the inner from the outer level of the media. The dissection can extend to a variable length of the aorta and blood either re-enters the true lumen distally or dissects outside the vessel, resulting in catastrophic bleeding (Figure 19.6).
- The site of entry is in the ascending aorta in just over half the cases and in the descending thoracic aorta adjacent to the subclavian artery origin in 40% of cases.
- Dissections are seen usually in patients with hypertension, medial

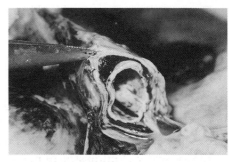

**Figure 19.6** Operative view of aortic dissection

degeneration, Marfan's syndrome and annuloectasia. Atherosclerosis is probably not an important risk factor.

- **Over 80% of dissections occur in people over 60 years of age.**

### Clinical features and diagnosis

Sudden death occurs due to:

- Rupture of the false channel into the thoracic cavity
- Rupture into the pericardium causing cardiac tamponade
- Occlusion of the coronary artery ostia and myocardial infarction.

Patients complain of severe sharp 'tearing' pain over the precordium or in the back.

As the dissection propagates, a variety of signs and symptoms are produced depending on which major blood vessels are occluded (e.g. subclavian, carotid, coeliac, etc.). These include:

- Cerebrovascular accident
- Paraplegia
- Bowel infarction
- Renal infarction
- Cold pulseless limb.

Chest x-ray shows a widened mediastinum and a possibly a left haemothorax. Aortography, CT scanning with contrast and trans-oesophageal echocardiography are used for diagnosis.

### Treatment

This condition has a high mortality – patients are often frail and unsuitable for major surgery. Dissections that re-enter can be managed conservatively by controlling hypertension. Surgical repair requires cardiopulmonary bypass.

## ACUTE TRAUMATIC AORTIC TRANSECTION

This is a **classic sudden deceleration** injury such as occurs in road traffic accidents. The forward motion of the aorta relative to the arch which is fixed by head and neck vessels causes tearing of the descending aorta, usually just distal to the origin of the left subclavian. **Pain is not a major feature.**

Whether a patient survives a complete transection depends on the integrity of the periaortic adventitia and mediastinal pleura. Bleeding into the mediastinum or pleural cavity causes hypovolaemic shock.

A small percentage will have paraplegia due to spinal cord ischaemia and, rarely, there will be lower body ischaemia.

The patient will always be at risk of sudden, fatal haemorrhage into the left hemithorax, maximally in the first 7 days, but also in later years.

### Diagnosis

- **Chest x-ray** shows upper mediastinal widening and possibly a left haemothorax.
- **Thoracic aortography, digital subtraction angiogram (DSA) and CT scan** are used to make the diagnosis and aortography is probably the better of the three.
- Trans-oesophageal echocardiography with colour flow Doppler is very accurate and can be performed in intensive care or in the operating theatre.

### Treatment

A descending aortic tear is repaired through a left thoracotomy. A shunt from left ventricular apex to the femoral artery without pump, or from the left atrium to the femoral artery with a pump, is used. Clamps are placed above and below and the tear repaired by end-to-end anastomosis or Dacron tube graft interposition.

Ascending aortas can be repaired by using cardiopulmonary bypass and, if necessary, deep hypothermia and circulatory arrest.

## PERICARDIAL DISEASE

### CHRONIC CONSTRICTIVE PERICARDITIS

This is an inflammatory process which leads to **adhesions, thickening of the pericardium and constriction of the heart.** The aetiology in most cases is unknown. Less than 3% have tuberculous pericarditis. Trauma and haemopericardium, radiation and cardiac surgery can all produce constrictive pericarditis.

### Clinical features and diagnosis

Fatigue, effort dyspnoea, neck vein distension, hepatomegaly, ascites and peripheral oedema are the usual signs and symptoms.

- **Pulsus paradoxus** (Figure 19.7) is seen in advanced cases.
- Chest x-ray is often unremarkable but may show some pericardial calcification.

### Treatment

Pericardectomy is performed through a median sternotomy or left thoracotomy.

**Pulsus paradoxus**

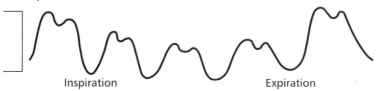

Inspiration                                    Expiration

**Figure 19.7** Pulsus paradoxus

### CHRONIC EFFUSIVE PERICARDITIS

Inflammatory reaction stimulates accumulation of pericardial fluid. Dense fibrinous coating of the visceral pericardium thickens it. Advanced **renal disease,**

**dialysis, malignant disease and trauma** are recognized causes. Infection is rarely the cause.

### Clinical features and diagnosis

Chest pain, fever, leucocytosis and pericardial friction rub are seen.

- Rarely, acute tamponade is found.
- Elevation of jugular venous pulse and pulsus paradoxus may be present.
- Chest x-ray shows an enlarged globular heart shadow.
- 2D echocardiography is diagnostic.

### Treatment

Pericardiocentesis directed by echo will alleviate immediate haemodynamic problems. A pericardial 'window' should be formed to drain the fluid either into the peritoneum (subxiphoid incision) or into the left chest (minithoracotomy or video assisted thoracoscopic surgery). For recurrence of the problem, a partial or complete pericardectomy is the definitive treatment.

## CONGENITAL HEART DISEASE

### ATRIAL SEPTAL DEFECT (ASD)

A defect in the atrial septum of variable size and position allows left-to-right shunting of blood and increased flow through the right ventricle and pulmonary tree. The commonest type of defect is:

- The fossa ovalis type (**ostium secundum defect**)
- When the atrioventricular septum is absent, there is a **primum septal defect** or AV caval defect. The tricuspid and mitral valve leaflets will be in continuity with an underlying membranous VSD.

The right atrium and ventricle hypertrophy and dilate as do pulmonary arteries. Pulmonary hypertension may develop in the third or fourth decade of life.

### Clinical features and diagnosis

- When the left-to-right shunt is small there are no symptoms or signs.
- When the shunt is large, symptoms appear after several decades and consist of effort dyspnoea, respiratory infections and atrial arrhythmias.
- Chest x-ray (Figure 19.8) shows right atrial enlargement, pulmonary artery prominence and plethoric lung fields.
- 2D echo will visualize the defect and colour flow Doppler will show the abnormal flow.
- Cardiac catheterization will quantify the shunt and assess pulmonary hypertension.

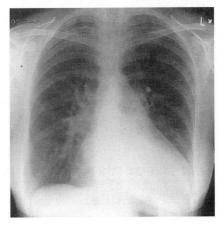

Figure 19.8 Chest x-ray showing upper lobe diversion in atrial septal defect

## Treatment

The natural history is of increasing shunt with age and up to 25% of people with a large ASD will die of it in late life.

- Repair of ASD is carried out on cardiopulmonary bypass. The right atrium is opened and a pericardial patch is usually used to close the defect.
- Normal life expectancy is restored in children and adults but in the older age group, although life expectancy is increased, it does not match the general population.

# VENTRICULAR SEPTAL DEFECT (VSD)

A VSD is a solitary or multiple defect in the interventricular septum.

- It can coexist with other intracardiac abnormalities.
- It can occur in any portion of the septum including the membranous septum.

### Clinical features and diagnosis

The size of left-to-right shunt will dictate the symptoms and signs.

- **In infants,** heart failure, tachypnoea, liver enlargement and a systolic murmur are diagnostic of a large VSD.
- Patients with small VSDs often have no signs apart from a pansystolic murmur.
- **Larger VSDs lead to pulmonary hypertension and RV hypertrophy.**
- Extreme pulmonary hypertension may lead to reversal of shunt and cyanosis – **Eisenmenger syndrome.**
- 2D echocardiography with Doppler is highly reliable in picking up even small defects.
- MRI can provide precise information about the morphology. These newer techniques have made cardiac catheterization and angiography unnecessary prior to the closure of primary VSDs.

### Treatment

- Small defects often close off spontaneously by 1 year and larger defects can narrow down and take much longer to close.
- Eighty per cent of large VSDs seen at 1 month of age will close spontaneously.
- Intractable heart failure with failure to thrive is the commonest indication for surgical repair of VSD during the first 2 years of life.
- Under cardiopulmonary bypass a Dacron patch is used to close the defect.
- Repair of VSD before the age of 2 is curative and can give normal life expectancy.
- Heart block, ventricular arrhythmia and progressive pulmonary hypertension are recognized causes of death.

# PATENT DUCTUS ARTERIOSUS

The fetal ductus arteriosus shunts blood from the pulmonary artery to the descending aorta and should close down when the baby is born. Muscular contraction closes the duct within 10–15 hours and usually by 2–3 weeks fibrosis causes permanent closure.

The incidence of isolated PDA (Figure 19.9) in term infants is about **1 in 2000**; female:male 2:1 live births.

### Clinical features and diagnosis

The size of the duct will dictate the magnitude of the left-to-right shunt and hence symptoms.

- In neonates, a large duct can cause severe congestive heart failure.
- A continuous murmur may be present and is usually loud and heard over the pulmonary artery.
- Chest x-ray shows cardiomegaly and a prominent ascending aorta.
- Echocardiography with colour flow Doppler is diagnostic.

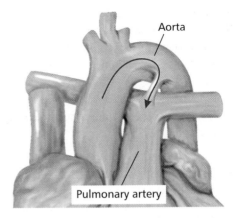

**Figure 19.9** Patent ductus arteriosus

### Prognosis

- Untreated PDA has a mortality of 30% in the first year of life.
- By the third to fourth decade, the death rate is 1–2% per year and rising.
- By 45 years of age, 42% will have died – usually from left ventricular failure.
- **Bacterial endocarditis is a potential complication.**
- Life expectancy is normal after surgical closure of PDA in infancy or childhood.

### Treatment

- Surgical closure of the duct is carried out through a left thoracotomy without cardiopulmonary bypass. The duct is double ligated.
- More recently, ducts have been closed **thoracoscopically** with a metal clip. This procedure allows a quicker recovery and discharge.
- **Percutaneous, transluminal closure of PDA** is finding increasing acceptance with a device which can be deployed to close the PDA. However, the success rate is still only 80% and the costs are higher than surgery.

## COARCTATION OF AORTA

This is a congenital narrowing of the descending thoracic aorta **in relation to the ductus arteriosus** (Figure 19.10):

- 25% of the cases have atresia (i.e. completely blocked)

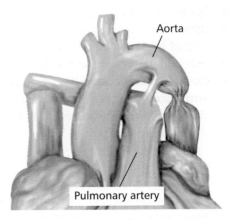

**Figure 19.10** Coarctation of the aorta

- 42% have a 'pinhole' lumen
- 33% have moderate narrowing
- The aorta appears to have a 'waist' externally and a 'shelf' of intima internally causes the narrowing. Male:female 2:1.

> - **Collateral circulation** between aorta above and below the coarctation is a striking feature and leads to **para-scapular pulsation** and **rib notching on chest x-ray**.

### Clinical features and diagnosis
### Neonatal presentation:
- Heart failure after a variable period (duct closure)
- A systolic murmur is heard over the heart and in the back
- There is a weakened, delayed femoral pulse
- If the coarctation is pre-ductal and the ductus stays open, lower body cyanosis appears
- Cardiomegaly with right ventricular hypertrophy is seen on a chest x-ray.

### Childhood:
- Hypertension is present in 90% and cardiomegaly in 33%
- Almost all childhood presentations are asymptomatic.

### Adult:
- Young adults are asymptomatic
- Heart failure may occur only after the age of 30 years
- Hypertension is more severe
- Most patients are found by chance with upper body hypertension and weak femoral pulses.

Aortography, measurement of pressure gradient across coarctation at rest and on exercise and two-dimensional echocardiography will diagnose this condition. Associated valve anomalies should also be looked for.

### Prognosis
- 10% of babies will die within 1 month if surgically untreated.
- 50% will die within the first 10 years.
- 25% of deaths occur in the 14–20 years age group with bacterial endocarditis, aortic rupture or intercranial haemorrhage.
- 25% die between 20 and 50 years from heart failure secondary to hypertension or valve heart disease.

### Treatment
Surgery is curative. Through a left thoracotomy, the ductus is ligated and the coarctation segment resected with an end-to-end anastomosis. Rarely, an inter-position of Dacron tube graft may be necessary. Long-term survival is good although marred by persistent hypertension in many.

# TETRALOGY OF FALLOT

This is the most common cause of cyanotic congenital heart disease and accounts for 8% of all congenital heart disease (Figure 19.11). The patient has:

1  Pulmonary stenosis
2  Ventricular septal defect
3  Overriding aorta which straddles the VSD and both ventricles
4  Right ventricular hypertrophy.

## Clinical features and diagnosis

- **Cyanosis** of variable degree.
- **Breathless when suckling** or other exertion.
- Children and adults develop clubbing.
- Marked reduction in arterial oxygen saturation.
- Mid-systolic pulmonary murmur.
- The heart is not enlarged.

In patients with severe cyanosis and polycythaemia, cerebral thrombosis may cause hemiplegia.

Chest x-ray shows a boot-shaped heart and rib notching due to collaterals.

Echocardiography is the definitive diagnostic procedure and will show the morphology.

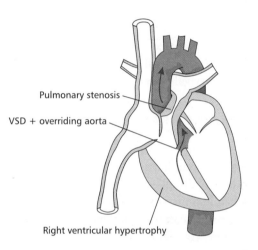

Pulmonary stenosis

VSD + overriding aorta

Right ventricular hypertrophy

**Figure 19.11** Fallot's tetralogy

## Prognosis

- 25% of surgically untreated infants will die within 1 year.
- 10% are dead by 10 years of age.
- 95% are dead by the age of 40 years.

## Treatment

The definitive procedure is performed on cardiopulmonary bypass and involves widening the pulmonary outflow with a pericardial patch and closure of VSD. The pulmonary valve is dilated and infundibular stenosis excised. Long-term survival is excellent and approaches that of the general population.

## COMPLETE TRANSPOSITION OF THE GREAT ARTERIES (TGA)

TGA is a congenital anomaly in which the aorta arises entirely or in large part from the right ventricle and the pulmonary artery from the left. The systemic and pulmonary circulations are in parallel.

- Life is unsustainable unless there is adequate mixing of blood between the right and left sides of the heart.
- When there is a high degree of mixing, arterial saturation may be near normal and the symptoms are minimal. With little mixing, hypoxia is severe.

Echocardiography defines the morphology of the defect and of the abnormal coronary arteries. Cardiac catheterization is not done routinely.

### Prognosis
- Only 15% of surgically untreated cases survive 6 months.
- Death is due to hypoxia, cerebrovascular events or congestive heart failure.

### Treatment
Under cardiopulmonary bypass, the aorta and pulmonary artery are divided and switched to the appropriate side of the heart. The coronary arteries are anastomosed to the neo-aorta.

Overall survival of over 80% at 5 years is now possible in most centres and over 95% survival is seen in selected centres. Long-term results are expected to be good.

## CARDIAC TRANSPLANTATION

Heart transplantation was carried out in many centres around the world following Christian Barnard's first procedure in 1966. However, due to poor outcomes, it largely disappeared from clinical practice only to be revived again in the 1980s when immunosuppression was better understood.

- For cardiac transplantation, the donor and recipient must have ABO (blood type) compatibility.
- Immunological compatibility is also studied by HLA typing, white blood cell antibody screen and lymphocyte cross-match.
- When a patient with brain death is young (<35 years old), without evidence of myocardial damage, sepsis or episode of hypotension, then he must be considered to be a potential donor and permission obtained from his/her family.
- The procurement of the donor heart is synchronized with the preparation of the recipient. The transplant co-ordination service will alert the appropriate centre to the availability of an organ and a harvesting team will procure the heart.
- The heart is preserved by cooling and plegia and transported rapidly to the recipient's hospital. On arrival of the donor organ in the operating theatre, the recipient is placed on cardiopulmonary bypass and his/her heart excised.
- The donor heart is connected to the recipient with four anastomoses – (1) left atrium, (2) right atrium, (3) pulmonary artery, (4) aorta.
- On removal of the aortic clamp, warm blood perfuses the coronaries and rhythm returns. Cardiopulmonary bypass is discontinued and the chest closed.

### Post-operative management
This is routine post-cardiac surgery management, including antibiotics, strict reverse isolation techniques in intensive care for 2–3 days, hand-washing and face masks for all who enter patient's room.

Immunosuppresive therapy is started in the peri-operative period and continued long term. Endomyocardial biopsy every week for 6 weeks is undertaken to identify possible rejection.

## Results

In the 1980s, 3-year survival was 65% and 10-year survival was 55% but in this decade 3-year survival is **83%**.

Causes of death are acute cardiac failure in 22%, infection in 22% and 15% rejection. Accelerated coronary artery disease is a common cause of death and need for retransplantation.

---

**CRIB BOX – CARDIAC SURGERY**

**Coronary artery disease**

- Most common cause of death in the UK
- Causes angina and myocardial infarction
- Surgery used for: (1) coronary insufficiency – PTCA or CABG; (2) sequelae of infarction – ventricular aneurysm; VSD; papillary muscle rupture

**Valve disease**

- Rheumatic heart disease is diminishing.
- Valves either stenose or become incompetent, causing **pressure loads** or **volume loads** on the ventricles and/or pulmonary vessels

**Thoracic aorta** is subject to **aneurysms, dissection, or traumatic transection**

**Pericardium** is subject to **constrictive pericarditis**, or **effusive pericarditis**

**Congenital heart disease**

- ASD
- VSD
- Patent ductus arteriosus
- Coarctation of the aorta
- Tetralogy of Fallot
- Transposition of the great arteries

# chapter 20

# DAY SURGERY

## DEFINITION

Day surgery may be defined as a surgical or other therapeutic procedure in which the post-operative recovery is sufficiently rapid and thorough that the patient may be safely allowed home the same day.

## THE PURPOSE OF DAY SURGERY

The purpose of day surgery is to provide surgical care that is as good, and preferably better, than in-patient care. Both surgical and anaesthetic techniques must be perfect, with few if any complications, since the patient will recuperate at home without any medical or nursing supervision.

For the **individual patient,** this ideal can be achieved due to:
- The skill of the surgeon
- The development of short-acting anaesthetic agents
- The improved use and knowledge of pain relief and pain prevention.

**To treat large groups of patients on a daily basis requires much more:**
- Multiskilled and trained day surgery nurses
- Careful and flexible day surgery management
- A thorough understanding by the surgeon and the anaesthetist of the real differences that exist between the management of in-patient and day surgery patients.

The practice of day surgery is blessed by two advantages over much of in-patient work:
- Most day surgery patients are fit and healthy
- Most fit and healthy patients would rather not stay overnight in hospital if they can avoid it.

## HISTORY

As with most developments in medicine, day surgery is not new. Nicoll, a paediatric surgeon, first described the benefits of day surgery for children and their parents in Glasgow in 1907.

The growth of day surgery in broader surgical practice occurred in the USA during the 1960s and 1970s. There, the need to keep the costs of health care under control made one-day surgery particularly attractive.

The Royal College of Surgeons of England's guidelines on day surgery were published in 1975 (and updated in 1985). Money was made available by the government for hospitals to build and equip new day surgery centres, so that day surgery may now account for **60% of elective surgery** in some hospitals.

Further developments in pain control, anaesthetic and surgical techniques, together with evening and weekend operating, are likely to result in further growth in day surgery early in the next century.

**Principles of day surgery**

- Safe surgery
- Efficient surgery
- Cost-effective surgery

# TYPES OF DAY SURGERY PROCEDURES

Day case procedures can be minor, intermediate or major (Table 20.1).

**Table 20.1** Day case procedures can be minor, intermediate or major (in parentheses)

| Procedures | | |
|---|---|---|
| **General surgery** | **Urology** | **Gynaecology** |
| Lumps & bumps | Circumcision | Termination of pregnancy |
| Anal polyps | Hydroceles | Laparoscopic sterilization |
| Inguinal hernias | Diagnostic cystoscopy | Infertility studies |
| Femoral hernias | Transurethral resection of | Minor gynaecological procedures |
| Umbilical hernias | bladder tumours | |
| Varicose veins (one leg at | Epididymal cysts | |
| a time) | (TURP) | |
| Breast lumps | (Lithotripsy) | |
| Skin grafts | | |
| (Haemorrhoids) | | |
| (Breast enlargement) | | |
| **Orthopaedics** | **ENT** | **Dental surgery** |
| Carpal tunnel | Grommets | Most procedures |
| Hand surgery | Septal surgery | |
| Diagnostic arthroscopy | Antral wash-outs | |
| (Therapeutic arthroscopy) | Tonsils & adenoids | |
| (Bunion surgery) | | |
| **Ophthalmology** | **Paediatrics** | |
| Most procedures | Circumcision | |
| | Testicular surgery | |
| | Hernia repairs | |

## PATIENT CRITERIA FOR DAY SURGERY

To be considered for day surgery a patient must satisfy three different sets of criteria: surgical, anaesthetic and sociodomestic.

**Suitability criteria for day surgery**

**Surgical**

- No post-operative impairment of independence or toilet functions
- Post-operative discomfort manageable with oral analgesia

**Anaesthetic**

- Normal, healthy people or mild systemic disease with no limitation on activity
- Minimal, if any, preoperative investigations required

**Sociodomestic**

- Accompanied by a responsible person for 24 hours
- Transport available to and from Centre (not public transport)
- Telephone available at home

## DIFFERENCES BETWEEN MAIN THEATRES AND DAY SURGERY CENTRES

### ADMINISTRATION

Within a centre it makes sense to devolve **all** patient administration to the centre, including **waiting list and contract management, operating list scheduling, follow-up appointments, coding and auditing.**

In many hospitals, day surgery now comprises 40–50% of all elective work:

- As day surgery procedures last for 60 minutes or less, most day lists contain larger numbers of patients than in-patient lists. Opportunities for inefficiencies and delays are therefore greater.
- If the organization of these lists is retained in the general office, the problems are compounded. Day surgery staff can not only plan, but anticipate and respond more quickly to organizational difficulties.
- The surgeon therefore loses some of his traditional operational control, but gains in having guaranteed lists arranged according to his preferences.

### PATIENT MANAGEMENT

The major differences between day surgery and in-patient management relate to the management of the patient outside the operating theatre, particularly in:

- Patient selection
- Patient information
- Preoperative assessment
- Hospital discharge
- Follow-up.

All these functions have evolved empirically in hospitals, and are usually organized by a variety of staff over several days and at several sites within the hospital.

Surgeons spend too little time in the day centre to be able to organize all this themselves. In addition:

- Different surgeons of differing grades will place different emphasis on various aspects of these processes: important information and advice may therefore be forgotten, leading to further complications and inefficiencies.
- Protocols governing all these matters need to be set up by clinicians and must relate to specific operative procedures.

## DAY SURGERY NURSES

The range of surgical and nursing specialities in most day centres is wide. Rather than employing traditional nurses with restricted skills many units have invested in training nurses to become **proficient in many skills**, e.g. theatre and anaesthetic assistance, recovery, administration, audit, designing protocols.

## PREOPERATIVE WORK-UP

### REFERRAL

Successful day surgery starts well before the day of operation.

- Care must be taken in selecting the correct patients and ensuring that the patient is both physically and mentally attuned to his/her treatment prior to its implementation.
- Some centres may have facilities for performing urgent surgery (e.g. hand trauma, ERPCs): these patients may be referred directly to the day surgery centre from the Accident and Emergency department.
- Some centres practise direct referrals from the GPs. This usually works best for minor procedures requiring local anaesthetic only – skin lesions, lipomas, ingrowing toenails, etc.

The administrative staff in the day centre send for the patients. Patients undergoing general anaesthetic procedures will need to attend for a pre-assessment visit. This pre-assessment visit allows:

- Suitability of the patient to be confirmed
- The operation to be explained in much greater detail
- A firm booking to be made at a time convenient for the patient.

## SUITABILITY

At the pre-assessment visit, patients are interviewed by a trained day surgery nurse. A care document is completed in which medical suitability is confirmed with reference to an appropriate algorithm (Figure 20.1).

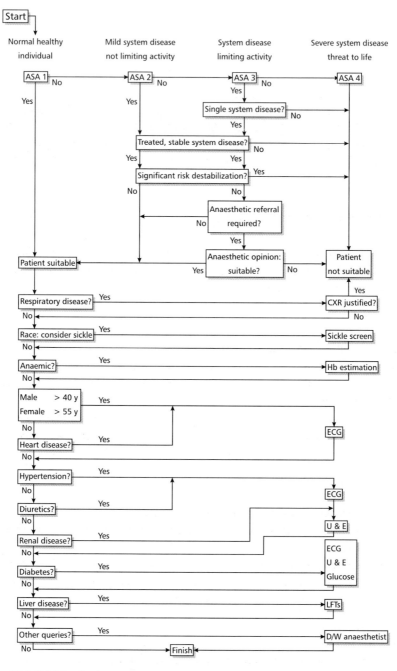

**Figure 20.1** Selection for day case surgery

## BOOKING AND PATIENT INFORMATION

Assuming the patient is deemed suitable, the patient is booked on to an appropriate list.

## PATIENT INFORMATION

This is very important: an uninformed patient will be more anxious, require more analgesia and is more likely to suffer from post-operative complications.

Most centres provide **written patient information,** but this must be supplemented by detailed discussion between the patient and the pre-assessment nurse at the time of their preoperative visit. The patient information leaflet should cover two aspects of day surgery – **a general overview** of what is likely to happen to the patient on the day of admission and **additional information which is procedure-specific,** i.e. related to their laparoscopic sterilization, varicose vein operation or arthroscopy. Some centres find it useful to use in-house videos which also cover common patient experiences.

## THE DAY OF OPERATION

The patients arrive at the day centre, having bathed and bringing with them their usual medication. If they are undergoing general anaesthesia they will not have eaten for 4 hours prior to admission.

## PREOPERATIVE CHECK

- The patient is checked on to the ward by the admitting nurse.
- The patient is visited by both the anaesthetist and surgeon, who will confirm the procedure to be performed, mark the site and arrange for the patient to sign a consent form for the operation.
- Post-operative pain relief is very important and this is often best dealt with before the operation. Many centres recommend the use of NSAIDs, usually in suppository form, either just before or after induction of anaesthesia.

## THE OPERATION

- The operative procedure will be similar to that performed in a main theatre setting.
- **Local anaesthetic** is infiltrated into wound sites to enable the patient to recover free of pain.
- Anaesthetic techniques allow for **rapid reversal** of sedation and concomitant reduction in recovery time. There has been an increase in the use of **sedoanalgesic** techniques and the use of the **laryngeal mask.**

## RECOVERY

The same criteria for recovery apply in day centres as for main theatres. Patients must be fully awake, alert and physiologically stable prior to returning to the ward area.

## DISCHARGE HOME

Once back in the ward, the patient recuperates and is usually given a light snack. Once seen by the operating surgeon and anaesthetist, the decision for discharge is frequently made by the ward nurse on the basis of a previously agreed protocol (Figure 20.2).

This ensures that the patient is fit enough to go home, fully understands the post-operative instructions and is aware of what to do in case of any post-operative problems.

## POST-OPERATIVE RECOVERY

- The speed of post-operative recovery will depend in part on the operative procedure performed and in part on the physical and mental state of the patient.
- All patients should eat and drink normally but avoid alcohol for the first few days.
- They should mobilize regularly, accepting that recovery occurs in fits and starts, and they will feel better some days than others.
- All centres prescribe post-operative analgesia for patients to take **regularly**. This is an important point, as the **aim is to prevent severe pain developing**, rather than treating it once it has occurred.
- A **contact number** should be available to all patients to phone in case of an emergency. Most queries can be answered over the phone and adequate reassurance given. If needed, day surgery staff can arrange for immediate contact of the patient with the relevant specialist surgeon.

> It should not be necessary for the patient to have to contact the community medical staff, be they general practitioners or nurses, other than for the removal of sutures.

## QUALITY ASSESSMENT

The number of patients treated in most centres is large, and continues to rise year by year. It is therefore very important to ensure that certain checks are built into the management process to monitor the quality of care that patients receive.

**Audit** of performance is therefore mandatory and should look at all aspects of patient care and safety. Topics should include:

- Wound infection rates
- Complication rates
- Admission to hospital rates
- Impact on the community
- Patient satisfaction questionnaires.

## DISCHARGE

The patient–

|  | YES | NO |
|---|---|---|
| 1. Has stable BP and pulse | | |
| 2. Can swallow and cough | | |
| 3. Can walk without feeling sick | | |
| 4. Has minimal nausea | | |
| 5. Can breath comfortably and exhibits no sign of respiratory distress | | |
| 6. Is fully conscious and orientated | | |
| 7. Has passed urine (where relevant) | | |
| 8. Has had something to eat or drink | | |
| 9. Has satisfactory operation site | | |
| 10. Has been given post-operative instructions and guidance (if ROS required, ensure advice given re: Practice Nurse) | | |
| 11. Has had post-operative drugs prescribed if required | | |
| 12. Has all appropriate discharge letters | | |
| 13. Is aware of outpatients follow-up if required | | |
| 14. Has a responsible adult to escort him / her home | | |
| 15. Has someone at home 24 hours | | |
| 16. Has completed patient satisfaction questionnaire (if relevant) | | |

SIGN ☐      PRINT NAME ☐

**Figure 20.2** Discharge protocol

## TEACHING AND TRAINING

The practice of day surgery differs sufficiently from that of in-patient surgery that it necessitates its own teaching and training. This includes the relevant skills required of junior anaesthetists and surgeons, as well as the variety of skills required of the nursing staff. In addition, the transfer of surgical activity from in-patient wards to day centres for much minor and intermediate elective surgical work is having an enormous impact on traditional surgical training of medical students. It is therefore equally important that medical students are welcomed into day surgery centres as part of their clinical training.

## THE FUTURE

- Day surgery has had an enormous impact on hospital surgical practice.
- New surgical, anaesthetic and nursing techniques will continue to be developed.
- Day surgery will continue to expand.
- Lessons learned from day surgery will be applied to in-patient surgery over the next decade.

---

**CRIB BOX – DAY SURGERY**

**Fifty per cent of elective surgery** is now performed in dedicated units

**Case selection is paramount** with patients with significant medical problems or those with anaesthetic risk excluded

**New anaesthetic techniques** and analgesic policies have broadened its usage

**Pre-assessment** clinics are important

**Sociodomestic** conditions must be suitable

**Senior** surgeons and anaesthetists must undertake the procedure

# chapter 21

# MINIMAL ACCESS SURGERY

## DEFINITION

The basic principle of minimal access surgery is to achieve a therapeutic objective by the least physiologically disturbing stimulus.

These procedures are practised by surgeons but also by physicians, endoscopists and radiologists.

## HISTORY

- Semm, a gynaecologist, performed the first laparoscopic appendicectomy in 1983.
- In the 1970s and 1980s gastroenterologists and radiologists developed ERCP, percutaneous cholangiography and percutaneous drainage of collections under ultrasound or CT scan guidance.
- The first reported laparoscopic cholecystectomy was performed by Muhe in 1986.

**Common characteristics of all minimally invasive procedures are:**
- They are performed with the aid of specially designed instruments that are inserted into natural lumens or cavities or through small keyhole incisions.
- Some form of imaging is used in the form of a direct vision scope (rigid or flexible), a video-endoscope or ultrasound/CT imaging.

The operations may be performed entirely with minimally invasive techniques, as in laparoscopic cholecystectomy (Figure 21.1), or part of the operation may require the creation of an incision and the application of open techniques (e.g. laparoscopic colectomy): so-called 'laparoscopically assisted procedures'.

Depending on the anatomical area and the approach, minimal access surgery may be classified as:
- Laparoscopic (cholecystectomy, appendicectomy, etc.)
- Endoluminal (sphincterotomy, polypectomy, etc.)
- Thoracoscopic (sympathectomy, etc.)
- Retroperitoneoscopic (nephrectomy, etc.)
- Radiological (nephrostomy, etc.)
- Mixed (combined PTC-ERCP for bypassing bile duct stricture).

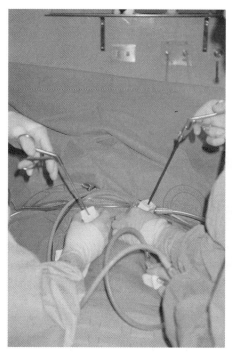

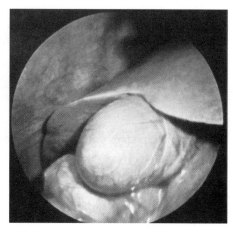

**Figure 21.1** Laparoscopic cholecystectomy: (a) general view; (b) laparoscopic view of gall bladder

(a)                                                                  (b)

### Advantages of minimal access surgery
- Less metabolic stress
- Fewer post-operative respiratory problems
- Reduction of wound infections
- Reduced length of hospitalization for many procedures as well as shorter time of home convalescence.

### Disadvantages of minimal access surgery
- There is evidence that laparoscopic hernia repair has a higher recurrence rate than the Lichtenstein open mesh repair.
- Reports concerning implantation of tumour at port sites have raised concern about the safety of laparoscopic surgery in patients with cancer.
- The benefit of an operation might be outweighed by the dangers, e.g. performing diagnostic laparoscopy in the obese or with a large midline incisional hernia.

## LAPAROSCOPIC SURGERY

The following equipment is necessary:

1 The rigid laparoscope
2 The computer chip camera
3 Two video monitors (Figure 21.2)

4  A light source (Figure 21.2)
5  A gas insufflator (Figure 21.2) which is at the same time a gas reservoir and a device that automatically controls the flow to keep intra-abdominal pressure constant
6  Trocars of appropriate diameter (10 mm for the camera, 5 mm for most dissecting instruments and diathermy, 12 mm for the endo-clip applicator, larger for other instruments such as staplers)
7  Laparoscopic instruments (depending on the operation); dissecting and grasping forceps, endoscopic scissors, hook diathermy, endoscopic clip applicators, tissue-holding forceps, laparoscopic knotting devices, staplers and many others
8  Suction and irrigation.

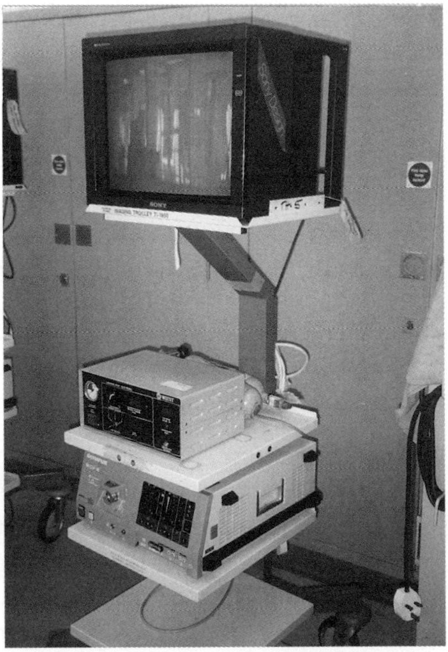

Equipment malfunction and particularly poor video picture quality increases the risk of complications.

**Figure 21.2** Gas insufflator, light source and monitor for laparoscopic operation

### Preoperative preparation
- Conversion to open operation should be explained to the patient and the consent signed appropriately.
- Preoperative haematological, biochemical, radiological and other investigations are carried out as indicated by the patient's fitness.
- Pre- and intraoperative antibiotics are prescribed with the same indications as with open procedures.
- Antithrombotic prophylaxis with subcutaneous heparin and thromboembolism deterrent (TED) stockings.

### Pneumoperitoneum
- Distension of the abdomen with gas is necessary to allow visualization of the viscera and manipulation of the instruments without the risk of accidental injury.
- An alternative technique which avoids the use of gas – abdominal wall retraction – is not widely practised in the UK at present.

  There are two ways to create a pneumoperitoneum:

1  **The Veress needle** technique. A special hollow needle with a spring-loaded blunt end to protect the viscera is inserted blindly immediately below the umbilicus. Once safely inserted, gas flow is commenced.
2  **The Hasson 'open technique'** using a blunt trocar avoids the complications of blind puncture.

The pneumoperitoneum is created through the port and after insertion of the camera the rest of the trocars are placed under direct vision from within the abdomen.

- Several gases ($CO_2$, helium, nitrous oxide, etc.) have been tried but $CO_2$ is the preferred one since it is not flammable and, although it is absorbed, usually its homeostasis is successfully regulated by the body.
- Prolonged pneumoperitoneum with $CO_2$ may occasionally result in hypercapnia and reduced pH, vascular collapse or diffuse vasodilatation. Gas embolism has been reported but it is usually subclinical.
- Intraperitoneal pressure is kept between 10 and 15 mmHg during the operation. Higher pressures may result in increased right shoulder pain (from phrenic nerve stimulation) and cardiorespiratory problems.

### Post-operative course

- **Post-operative pain is much less after laparoscopy** than after laparotomy and is mainly in the form of mild abdominal discomfort and right shoulder pain which is easily controlled with oral analgesics.
- Respiration is not inhibited by pain and since mobilization usually is immediate, respiratory complications are rare.
- The stomach and small bowel regain their motility rapidly and most patients can tolerate fluids initially and then food 3–6 hours later.
- Early mobilization reduces the risk of deep venous thrombosis and pulmonary embolism.
- Pneumoperitoneum creates a degree of venous stasis in the legs during the procedure – intermittent calf compression and subcutaneous heparin are indicated.
- Wound infections are much rarer than with open procedures but they still occur, especially at umbilical wounds.

### Complications

Laparoscopic surgery is not free of complications. They can, however, be minimized by ruling out patients with contraindications for laparoscopy and ensuring that surgeons are formally trained in the method. Table 21.1 lists the main contraindications.

**Table 21.1** Contraindications for laparoscopic surgery

| Absolute | Relative |
| --- | --- |
| Intestinal obstruction | Morbid obesity |
| Generalized peritonitis | Ascites |
| Abdominal wall infection | Extensive prior abdominal surgery |
| Coagulopathy | Large umbilical hernia |

- The most serious complication is injury of the bowel or a major vessel (aorta, vena cava, iliac vessels) at the time of creation of the pneumoperitoneum on blind insertion of the trocar.
- This can be prevented by using the open technique with the blunt trocar and by avoiding puncture near surgical scars where small bowel adheres.
- Injury of the bladder is prevented by temporary catheterization.
- A nasogastric tube prevents puncture of a distended stomach.

Usually all injuries can be repaired without major consequences if they are recognized. **Disasters occur from unrecognized injuries:**

- Subcutaneous, preperitoneal or omental emphysema results from misplacement of the Veress needle.
- **Tension pneumoperitoneum** occurs if $CO_2$ pressure rises above 30 mmHg.
- **Hypercapnia and acidosis** may develop occasionally from excessive $CO_2$ absorption.
- In laparoscopic cholecystectomy where **diathermy** is used to remove the gall bladder, injuries occur from accidental contact of the hook diathermy with other instruments or clips.
- Unrecognized injury of the epigastric vessels at the sites of the trocars may result in post-operative bleeding.
- Intraoperative **bleeding** is a complication that can occur during any laparoscopic procedure and may itself lead to further complications. If it is not controlled easily, multiple clip application and excessive use of diathermy may result in injuries of adjacent structures.
- A worrying late complication that has been recently reported is **port site implantation of malignant tumours**. This has raised concern that laparoscopic surgery may not be safe for patients with abdominal cancer.
- Incisional hernias, although uncommon, have been reported at trocar sites.

## LAPAROSCOPIC OPERATIONS IN GENERAL SURGERY

Almost every operation in general surgery has been attempted laparoscopically.

- A few have become rapidly established and largely replaced the open procedure, e.g. laparoscopic cholecystectomy.
- Others, such as laparoscopic adrenalectomy and fundoplication, are performed in specialized centres.
- A third group of operations such as laparoscopic pancreatectomy and hepatectomy have been performed in isolated cases but face strong scientific and ethical objections.
- The wide spectrum of minimally invasive surgery is shown in Table 21.2.

**Table 21.2** Common minimally invasive surgery procedures

| **Laparoscopic** | **Retroperitoneoscopic** |
|---|---|
| Cholecystectomy | Nephrectomy |
| Common bile duct exploration | Pyeloplasty |
| Inguinal hernia repair | |
| Appendicectomy | **Vascular** |
| Colectomy | Stenting of aortic aneurysm |
| Splenectomy | Endoscopic angiosurgery |
| Nissen's fundoplication | |
| Rectopexy | **Endoscopic** |
| Vagotomy/seromyotomy | ERCP: sphincterotomy and stenting |
| Gastrojejunostomy | Polypectomy |
| Ileostomy/colostomy | Palliative laser resection of tumours |
| Diagnostic laparoscopy (trauma, sepsis) | |

**Thoracoscopic**

Sympathectomy
Pulmonary resection
Heller's myotomy
Pericardial window
Correction of congenital anomalies

# LAPAROSCOPIC CHOLECYSTECTOMY

- Laparoscopic cholecystectomy is the operation most commonly performed today by general surgeons.
- Indications for surgery are:
  - Chronic uncomplicated cholelithiasis
  - Acute cholecystitis
  - Empyema
  - Common bile duct stones.
- Today only small contracted calcified gall bladders and pericholecystic abscesses are absolute contraindications.
- 2–10% of procedures started laparoscopically are converted to open operations, for various reasons.

### Preoperative assessment
- Ultrasound scan of the liver/biliary tree
- Liver function tests
- Preoperative ERCP (Figure 21.3) to confirm the presence of the stones and allow endoscopic extraction before cholecystectomy. (The alternative is to perform an intraoperative cholangiogram during laparoscopic cholecystectomy.)
- If ductal stones are confirmed, then **laparoscopic common bile duct exploration** or **conversion to open** exploration can be performed.

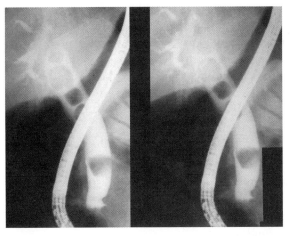

**Figure 21.3** ERCP showing common bile duct stones

**Post-operative period**

Recovery is rapid. Hospital stay is usually 24–48 hours as opposed to 5–7 days for the open procedure, and some centres do selected patients as day cases.

**Complications**

- The most serious injury is to the extra-hepatic bile ducts.
- This may produce a leak of bile which leads to **biliary peritonitis** or **complete or partial obstruction** of the bile duct.
- This presents in the immediate post-operative period with **obstructive jaundice** or weeks to months later with **cholangitis**.
- One cause of such injuries may be unrecognized **anatomical anomalies** of the bile ducts or **distortion** of normal anatomy by traction.
- Bile duct injuries occur during **open cholecystectomy** with a frequency of 0.2–0.3% (Figure 21.4). The incidence was undoubtedly higher when laparoscopic cholecystectomy was first introduced and has subsequently fallen to 0.3%. It is hoped that improvements in technique, instrumentation and training will reduce the scale of this problem still further.

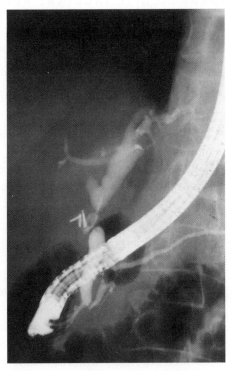

**Figure 21.4** ERCP of ductal injury following laparoscopic cholecystectomy

## LAPAROSCOPIC APPENDICECTOMY

- The mesentery and the appendix are ligated using either an endoscopic loop or an endoscopic stapler and the appendix is retrieved in a bag.
- The value of laparoscopic appendicectomy is greater if there is uncertainty about the diagnosis (the negative appendicectomy rate is approximately 20%).

## LAPAROSCOPIC NISSEN'S FUNDOPLICATION

- The indication is hiatus hernia and severe oesophagitis unresponsive to medical treatment.
- The principles of the technique are:
  - Mobilization of the gastric fundus
  - Suturing of the diaphragmatic crura
  - Wrapping of the fundus around a 50 mm bougie.
- It is a cost-effective operation when compared with long-term proton pump inhibitor therapy, but requires advanced laparoscopic skills and training.
- The most serious complication is perforation of the oesophagus.

## LAPAROSCOPIC INGUINAL HERNIA

- This may be performed intra- or preperitoneally.
- After the pneumoperitoneum or preperitoneal space has been created, the hernial sac is visualized.
- The sac is dissected and a **mesh** is applied to the defect and either fixed with staples on to the pubic tubercle and Cooper's ligament or held in the preperitoneal space.
- **Complications** include bleeding, bladder injury, femoral nerve injury and intestinal obstruction.
- Laparoscopic repair is not widely accepted in the UK because it carries a **higher recurrence rate** than the open techniques and is **expensive.**
- Its main indications are **bilateral and recurrent hernias.**

## LAPAROSCOPIC COLECTOMY

- Indications are benign conditions (inflammatory bowel disease, polyposis, diverticular disease) or colonic cancer.
- Dissection is performed as with the open procedure with recognition of the ureters and removal of the mesenteric lymph nodes.
- The anastomosis is fashioned either **extracorporeally** through a small incision or **intracorporeally** with the endoscopic stapler.
- Port site recurrences have been reported. These are believed to occur because of **spillage of cancer cells** and **increased intraperitoneal pressure** that leads to malignant cells being implanted along the port tracks.

## THORACOSCOPIC SYMPATHECTOMY

- Performed for hyperhidrosis of the hands and axillae.
- It entails visualization of the thoracic ganglion chain and ablation of T2–T3 ganglia with diathermy (Figure 21.5).
- Care must be taken to avoid T1 damage which will result in **Horner's syndrome.**
- Other complications include pneumothorax and compensatory hyperhidrosis of the trunk.

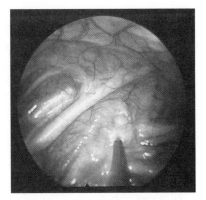

**Figure 21.5** Thoracoscopic sympathectomy

## THE FUTURE OF MINIMAL ACCESS SURGERY

- Well-established procedures such as laparoscopy, ERCP, thoracoscopy, percutaneous drainage of collections, angioplasty, etc., will continue.
- Operations such as Nissen's fundoplication, rectopexy, common bile duct exploration will be performed in specialist centres.
- Since minimal access surgery was developed, smaller cameras and instruments have given birth to **needlescopic surgery**, which allows removal of the gall bladder through three incisions of 1.7 mm.
- The combination of lasers with microscopic angioscopes may reduce the number of vascular bypasses.
- Aortic stenting is developing and may replace the majority of elective open aortic aneurysm repairs.
- Laparoscopic ultrasound as a diagnostic aid to laparoscopy may obviate exploratory laparotomies, particularly for cancer staging.
- Robots as camera men may replace trained assistants if they prove cost-effective.
- **Virtual reality** and **telepresence** may soon give the opportunity to the surgeon to visualize the abdominal cavity and operate on patients thousands of miles away.

## CRIB BOX – MINIMAL ACCESS SURGERY

**Principle** – to achieve the therapeutic objective with the least physiologically disturbing stimulus and with minimal physiological consequences

### Methods

- Specially designed equipment/instruments
- Some form of imaging
- Specialized personnel

### Wide spectrum

- Laparoscopic
- Retroperitoneoscopic
- Thoracoscopic
- Endoluminal
- Endovascular
- Radiological
- Combined

### Advantages

- Less trauma
- Fewer metabolic consequences
- Fewer post-operative complications
- Shorter hospitalization

### Disadvantages

- Expensive technology
- Increased need for sub-specialization
- Iatrogenic complications when performed by poorly trained surgeons

**Future** – a significant percentage of open operations will probably be permanently replaced by minimally invasive procedures

# chapter 22

# PAEDIATRIC SURGERY

General surgical pathology in infants and children is relatively common and can arise because of a pre-existing congenital or developmental defect (e.g. hernias). Surgical problems in neonates are much less common. For example, congenital oesophageal atresia and duodenal atresia have a frequency of around 1 in 3000–5000 births compared with a frequency of about 1 in 250 births for pyloric stenosis.

## HERNIAS

Umbilical (Figure 22.1) and **inguinal** are the most common hernias in children and both have their origin in developmental anomalies.

### UMBILICAL HERNIA

- In the early weeks after birth there is potential for hernia formation through the umbilical scar.
- An active fibrous reaction after birth obliterates the umbilical vessels. If this process is incomplete, herniation of underlying omentum and bowel may occur.
- Umbilical hernias are most obvious when the child cries or strains.
- They **rarely** become irreducible or obstructed.
- The defect can be felt easily with the fingertip – its diameter can predict those that will close spontaneously and those that will need surgery.
- **90% of those with a defect under 1 cm** in diameter at presentation will **close before the first birthday**.
- There is a clear racial predilection for children of **Afro-Caribbean** origin although the reason is not known.
- Rarely, umbilical hernias are associated with congenital hypothyroidism.

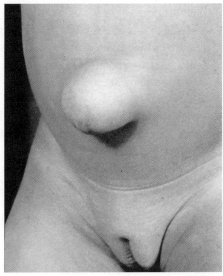

**Figure 22.1** Umbilical hernia (Courtesy of The Wellcome Trust)

## INGUINAL HERNIA

- **Always indirect** in children and traverse the deep and superficial inguinal rings.
- Boys are more often affected than girls (5:1).
- Hernias are more frequent in the premature.
- Rarely, inguinal hernias are due to a sustained higher intra-abdominal pressure (e.g. liver disease, ascites and cystic fibrosis).
- **Irreducibility is a serious sign** and should prompt an attempt at reduction under sedation (**taxis**) or, if this fails, urgent surgical repair.
- Inguinal hernia repair in children differs from that in adults – the hernia sac is separated from the vas and testicular vessels and simply excised at the internal ring (i.e. **inguinal herniotomy** only).

# CONGENITAL HYPERTROPHIC PYLORIC STENOSIS

This condition arises **some weeks after birth** and is characterized by **hypertrophy and hyperplasia of the smooth muscle of the pylorus** that causes gastric outlet obstruction.
- The aetiology is unclear although there is a definite genetic predisposition.
- The male to female ratio is about 4:1 and there may be a predisposition for the first-born.
- The frequency of pyloric stenosis is 1 in 250 births.

### Clinical features
- Symptoms usually arise at **2–3 weeks** of age in otherwise normal infants.
- Gastric outlet obstruction and work hypertrophy of the stomach causes vomiting which is forceful and **projectile** but **WITHOUT BILE**.
- The baby feeds hungrily but vomits soon after, producing weight loss and dehydration.
- The diagnosis is established by observing gastric peristalsis and **palpating the hypertrophied pyloric 'tumour'**. This is felt just to the right of the midline and has the size and consistency of a small olive.
- Palpation is most easily achieved by feeding the infant and hence relaxing the abdominal wall.
- Gastric outlet obstruction results in loss of water and HCl. This causes dehydration and **hypochloraemic metabolic alkalosis** with a high serum bicarbonate and low chloride.
- The electrolyte disturbance and dehydration need correcting with intravenous **saline** before surgery. Usually about 24 hours of rehydration and restitution of electrolyte imbalance is needed.
- A nasogastric tube keeps the stomach empty.

---

**IMPORTANT LESSON**
The biochemistry of pyloric stenosis (adult or infantile) is a common examination question. Remember '**dehydration and hypochloraemic alkalosis with an inappropriate acid urine**'. Now look it up in a biochemistry textbook.

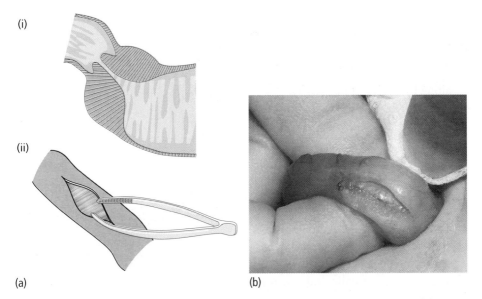

(i)

(ii)

(a)                                              (b)

**Figure 22.2** Ramstedt's pyloromyotomy: (a) (i) hypertrophic pyloric stenosis; (ii) splitting of the hypertrophied pyloric smooth muscle (Ramstedt's operation); (b) operative photograph

### Surgery

- The condition is treated with a **Ramstedt's pyloromyotomy** (Figure 22.2).
- There are a number of possible surgical approaches to the pylorus in these infants, but the most commonly used is a small transverse right upper quadrant incision.
- A longitudinal incision into the pylorus splits the hypertrophied muscle but leaves the mucosa intact and relieves the gastric outlet obstruction.
- This is virtually certain to cure the vomiting and is seldom associated with further problems.

## INTUSSUSCEPTION

- In this condition one portion of the bowel **invaginates** into an adjacent distal portion and is carried along by waves of peristalsis (Figure 22.3).
- Any part of the mobile and unfixed gastrointestinal tract can be involved. Most commonly it is the terminal ileum which intussuscepts into the ascending and transverse colon.
- It occurs in infants between **6 months and 2 years** and is probably precipitated by swelling of lymphoid tissue (**Peyer's patches**) in the distal ileum caused by viral infection.
- Intussusception causes **small bowel obstruction** and, furthermore, because the mesenteric vessels are also intussuscepted and compressed **the invaginated bowel rapidly becomes ischaemic**.

- Intussusception in infants is invariably idiopathic (primary). Secondary causes involve an intrinsic anomaly of the bowel mucosa that starts the invagination process by being caught up and swept along by waves of peristalsis.

The classification of intussusception in shown in Table 22.1.

### Clinical features

- It presents typically in an overweight baby who has recently been weaned.
- The infant develops sudden, severe abdominal colic and inconsolable screaming episodes.
- The episodes of colic and screaming occur every 10–15 minutes and cause great distress to the mother and child.

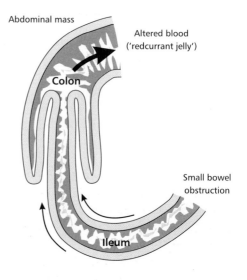

**Figure 22.3** Intussusception. The lead point in the terminal ileum prolapses within the adjacent ascending colon

**Table 22.1** Classification of intussusception

|  | Age group | Underlying cause |
|---|---|---|
| Primary | Infants | Hyperplasia in Peyer's patches |
| Secondary | All ages | Meckel's diverticulum |
|  |  | Lymphoma |
|  |  | Polyps (e.g. Peutz–Jegher's syndrome) |
|  |  | Henoch–Schönlein purpura |
|  |  | Duplication cysts |

- Blood and mucus are passed per rectum ('**redcurrant jelly stool**') due to congestion and infarction of the intussuscepted bowel mucosa.
- It is often possible to feel the intussusception as a '**sausage-shaped**' **mass** in the upper abdomen (Figure 22.4). Rarely, the apex of bowel protrudes through the anus with all the appearances of a rectal prolapse.

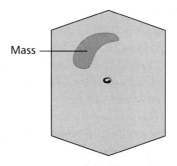

**Figure 22.4** Sausage-shaped mass of intussusception in an infant

**Abdominal ultrasound** may show the soft tissue mass which in cross-section has a 'target'

appearance and a **barium enema** shows the filling defect within the colon. The contrast outlines the gap between the two layers of bowel giving a **'watch'** or **'clock spring'** appearance.

### Treatment

There are two complementary methods of management – **hydrostatic reduction and/or surgery.**

- An air or barium enema under radiological screening control (Figure 22.5) can reduce the intussusception with hydrostatic pressure. Successful reduction is demonstrated by reflux of contrast into the terminal ileum. Recurrence of the intussusception is rare, probably because oedema of the bowel wall initially and subsequent adhesions maintain the reduction.
- Surgery is needed for failed reduction enemas and complicated cases. Occasionally bowel resection is required if the intussuscepted bowel has perforated or infarcted.

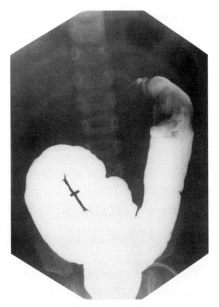

**Figure 22.5** Radiological appearance of contrast enema in intussusception. There is a filling defect within the splenic flexure and contrast is being forced between two layers of intussuscepted bowel wall

## MECKEL'S DIVERTICULUM

- This is an embryological remnant of the **vitello-intestinal duct** which represents the midpoint and apex of the fetal midgut (Figure 22.6).
- Normally the duct from the umbilicus to the gut obliterates before birth.
- Rarely, it remains wholly patent, producing a **faecal fistula** at the umbilicus.
- More commonly the proximal portion stays patent to produce a Meckel's diverticulum of variable length in the terminal ileum.
- It is a **true** diverticulum which arises from the **anti-mesenteric border** of the ileum and is composed of all three layers of bowel wall.
- It is lined by intestinal mucosa, sometimes with islands of **ectopic gastric or pancreatic tissue.** A **peptic ulcer** (with attendant complications) may arise adjacent to islands of gastric acid-producing cells.
- Occasionally a fibrous cord connects the tip of the diverticulum to the umbilicus.

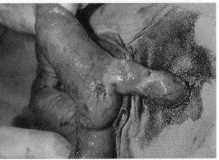

**Figure 22.6** Meckel's diverticulum

## Clinical features

- Most Meckel's are uncomplicated and asymptomatic.
- They may become **inflamed** and mimic acute appendicitis.
- They may **perforate** to give rise to peritonitis.
- Ectopic gastric mucosa can cause recurrent post-prandial pain and **gastrointestinal bleeding** due to peptic ulceration.
- The diverticulum can form the lead point of a secondary **intussusception**.
- **Volvulus** can occur around the fibrous cord if present.

> **Meckel's diverticulum**
>
> - 2% of population
> - 2 inches long
> - 2 feet from ileocaecal valve

# INTESTINAL OBSTRUCTION OF THE NEWBORN

All babies may regurgitate or vomit a little of their feed – this is normal. **Vomiting which is bile-stained is caused by intestinal obstruction.** Although rare, intestinal obstruction in the neonate presents in the same way as at any other age with:

- **Vomiting** – bile-stained
- **Dehydration** – depressed fontanelle; oliguria; inelastic skin
- **Abdominal distension** – gross if the obstruction is low; minimal if it is high
- **Absolute constipation** – failure to pass meconium within 18 hours of birth.

In addition, **visible peristalsis** is often very obvious.

The most important investigation is a plain abdominal x-ray; the position of gas and fluid levels in the bowel indicating the site of obstruction.

The most common causes of neonatal intestinal obstruction are **malrotation, Hirschsprung's disease, meconium ileus, intestinal atresia and anorectal atresia.**

## MALROTATION OF THE MIDGUT (VOLVULUS NEONATORUM)

### Embryology

- The gastrointestinal tract is divided into three parts, **the foregut, the midgut and the hindgut,** corresponding to the vascular territory of the coeliac trunk, the superior mesenteric and the inferior mesenteric arteries, respectively.
- During the first few weeks of organ development the midgut loop leaves the abdominal cavity at the umbilicus, forced out by the rapidly enlarging liver.
- On its return, it rotates in an anticlockwise direction (180°) so that the distal part (what will become the transverse colon) is now above the proximal part (the third and fourth parts of the duodenum).
- There is then a final 90° of rotation when the caecum and ileocaecal segment descends down the right paracolic gutter to lie in the right iliac fossa.

The commonest variant of malrotation occurs when this final 90° descent fails to happen.

- **The caecum lies high in the right upper quadrant next to a right-of-midline duodeno-jejunal (DJ) flexure.** The resulting narrow mesenteric midgut base produces an intrinsically unstable arrangement of bowel that is liable to twisting (**volvulus**).

### Clinical features
- About half of all malrotations will present within the first week of life.
- The **duodenum is obstructed**, either from thickened peritoneal bands of connective tissue (**Ladd's bands**) traversing it from the caecum or from kinking and twisting as it goes into the midgut loop.
- Failure to establish feeds and **bile vomiting** are the predominant symptoms.
- The midgut is at risk of **ischaemia** and **infarction** if a volvulus has occurred and to these symptoms will be added the signs of an **abdominal catastrophe** (shock, collapse, generalized abdominal tenderness and eventually peritonitis).
- The diagnosis of malrotation can be made by a contrast **meal and follow-through** which will show the dilated duodenum, a right-sided DJ flexure and right-sided jejunal loops.
- An **abdominal ultrasound** may also be suggestive as it can show the abnormal positions of the superior mesenteric artery and vein.

### Surgery
The principles of surgery are:
- Untwist any volvulus.
- Correct duodenal obstruction by dividing Ladd's bands.
- Prevent any future tendency to twist by separation of the two limbs of the midgut loop and completely un-rotate the bowel.

This ensures that all the large bowel then lies on the left and all the small bowel on the right (**Ladd's operation**). The appendix will, of course, then be a left-sided organ and this **information should always be given to the parents.**

## HIRSCHSPRUNG'S DISEASE

Harald Hirschsprung, a Danish paediatrician, described the clinical features of this disease in 1886, although the characteristic histological features were not recognized until later (Figure 22.7).

### Pathology
- 1 in 5000 infants and children.
- The characteristic histological feature of Hirschsprung's disease is **an absence of ganglion cells in the submucosa of the intestine.**
- This leads to a **propulsive failure** of the distal bowel and a functional bowel obstruction.
- Ganglion cells are an integral component of the

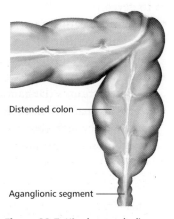

Distended colon

Aganglionic segment

**Figure 22.7** Hirschsprung's disease

enteric nervous system and originate from neural crest epithelium lying adjacent to the embryonic neural tube.

- Before birth, such cells migrate distally along the gastrointestinal tract towards its caudal end.
- In Hirschsprung's disease, this migration fails and **the distal bowel remains aganglionic and dysfunctional**.
- The affected segment is usually the **rectum and distal sigmoid** although in severe cases the whole of the colon is involved.
- The normal ganglionic bowel responds to the functional distal obstruction by work hypertrophy and dilatation. The normal ganglionic bowel, therefore, appears **abnormal** whereas the aganglionic segment looks normal.

### Clinical features

Hirschsprung's disease presents:

- In the **neonatal period** as an acute intestinal obstruction, with failure to pass meconium.
- In **childhood** with severe, persistent constipation.
- In **older children**; constipation has usually dated from infancy and is resistant to all laxative regimens. The abdomen is distended, often with gross enlargement of the proximal colon.

A **barium enema** in both neonates and children may show a marked 'transition' zone between ganglionic and aganglionic bowel but should not be regarded as diagnostic (Figure 22.8). **Formal biopsy and histological examination** of the rectal mucosa and submucosa must be performed and confirms aganglionosis.

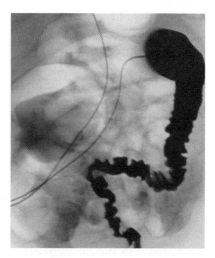

### Treatment

- A defunctioning colostomy proximal to the aganglionic segment allows an infant to develop normally.
- Definitive treatment at a later date requires surgical excision of the affected aganglionic bowel (usually recto-sigmoidectomy) and a so-called 'pull-through' reconstruction (**Duhamel operation**) where normal proximal ganglionic bowel is pulled through the anal sphincter and anastomosed to the anorectum.

**Figure 22.8** Barium enema in a newborn with Hirschsprung's disease. There is a radiological 'transition' zone in the descending colon between normal and ganglionic but dilated bowel, and aganglionic but non-dilated bowel

## MECONIUM ILEUS

- This is the neonatal manifestation of cystic fibrosis (fibrocystic disease; mucoviscidosis).

- It occurs in about 10% of neonates affected with CF.
- The terminal ileum is **obstructed** by viscid putty-like meconium.
- The obstruction may be complicated by volvulus, gangrene or perforation.
- In uncomplicated cases the sticky meconium can be displaced with Gastrografin enemas administered under radiological control.
- Surgical treatment requires manual removal of the meconium and lavage of the bowel. Gangrenous bowel is resected.
- These children require long-term oral pancreatic enzyme supplements (Pancrex).

## CONGENITAL INTESTINAL ATRESIA

Atresia is defined as **congenital imperforation of a normal channel or opening**. Atresia in the bowel can take the form of a simple stenosis, an obstructing diaphragm, or complete agenesis of segments of intestine.

### Duodenal atresia
- Atresia or stenosis of the duodenum usually occurs distal to the ampulla of Vater (75%).
- The vomit is therefore bile-stained and the upper abdomen distended.
- An erect plain x-ray shows a classical 'double bubble' appearance of air on top of fluid levels in the distended stomach and duodenum (Figure 22.9).
- Volvulus neonatorum can present similarly (due to duodeno-jejunal obstruction).
- There is an association with Down's syndrome.
- Treatment entails bypassing the atresia with a duodeno-duodenostomy.

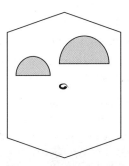

**Figure 22.9** Plain x-ray appearance of duodenal atresia showing 'double bubble'

### Jejuno-Ileal atresia
- Atresia of the small bowel presents similarly to duodenal atresia with bile-stained vomiting.
- There may be one single or multiple segments of atresia with the bowel resembling a string of sausages.
- Treatment involves resection of the underdeveloped segments and anastomosis. This can be difficult due to disparity in size between the proximal grossly distended bowel and the collapsed distal bowel.

## IMPERFORATE ANUS (ANORECTAL ATRESIA)

- 1 in 5000 live births.
- Caused by failure of fusion of the embryological proctodaeum with the rectum (Figure 22.10).
- Two degrees of severity – **low** and **high** atresia.
- The least severe (low) is best described as a **'covered'** anus – a thin membrane which obstructs the passage of meconium can be perforated to produce a fairly normal anus.

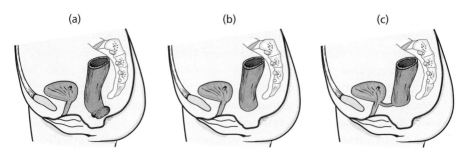

**Figure 22.10** Imperforate anus: 1, low; 2, high; and 3, fistula into bladder

- Almost all high anorectal atresias have a fistulous communication with the next available epithelial surface (vagina in a girl and bladder or urethra in a boy).
- Most high anorectal atresias are treated by initial diversion (e.g. sigmoid colostomy) with a later anorectal reconstruction and division of the fistula.
- Other congenital anomalies are common (particularly renal anomalies).

## OESOPHAGEAL ATRESIA AND TRACHEO-OESOPHAGEAL FISTULA

- Relatively common – 1 in 3000 live births.
- Fetal swallowing of amniotic fluid is impaired so maternal polyhydramnios may develop.
- Presents with swallowing difficulties of own saliva (looks 'mucousy' or 'bubbly') and if feeding is attempted, respiratory distress and cyanosis may occur due to aspiration into the lungs.
- The diagnosis is confirmed by attempted passage of a nasogastric tube which is arrested in the upper oesophagus.
- Gas in the bowel on x-ray demonstrates that the distal oesophagus is connected to the trachea.
- The most common variety is a **blind proximal pouch and distal tracheo-oesophageal fistula** (Figure 22.11).
- There may be other congenital abnormalities.

### Treatment
- Usually instigated within 24 hours to prevent aspiration pneumonia.
- Through a right thoracotomy the two ends of the oesophagus are mobilized and anastomosed with closure of the tracheal fistula.
- Strictures can occur at the suture line at a later date and require dilatation.

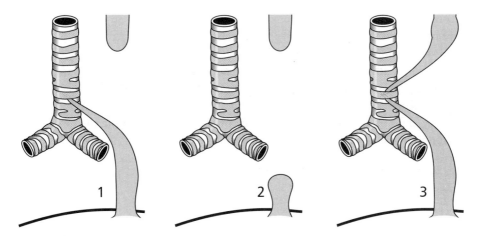

**Figure 22.11** Tracheo-oesophageal fistula: 1, proximal atresia and distal tracheo-oesophageal fistula; 2, long-gap oesophageal atresia and no fistula; and 3, proximal atresia and double fistula

## CONGENITAL DIAPHRAGMATIC HERNIA

- Caused by a defect in development of a hemidiaphragm from the pleuro-peritoneal membrane.
- It occurs normally on the left side; bowel herniates into the chest through the defect (**foramen of Bochdalek**).
- The lung on the affected side is invariably hypoplastic.
- Presentation is neonatal cyanosis and respiratory distress with poor or absent breath sounds on the affected side.
- Chest x-ray confirms the diagnosis.

### Treatment
Surgery to repair the defect is usually undertaken within 2 or 3 days of birth. Malrotation of the gut may be an additional complication.

## ABDOMINAL PAIN IN CHILDREN

Although abdominal pain is common in children, a relatively small proportion have surgical pathology. Only about **70% of all children** admitted to hospital with abdominal pain are eventually shown to have a specific cause (surgical or medical), with about 30% being cases of acute appendicitis.

There are **few specific signs** of serious underlying disease and discrimination can often be very difficult. The younger the child the more difficult it can be for him/her to localize the pain. A number of non-surgical conditions (e.g. tonsillitis, pneumonia) may present with entirely abdominal symptoms. **Pain is frequently** accompanied by vomiting but again this is rarely specific for surgical disease, although the presence of bile is highly suggestive.

An **abdominal examination** in children should always be carried out despite obvious difficulties and reluctance. The examiner should be **gentle, patient and careful** to gain the confidence of the child (and the parent). It is not necessary to do this formally on an examination couch and more information may be gained with the **child on the mother's knee**, lying or even standing facing the mother.

**Abdominal palpation should be slow** and begin well away from the affected area to gain the confidence of the child. Using the child's own hand to palpate is a useful ploy since resistance to movement of the hand will be felt over tender areas.

There are no investigations specific to childhood abdominal pain:

- Urine microscopy and culture should be routine.
- **Abdominal ultrasound** will be diagnostic in intussusception and may be helpful in pelvic pathology (appendicitis or tubo-ovarian disease in teenage girls).
- The most important part of the diagnostic evaluation of abdominal pain in children is simply **admission and re-evaluation** several hours later. Abdominal re-examination will confirm or refute persistent peritoneal signs and allow those of a more non-specific character to settle without the need for surgical exploration.

## MESENTERIC ADENITIS

This is a poorly defined condition that occurs primarily in children and is almost certainly caused by a viral infection. The most striking feature is inflamed and swollen lymph nodes throughout the gut mesentery but particularly in the right iliac fossa. It is of importance simply because it presents like appendicitis.

- The characteristic clinical features are **poorly localized abdominal pain**, with usually right iliac fossa tenderness (but seldom guarding or rigidity) and a **high temperature** (occasionally up to 40°C).
- Often there is a history of recent sore throat or upper respiratory tract infection.
- The child is usually flushed and has **generalized enlarged palpable lymph nodes** (e.g. neck, axillae, groins).
- It is treated with analgesics, antipyretics and serial re-examination to ensure that the abdominal signs have not changed.
- Occasionally surgical exploration via an appendix incision or laparoscopy is necessary to exclude appendicitis. In such cases the appendix is removed.

## CRIB BOX – PAEDIATRIC SURGERY

### Umbilical hernia

- Common, particularly in Afro-Caribbeans
- 90% close spontaneously
- defect >1 cm will probably require surgery

### Inguinal hernia

- Common, esspecially pre-term infants and boys
- Always indirect
- Always need repair

### Congenital hypertrophic pyloric stenosis

- 1 in 250 infants. More common in boys (4:1)
- Projectile vomiting WITHOUT bile
- Presents from about the second week of life
- Palpable tumour and visible peristalsis
- Hypochloraemic metabolic alkalosis
- Ramstedt's pyloromyotomy

### Intussusception

- Usually primary; ? hypertrophied Peyer's patches
- Presents after weaning; screaming colic; redcurrant jelly stools
- Treat with hydrostatic reduction or surgery

### Meckel's diverticulum

- Embryological midpoint of gut
- Remnant of vitello-intestinal duct
- 2%; 2 inches long; 2 feet from ileocaecal valve
- Mainly asymptomatic
- Complicated by diverticulitis; peptic ulcer; intussusception; volvulus

### Neonatal intestinal obstruction

- Presents with BILIOUS vomiting
- Caused by malrotation (remember Ladd's bands); Hirschsprung's (aganglionosis); meconium ileus (cystic fibrosis); intestinal and anorectal atresia

### Abdominal pain

- Specific diagnosis made in only 70% of children
- 30% of these have appendicitis
- Abdominal pain is a very common symptom in non-surgical conditions

# chapter 23

# ABDOMINAL HERNIA

## DEFINITION

A hernia is the abnormal protrusion of an organ through a defect in the wall of the cavity in which it lies, or into a subsidiary compartment of that cavity.

An abdominal hernia is the protrusion of peritoneum with its contents through an abnormal abdominal opening.

### Common sites (Figure 23.1)

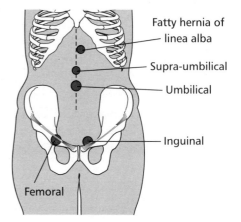

- The commonest hernia is **inguinal**, constituting 75% of all hernias. Inguinal hernias occur predominantly in men.
- **Femoral** hernia is the next commonest and **para-umbilical** hernias account for 10%.
- Abdominal incisions may break down to produce an **incisional** hernia.
- A hernia can be intra-abdominal (**internal**) rather than external, e.g. hiatus hernia. Rare internal hernia sites include obturator, paracaecal, paraduodenal, and diaphragmatic.

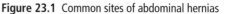

**Figure 23.1** Common sites of abdominal hernias

### Differential diagnosis

A number of masses in the groin may mimic a hernia (**this is a common examination question**):

- Skin – epidermoid cyst; fibroma; haemangioma
- Fat – lipoma
- Lymph nodes – reactive or malignant
- Vessels – femoral artery aneurysm; saphena varix
- Nerves – neuroma
- Scrotum – hydrocele; epididymal cyst.

An inguinal hernia must be differentiated from a femoral hernia by its position.

### Diagnosis

To ensure confident diagnosis of a groin hernia:

1 **The patient is asked to stand!** Is there a **visible swelling**, or does a swelling appear on straining or coughing?
2 Is there a **'cough impulse'** palpated over the hernial site or swelling when the patient strains or coughs?
3 **The patient is asked to lie down.** Does the hernia **reduce** spontaneously or with gentle manipulation? Does it reappear on straining or coughing? (One should **never** attempt to reduce a hernia with the patient standing – especially in a clinical examination).
4 Is it an inguino-scrotal hernia or a hydrocele? One can 'get above' a hydrocele and it transilluminates.

## GROIN ANATOMY

The three-dimensional anatomy of the inguinal and femoral canal confuses students. The key is the inguinal ligament that lies between the anterio-superior iliac spine and the pubic tubercle (Figure 23.2).

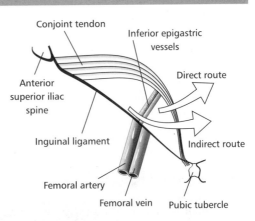

Beneath the ligament and running vertically are the femoral artery and vein. The anterior abdominal wall in this area comprises external oblique, internal oblique and transversalis muscles, which are all attached to the inguinal ligament. The inferior epigastric artery and vein branch from the femoral vessels and run upwards behind the muscles.

**Figure 23.2** Inguinal anatomy

The inguinal canal passes obliquely through the muscles with the conjoint tendon arching over it. Through this canal **indirect and direct inguinal hernias** may occur, the only restraint being the transversalis fascia, which is usually strong in this area.

A **femoral hernia** occurs in the femoral canal which lies medial to the vessels as they pass under the inguinal ligament. The femoral canal borders are:

- Anterior – inguinal ligament
- Posterior – pectineus and pubic bone
- Medial – lacunar ligament
- Lateral – femoral vein.

## CLASSIFICATION OF HERNIAE

### REDUCIBLE

The contents of the hernia, which may be bowel, omentum or other viscera, will return to the abdominal cavity either spontaneously or by gentle manipulation.

## IRREDUCIBLE

The contents of the hernia cannot be returned to the abdominal cavity. This may progress to strangulation.

## STRANGULATED

The blood supply to the contents of the hernia is compromised by **pressure** and **oedema** at its neck. This may progress to gangrene of the incarcerated tissue (usually bowel), causing toxaemia and **peritonitis**.

Strangulation is recognized by **irreducibility, excessive pain** and **tenderness** over the hernia, inflammation of the overlying skin, and generalized toxicity (hypotension, tachycardia, fever and leucocytosis). It requires urgent surgical intervention once appropriate resuscitation is complete.

- The most likely herniae to strangulate are femoral and para-umbilical.

- Occasionally a knuckle of the side wall of bowel is caught in a hernial sac, but continuity of the lumen is maintained (Richter's hernia). In this case, the bowel wall may strangulate but there is no intestinal obstruction.

## INGUINAL HERNIA

An inguinal hernia may be **direct** or **indirect**. These two varieties are distinguished anatomically at operation by whether the sac is **medial** or **lateral** (respectively) to the inferior epigastric vessels. In adults they cannot be distinguished with certainty on clinical examination alone. Hernias in children are invariably indirect.

- The **commonest** (70%) is an **indirect** hernia which lies within the spermatic cord and follows it down the inguinal canal, often into the scrotum (inguino-scrotal hernia) (Figure 23.3). Most can be considered as **congenital** in that the sac is a patent processus vaginalis (see Chapter 34).
- A **direct** hernia is due simply to a weakness in the posterior wall (transversalis fascia) of the inguinal canal medial to the inferior epigastric vessels.
- A 'sliding' (en glissade) hernia can occur, usually in older men. The peritoneal sac contains caecum (on the right) and sigmoid colon (on the left) which slide into the hernia because of their posterior peritoneal attachment.

### Precipitating factors

Inguinal hernias are common and may be precipitated by:

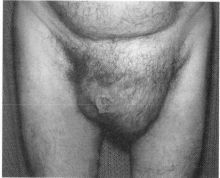

**Figure 23.3** Large left inguinal scrotal hernia

1 **Straining** to lift a heavy weight (manual labourers)
2 Repeated **coughing** (bronchitis; smokers)
3 Straining at **stool** (constipation; rectal tumours)
4 Straining to **pass urine** (prostatism).

> **IMPORTANT LESSON**
> Note the important association with prostatism and rectal tumours. Ask about job, chest
> symptoms, bowel and bladder function.

### Symptoms

Inguinal hernias may occur at **any age** including infancy and childhood. The patient presents with a swelling in the groin that may be symptomless or cause an uncomfortable **dragging** sensation. Strangulated hernias present acutely with bowel obstruction and severe pain at the hernia site.

### Management

- Most inguinal hernias should be repaired while they are still small and relatively asymptomatic.
- **Elderly men** with easily reducible wide-necked **direct** inguinal hernias and little risk of strangulation but significant perioperative morbidity, may be treated conservatively.
- Inguinal hernias can be repaired under general or local anaesthesia. Most are done in day surgery centres.
- Some men prefer a truss to an operation, the truss providing pressure over the deep inguinal ring, thereby holding the hernia reduced.
- Babies may be admitted with what may appear to be irreducible hernias. These will usually reduce with suitable sedation, but the parents should be offered surgery for their child on the next elective list.

Before surgery is considered, patients should be encouraged to **give up smoking** and **lose weight**, in an attempt to reduce infection and the risk of recurrence.

## INGUINAL HERNIA REPAIR

The operation entails excision or inversion of the peritoneal sac (**herniotomy**), followed by some method of repairing the posterior wall of the inguinal canal (**herniorrhaphy**) to narrow the dilated deep ring and strengthen the transversalis fascia.

The **criteria** for the preferred method of repair are:

1 Ease of performance
2 Degree of post-operative pain
3 Fastest return to work
4 Recurrence rates.

> - The 'no tension' mesh repair (**Lichtenstein**) uses a sheet of non-absorbable plastic mesh
> (Figure 23.4). It is sutured to the inguinal ligament and pubic tubercle, encircles the spermatic
> cord at its emergence from the deep ring and finally is secured to the surface of the internal
> oblique. This technique reduces post-operative pain and has a low recurrence rate (0.5%).

- Older methods of repair such as **Bassini** (suture approximation of conjoint tendon to inguinal ligament), and **Shouldice** (plication of transversalis fascia) have largely been abandoned in favour of mesh implants.
- **Laparoscopic repair** is also practised. The approach may be either intraperitoneal or pre-peritoneal with a mesh sutured across the defect or pushed into the defect as a plug. The greatest value of this technique is in **recurrent and bilateral herniae.**
- In **infants** and **children**, herniotomy (removal of the indirect sac) is all that is required.

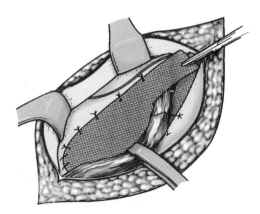

**Figure 23.4** Lichtenstein repair showing mesh insertion

## FEMORAL HERNIA

- Femoral hernia (Figure 23.5) carries a **high risk of strangulation** and the diagnosis is often missed.
- Femoral hernia is more common in women due to the wider angle between inguinal ligament and pubic bone. They appear initially below the inguinal ligament and **below and lateral to the pubic tubercle.** Large femoral hernias spread upwards over the inguinal ligament and may be confused with inguinal hernias.

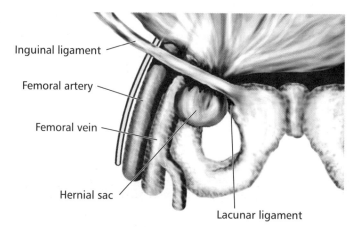

Inguinal ligament

Femoral artery

Femoral vein

Hernial sac

Lacunar ligament

**Figure 23.5** Femoral hernia anatomy

- Because of the risk of strangulation they should be repaired as soon as is practicable after diagnosis.
- In an elderly woman with unexplained intestinal obstruction, the femoral canals should be carefully examined for a hernia.

## FEMORAL HERNIA REPAIR

There are two surgical approaches:

1 **Below the inguinal ligament** – through an incision below the inguinal ligament the hernia is identified and its contents returned to the abdominal cavity. Once the sac has been excised, the canal is obliterated with sutures or insertion of a mesh.
2 **Above the inguinal ligament** – an incision through the conjoint tendon or transversalis fascia allows inspection of the upper end of the femoral canal in the extraperitoneal plane. This approach is used for repair of a strangulated or obstructed hernia since the peritoneum can be opened and the bowel inspected for viability and resected if necessary. The canal is obliterated using sutures or mesh.

## PARA-UMBILICAL HERNIA

True umbilical herniae are congenital and occur in infants. Para-umbilical herniae (Figure 23.6) are acquired and occur in adults just above or below the umbilical scar. They are seen most often in obese multiparous women with weak abdominal muscles and may achieve a considerable size. They **commonly become irreducible and strangulate.**

## PARA-UMBILICAL HERNIA REPAIR

- Weight loss is mandatory before elective repair.
- The sac is dissected clear, opened and then emptied of loops of bowel and omentum.
- The repair is achieved by overlapping layers of rectus sheath and securing with non-absorbable sutures, usually incorporating a mesh.

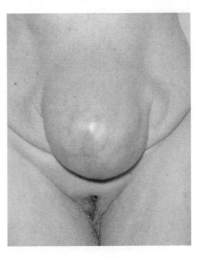

**Figure 23.6** Para-umbilical hernia (Courtesy of The Wellcome Trust)

## EPIGASTRIC AND SPIGELIAN HERNIAE

Both these uncommon hernias occur through defects in the anterior abdominal wall.

- An **epigastric** hernia is through a midline defect in the linea alba above the umbilicus. It usually contains a knuckle of extraperitoneal fat.
- A **Spigelian** hernia lies at the lateral edge of the rectus muscle at the lower level of the posterior rectus sheath.

Epigastric and Spigelian hernias present usually as small swellings which cause discomfort that is worse on exertion. They are **often mistaken for lipomata** (the examiner should feel for a cough impulse; does it reduce?). Both are repaired by excising the sac and closing the defect with non-absorbable sutures or mesh.

## INCISIONAL HERNIA

Some of the most severe and grotesque hernias follow weakening or disruption of an abdominal incision. An incisional hernia (Figure 23.7) may not appear for months or years after the original operation. Once present, the hernia tends to increase in size until a considerable part of the abdominal contents is contained within it.

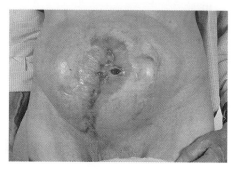

**Figure 23.7** Incisional hernia

### Predisposing factors
- Inadequate or insecure closure of the initial incision
- Infection or haematoma in the surgical wound
- Gross obesity
- Chronic coughing or straining

### Treatment
Surgical repair may be impossible and these patients should be offered a firm **abdominal belt or corset.**

Operations can be difficult and complex. Once the sac has been mobilized, various techniques can be employed to close the muscle defect:
- Deep tension nylon sutures
- Flaps of anterior rectus sheath can be mobilized across the defect and sutured
- Non-absorbable mesh is popular and this may be used to buttress deep tension sutures or laid across a defect.

Reduction of a large long-standing hernia back into the abdomen can cause severe **respiratory problems** due to pressure on the diaphragm. Chest physiotherapy is important.

## STRANGULATED HERNIA

The contents of any hernia can strangulate (Figure 23.8). Occasionally only fat or greater omentum is involved, but most often it is a length of bowel.

- A strangulated hernia is an emergency.
- Patients are septic, dehydrated and intestinally obstructed.
- Resuscitation with intravenous fluids and intensive monitoring are needed.
- Broad spectrum antibiotics and metronidazole should be given intravenously and the patient prepared for surgery.

## Procedure

At operation the hernia is opened and its contents reduced. Any bowel is assessed for **viability** and wrapped in warm saline packs for 5 minutes to increase blood flow. If the colour improves and a pulse can be felt in the adjacent mesentery, the bowel can safely be left in the abdominal cavity. If the bowel remains a deep purple or blackish colour, it must be resected before repair of the hernia.

A strangulated hernia should be treated with care in the preoperative phase – vigorous palpation may lead to a hernia reduction *en masse*, whereby the hernial swelling has disappeared but the strangulated bowel is still encased within its constricting sac and remains obstructed with a compromised blood supply.

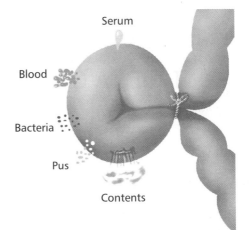

**Figure 23.8** Effects of strangulation

---

**CRIB BOX – ABDOMINAL HERNIA**

- **Remember the definition** of a hernia
- Commonest surgical problem in UK
- Inguinal, femoral, para-umbilical and incisional most common
- Examine the patient **standing** and then **ask him/her to lie down** to check for reduction
- Be able to **distinguish between femoral and inguinal** hernia anatomically and clinically
- Herniae are **reducible, irreducible, strangulated**
- Pain, irreducibility and toxaemia equals strangulation
- Femoral and para-umbilical most commonly strangulate
- Non-tension **mesh repair (Lichtenstein)** is most popular method for inguinal hernia

# chapter 24

# THE ACUTE ABDOMEN

## DEFINITION

Acute abdomen is defined as undiagnosed abdominal pain of duration less than 7 days, excluding abdominal trauma. Classification is by pathological process, such as **obstruction, inflammation, haemorrhage** and **infarction**. Careful history taking and examination are mandatory.

## HISTORY

### Pain

Patients describe abdominal pain with a variety of usually unhelpful adjectives, e.g., burning, sharp, dull, knife-like, etc. Interpreting these terms is made easier with the knowledge that **there are only two types of abdominal pain:**

> 1 **Colic** – signifies obstruction to a hollow viscus (gut; gall bladder; ureter). The patient rolls around in spasms or waves of intense pain caused by smooth muscle contraction. In between each wave of pain there may be no symptoms.
> 2 **Continuous** – signifies infection, inflammation or ischaemia (e.g. appendicitis; ulceration; strangulation). The patient lies still because movement exacerbates the pain.

It is vital to be able to interpret the patient's story and decide which pathological process is being described. Other clues in the history are:

- **Onset** – gradual in inflammatory conditions, sudden in infarction and perforation.

> - **Site** – depends upon the innervation of the peritoneum or organ involved. The bowel is supplied segmentally by visceral nerves because of its embryonic development from foregut, midgut and hindgut. The site of visceral pain is shown in Figure 24.1. The parietal peritoneum is innervated by **somatic nerves**. The pain of local peritonitis due to inflammation of the parietal peritoneum overlying an affected organ is more intense and well localized. Localization of pain in three common inflammatory conditions affecting the foregut, midgut and hindgut is shown in Table 24.1.

- **Radiation** – pain may be referred to a remote place far from the diseased organ. This depends on the dermatome segments of the nerves conducting the pain impulses, for example:

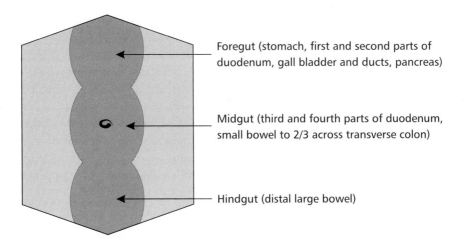

Foregut (stomach, first and second parts of duodenum, gall bladder and ducts, pancreas)

Midgut (third and fourth parts of duodenum, small bowel to 2/3 across transverse colon)

Hindgut (distal large bowel)

**Figure 24.1** Common distribution of visceral pain

**Table 24.1** Localization of somatic pain

| |
|---|
| Cholecystitis – Epigastrium → right hypochondrium |
| Appendicitis – Para-umbilical → right iliac fossa |
| Diverticulitis – Suprapubic → left iliac fossa |

- **cholecystitis** can cause hyperaesthesia below the right scapula (9th, 10th, 11th intercostal nerves);
- **diaphragmatic irritation** which may be caused by bleeding from a ruptured ectopic pregnancy can produce shoulder tip pain (3rd, 4th, 5th cervical nerves – same segments as phrenic nerve);
- **ureteric colic** and retroperitoneal bleeding produce pain in the groin, inner thigh and scrotum (1st lumbar nerve).
- **Relief** – patients lay still with shallow respirations in inflammatory conditions, whereas colic produces restless patients who roll about and may walk around.

### Associated symptoms
- **Nausea and vomiting** – may be the first symptom of high small bowel obstruction. Initially vomit may contain bile but with time it becomes thick, brown and offensive (**faeculent vomiting**). Patients with localized inflammatory conditions may only vomit once or twice. Vomiting may be due to mechanical obstruction, the toxaemia of inflammation, severe pain or may even result from opiate injections unless antiemetics are also administered.
- **Anorexia** – this is significant in children.
- **Bowel function** – constipation is usual in inflammatory conditions. However, diarrhoea may occur due to irritation of the colon or rectum by pelvic peritonitis or abscess. Constipation for faeces **and** flatus is a feature of large bowel

obstruction (**absolute constipation**). Alternating constipation and diarrhoea may be a feature of incomplete colonic obstruction.

- **Indigestion** – suggests a past history of peptic ulcer disease.
- **Jaundice** – may support a diagnosis of acute cholecystitis or biliary colic.
- **Genitourinary symptoms** – information about the frequency of micturition, dysuria or haematuria should be sought, as well as a careful menstrual history with details of the frequency and regularity of periods and the date of the last period. Vaginal discharge may indicate inflammation in the genital tract.
- Details of all **previous operations**, hospital admissions and a careful **drug history** with allergies and details of **smoking** and **alcohol** intake are important.

## EXAMINATION

The general appearance can give helpful clues as to the seriousness of the condition.

- A cold clammy skin indicates hypovolaemic shock due to dehydration or haemorrhage.
- A high fever with rigors suggests abscess formation, cholangitis or urinary tract infection.
- Evidence of anaemia and jaundice.
- In the presence of intra-abdominal sepsis a pronounced foetor is usually found.
- The extreme toxaemia and dehydration of advanced peritonitis produces an ashen countenance, drawn features and sunken eyes, the so-called '**Hippocratic facies.**'
- Serious medical conditions, such as lower lobe pneumonia, myocardial infarction and diabetic ketoacidosis, all of which can present with abdominal pain, should be excluded.

## ABDOMINAL EXAMINATION

The area from nipple to mid-thigh is exposed. Ideally the patient should be flat with the head supported by one pillow. The examiner should get down to the level of the abdomen, if necessary on one knee, taking time to win the confidence of the patient (particularly children) before touching the abdomen.

### Inspection
Time should be taken to look first, not forgetting to inspect the groins and external genitalia.

- Look for scars, masses, hernias, asymmetry and visible peristalsis.
- Distension of the small bowel is usually centred around the umbilicus.
- Distension of the colon causes a fullness in the flanks.

### Palpation
This is performed with the flat of the hand with flexion of the metacarpophalangeal joints.

Initially palpation is begun furthest from the painful area, passing through all the quadrants, eliciting slight degrees of local tenderness and guarding. This sign is good evidence of local peritonitis due to inflammation of the parietal peritoneum over an affected organ.

Deep palpation in a non-tender area of the abdomen followed by sudden release of pressure from the hand sends a shock wave through the abdominal cavity which causes pain at any site of inflammation – **rebound tenderness.**

In diffuse peritonitis the whole abdominal wall is **rigid, board-like and intensely tender.**

### Percussion

This is a useful test to detect fluid or gas. Patients with ascites have shifting dullness. Gentle percussion is a kinder and more accurate way of testing for rebound tenderness.

### Auscultation

Background noise is reduced to a minimum and time taken to listen. A silent abdomen suggests general peritonitis although the patient's respiration and heart sounds are easily heard. Loud hyperactive bowel sounds suggest mechanical obstruction. High-pitched tinkling sounds suggest paralytic obstruction.

## INVESTIGATIONS

### Urinalysis

The urine is tested for albumin, blood, sugar and a pregnancy test performed on women of child-bearing age. Send urine for microscopy if a urinary tract infection is suspected.

### Serum analysis

Blood is taken for a full blood count, urea and electrolytes. The presence of a **leucocytosis** suggests infection. The haematocrit will help to estimate the level of dehydration. It is important to identify the presence of gross anaemia before anaesthesia. A **sickle cell screen** is performed in Afro-Caribbeans. A serum **amylase** which is 2–3 times above the upper limit of normal confirms acute pancreatitis. A urea and electrolyte estimation helps to confirm dehydration, any unsuspected renal problems and electrolyte imbalance. Blood is also taken for **group and save** and an urgent **cross-match** of 2 units is requested before any laparotomy.

### Radiology

Unnecessary radiology is avoided, particularly in children and young women with suspected appendicitis. Two x-rays are needed in most adults with an acute abdomen:

1  **Erect chest x-ray** – used to look for gas under the diaphragm, indicating perforation. It is important to prop the patient up at 45° for 5 minutes before this film is taken to allow gas to move up under the diaphragm. Free peritoneal gas is also seen on supine abdominal films as areas of lucency between loops of bowel. It is unkind to ask a patient with an acute abdomen to stand up for an erect abdominal x-ray and it yields no added information in patients with

perforation. The chest x-ray also assesses the cardiopulmonary state of the patient before anaesthesia and rules out any unsuspected lung pathology such as a lower lobe pneumonia.

2 **Supine abdominal x-ray** – gas patterns in the small and large bowel can be used to diagnose intestinal obstruction. An erect abdominal film demonstrates fluid levels in obstruction but is unnecessary.

Contrast studies of the small or large bowel are sometimes required to determine the nature and location of an obstruction, and for treatment (hydrostatic reduction of intussusception).

An abdominal **ultrasound** may be helpful in the diagnosis of right iliac fossa pain in young women to look for tubular-ovarian pathology and free fluid in the pelvis.

## INTESTINAL OBSTRUCTION

### DEFINITION

Intestinal obstruction (Figure 24.2) is failure of normal transit of bowel contents. This may be due to:

1 **Mechanical obstruction**, i.e. a physical blockage
2 **Paralytic (functional) obstruction**, i.e. absence of peristalsis.

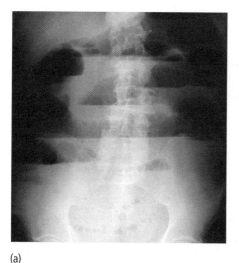

(a)

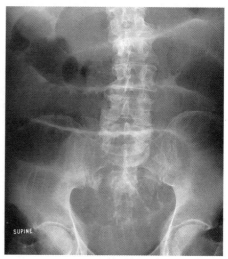

(b)

**Figure 24.2** (a) Erect film showing fluid levels. (b) Supine film showing dilated small bowel in intestinal obstruction

## IMPORTANT QUESTIONS

1 Is the diagnosis intestinal obstruction?
2 What type of obstruction is it?
3 Does this patient need an emergency operation or conservative treatment?

### Is the diagnosis intestinal obstruction?

There are four cardinal features of intestinal obstruction:

1 Vomiting
2 Dehydration
3 Distension
4 Constipation.

- **Vomiting** initially is of gastric contents and recently ingested food. As obstruction continues the vomit is yellowish-green fluid from the upper small bowel. Finally, the vomit turns **'faeculent'** (dark brown and offensive) due to bacterial overgrowth in the stagnant intestinal fluid.
- **Dehydration** is due to vomiting and loss of fluid into the distended gut from where it cannot be absorbed. It occurs early in high mechanical obstruction and late in low obstruction. Electrolyte losses depend on their concentration in the fluid lost (e.g. in pyloric stenosis, water and HCl only).
- **Distension** of the abdomen depends on the level of obstruction. It may be gross with low colonic obstruction or minimal with high small bowel obstruction.
- **Constipation** is similarly variable. An obstructing lesion in the distal large bowel usually leads to early constipation and eventually absence of flatus (absolute constipation). In small bowel obstruction patients may continue to pass flatus and faeces intermittently. Patients with incomplete obstruction may experience diarrhoea.

---

**PAIN IS VARIABLE and may be present (colicky or continuous) or absent, depending on the cause, time of presentation and type of obstruction.**

For example, after major abdominal surgery a state of paralytic obstruction (**paralytic ileus**) exists for a period of several days – if fed the patient will **vomit**; without intravenous fluids **dehydration** occurs; the abdomen **distends** and there is absolute **constipation**; but pain (other than discomfort from the incision) is absent. Passage of flatus and return of bowel sounds signals resolution of the paralysis.

Conversely, a strangulated hernia presents initially with colic and hyperactive bowel sounds due to mechanical obstruction. Eventually the bowel stops contracting and the colicky pain disappears. If ischaemia and perforation supervene the pain becomes continuous and the abdomen silent due to generalized peritonitis and paralytic obstruction.

## What type of obstruction is it?

- **Mechanical** obstruction (Figure 24.3) is often called 'dynamic' because peristalsis of the bowel continues in an attempt to overcome the obstruction. This results in colic, visible peristalsis and increased bowel sounds.
- **Paralytic, functional** or **adynamic obstruction** has no peristalsis and auscultation reveals a silent abdomen or tinkling bowel sounds. The latter is caused by intestinal contents pouring from one distended loop of flaccid bowel to another under the effects of gravity or general body movements. There may be no pain, or the continuous pain of ischaemia or peritonitis.

Causes of **mechanical obstruction** are shown in Table 24.2. Overall, hernias and adhesions are the most common.

Causes of **functional obstruction** are varied and include:

- Peritonitis (calor, rubor, dolor, tumour and *loss of function*)
- Post-operative paralytic ileus
- Ischaemia
- Electrolyte imbalance (including metabolic causes, e.g. diabetic ketoacidosis)
- Retroperitoneal haematoma
- Pancreatitis
- Prolonged bed rest
- Malignant infiltration
- Long-standing mechanical obstruction.

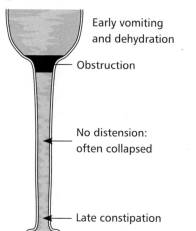

**High obstruction**

- Early vomiting and dehydration
- Obstruction
- No distension: often collapsed
- Late constipation

**Low obstruction**

- Late vomiting and dehydration
- Marked distension
- Early constipation

**Figure 24.3** Signs of mechanical obstruction

**Table 24.2** Causes of mechanical obstruction

| Neonate | Child |
|---|---|
| Hernia | Intussusception |
| Volvulus neonatorum | Meckel's diverticulum |
| Hirschsprung's | Bezoars |
| Intestinal atresia | Hernia |
| Congenital bands | |

| Adult | Elderly |
|---|---|
| Adhesions | Colonic tumours |
| Hernia | Hernia |
| Crohn's disease | Volvulus |
| Small bowel tumours | Pseudo-obstruction |
| | Gall stone ileus |

Long-standing mechanical obstruction appears out of place but is included because mechanically obstructed bowel will eventually stop contracting due to gross distension, compromising blood flow in the bowel wall – the relative ischaemia results in paralysis. **Thus mechanical (dynamic) obstruction will eventually become paralytic (adynamic).**

Where there is uncertainty, contrast studies of the bowel will show the presence of a mechanical obstruction.

### Does the patient need an emergency operation or conservative treatment?

Many causes of intestinal obstruction obviously need urgent surgery, e.g. obstructed hernia; generalized peritonitis. Difficulty arises in differentiating between simple and complicated mechanical obstruction.

- In **simple obstruction** the abdomen is distended but soft. There may be visible peristalsis but tenderness and guarding are absent, the patient is afebrile and generally well. Simple obstruction is often seen with intra-abdominal adhesions and initially may be treated conservatively.
- In **complicated obstruction** the blood supply of the bowel wall is impaired and **ischaemia, strangulation** and **perforation** occur. The colicky abdominal pain is superseded by the **continuous pain** of ischaemia and eventually peritonitis as bacteria and bowel contents escape from the necrotic bowel into the peritoneal cavity.

Indications of complicated obstruction are **continuous pain, abdominal tenderness, tachycardia, fever** and **leucocytosis** – any or all of which mean urgent laparotomy is required to prevent perforation and peritonitis. A period of observation and regular examination is permissible if the initial situation is unclear.

## Conservative management

Patients with simple obstruction and suspected intestinal adhesions can be treated conservatively in the expectation of spontaneous resolution. The essence of this treatment is adequate **analgesia, nasogastric aspiration and intravenous fluids** – so-called 'drip and suck'.

- **Analgesia** – requirements are usually nil or minimal using NSAIDs and opiates. **Continuous pain** or **unremitting colic** are indications for surgery.
- **Nasogastric aspiration** – avoids repeated vomiting which demoralizes the patient and carries a risk of aspiration of gastric contents into the lungs. The volume of nasogastric aspirate monitors fluid losses and assesses the progress of conservative treatment.
- **Intravenous fluid and electrolyte replacement** – normal daily requirements **plus** aspirate losses. Patients with profound dehydration may require a **central venous pressure line** for accurate fluid replacement, particularly in the elderly with cardiopulmonary disease.

Success of conservative treatment is heralded by reduced nasogastric aspirate, passage of flatus ('Have you passed any wind today Mrs Bloggs?'), reduced distension and return of normal bowel sounds.

## PERITONITIS

Inflammation of the peritoneum encompasses a wide range of clinical conditions from local peritonitis with minimal systemic upset to gross generalized faecal peritonitis and impending multi-organ failure. Peritonitis can be classified as primary or secondary.

- **Primary** bacterial peritonitis is extremely rare and seen in young girls, the bacteria (streptococci) probably gaining access to the peritoneum via the genital tract.
- **Secondary** bacterial contamination is the result of bacteria spreading from a focus such as **appendicitis or salpingitis** or escaping from the bowel lumen as in **perforation** or **ischaemic necrosis** of the bowel wall.

## Causes of peritonitis

Peritonitis can be **local** or **generalized**.

Local:

- Epigastrium – pancreatitis
- Right hypochondrium – cholecystitis
- Right iliac fossa – appendicitis, diverticulitis, gynaecological causes
- Left iliac fossa – diverticulitis
- Suprapubic – cystitis, gynaecological causes.

Gynaecological causes include salpingitis, ectopic pregnancy, ruptured follicle and torsion of an ovarian cyst.

Generalized:

- Perforations of – stomach (benign and malignant ulceration); duodenum (benign ulcer disease); gall bladder (unusual); small bowel (Meckel's, intussusception, Crohn's); appendix; caecum (carcinoma, diverticular disease); sigmoid (carcinoma, stercoral, diverticular disease); bladder (traumatic).

- Haemorrhage from – abdominal aortic aneurysm; ruptured ectopic pregnancy; trauma (spleen).

### Peritoneal defences

- The surface area of the peritoneum is equivalent to that of the skin and it therefore has a great propensity to absorb and neutralize any bacterial infection.
- Any local peritonitis causes a local paralysis of the bowel. Normal peristalsis occurring elsewhere has the effect of pushing the greater omentum (the 'abdominal policeman') into the area of least activity, with the result that the inflammation tends to be effectively isolated. Fibrinous adhesions between the omentum and inflamed peritoneum hold the omentum in place.

### Symptoms and signs

The severity of symptoms and signs are proportionately related to the extent of the peritonitis. Generalized peritonitis presents with:

- **Pain** – constant and burning. The patient lies motionless with shallow respirations since any movement exacerbates the pain. The abdomen is silent with 'board-like' rigidity.
- **Dehydration, hypotension** and **hypovolaemic shock** – occurs rapidly as large volumes of peritoneal inflammatory exudate enter the peritoneal cavity from the circulation.
- **Toxaemia.**
- **Abdominal distension** – increases as paralytic obstruction develops.
- **Hypoxia, pulmonary collapse** and **hypostatic pneumonia** – result from diaphragmatic splinting and shallow respiration.

### Treatment

- Local peritonitis due to cholecystitis, diverticulitis and pancreatitis is treated conservatively unless repeated examination shows signs of spreading inflammation.
- Local peritonitis from appendicitis is treated by surgery.
- Generalized peritonitis is an absolute indication for surgery after adequate resuscitation.

### Resuscitation

All patients requiring surgery will need an initial period of resuscitation. A checklist is helpful:

- **Opiate analgesics** – given intravenously, as intramuscular injections are poorly absorbed due to the poor peripheral circulation in shock and toxaemia.
- **Intravenous fluids with a central venous pressure line** for close monitoring of all patients with general peritonitis, especially elderly patients.
- **Oxygen therapy.**
- **Antibiotics** – broad spectrum intravenously.
- **Urethral catheter** – adequate resuscitation gives a urine output of at least 0.5 ml/kg/h (before laparotomy if possible).

- **Blood sample** for full blood count, urea and electrolytes, serum amylase, cross-match 2 units.
- **Arterial blood gases**.
- **Radiology** – erect chest and abdominal x-ray.
- **Electrocardiograph**.
- **Informed consent** and discussion with relatives.
- **ITU or high dependency** placement to facilitate resuscitation before theatre.

### Surgery

**Emergency operations** are usually performed through a midline incision. The cause of the peritonitis is sought and dealt with appropriately by removal of the inflamed organ, closure of perforations or resection of gangrenous bowel. The peritoneal cavity is then cleaned with several litres of warm saline.

## HAEMORRHAGE

Significant intraperitoneal bleeding produces obvious signs of shock such as pallor, sweating, thirst, faintness, tachycardia and hypotension. Blood is an irritant and within the peritoneum produces signs of peritonism with tenderness, guarding and absent bowel sounds. Diaphragmatic irritation from blood **commonly produces referred pain in the shoulder** tip and this is an important sign in someone who is shocked with no obvious source of bleeding. With minor bleeding the signs are less obvious and consist of niggling shoulder tip pain and fatigue.

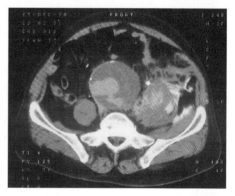

**Figure 24.4** CT scan of ruptured abdominal aortic aneurysm

Common causes of intraperitoneal bleeding include:
- Trauma – especially to the spleen and liver
- Ruptured abdominal aortic aneurysm (Figure 24.4)
- Gynaecological bleeding – ectoptic pregnancy and ruptured ovarian or corpus luteal cysts.

Intraperitoneal haemorrhage can clearly range from catastrophic to relatively trivial. Treatment requires appropriate resuscitation with blood, followed by surgery.

## INFARCTION

Interruption of the blood supply to the bowel is produced by:
- **Extrinsic pressure** on the bowel or mesentery, causing **strangulation**
- **Thrombosis or embolus** in the mesenteric vessels.

The causes are therefore:

- Bowel strangulation in a hernia
- Bowel strangulation by adhesions
- Occlusion of the mesenteric vessels in a volvulus or intussusception
- Embolization or atherosclerotic thrombosis of mesenteric vessels.

Strangulation generally occurs in association with a mechanical obstruction. If the bowel becomes ischaemic but without strangulation, a localized ileus and paralytic obstruction follow.

### Clinical features

- **Acute inflammation and tenderness**, e.g. over a groin hernia
- **Generalized peritonitis** and secondary ileus. Often the signs are masked and not as well marked as would be expected by the severity of the pain
- **Tachycardia and hypotension** as a result of fluid sequestration and vomiting
- **Septicaemic shock.**

### Investigations

- High **white cell count**
- **Haemoconcentration** with a high haematocrit and haemoglobin
- **Dilated small bowel loops** on x-ray with intramural gas at a later stage.

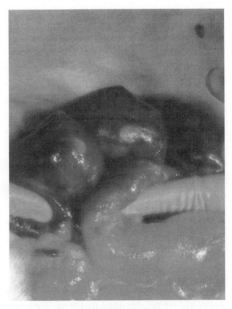

Bowel infarction (Figure 24.5) is most commonly diagnosed at surgery for generalized peritonitis. Small lengths of infarcted bowel can be resected without long-term consequences of malabsorption. Occasionally the whole small bowel is infarcted from thrombosis or embolism of the superior mesenteric artery – the patient is often elderly and the condition terminal. Successful resection of the whole small bowel requires subsequent permanent parenteral nutrition.

**Figure 24.5** Infarcted small bowel

## GYNAECOLOGICAL CAUSES OF PAIN

### RUPTURED ECTOPIC PREGNANCY

- Pain in the lower abdomen is also referred to the shoulder tip.
- There is often a history of vaginal bleeding and of a missed period.
- Patients may be normotensive or extremely pale and shocked.

- Abdominal signs may be absent or show tenderness and guarding across the lower abdomen.
- Vaginal examination produces severe pain on movement of the cervix.

## TWISTED OVARIAN CYST

This presents with sudden onset iliac fossa pain and vaginal examination produces pain on movement of the cervix. There may be a mass in the right or left iliac fossa or on rectal examination. It is a differential diagnosis in acute appendicitis.

## ACUTE SALPINGITIS

Abdominal pain may be in the right iliac fossa but is often bilateral and suprapubic. Urinary symptoms and vaginal discharge are often present and movement of the cervix is painful.

## RUPTURED CORPUS LUTEUM CYST

There is sudden onset of low abdominal pain due to rupture of an ovarian follicle releasing a little fluid and blood into the peritoneal cavity. This occurs midway between the periods, hence the name of Mittelschmerz. Rarely, there is severe bleeding.

# ABDOMINAL PAIN WITHOUT INTRAPERITONEAL PATHOLOGY

## ABDOMINAL WALL

Occasionally patients presenting with severe abdominal pain have pathology within the abdominal wall. Tenderness is most marked over the area involved **and increases on tensing the anterior abdominal wall muscles**; this normally causes a decrease of tenderness in those with intra-abdominal pathology.

## MEDICAL CONDITIONS

Many medical problems present with real or referred abdominal pain. The surgeon needs to avoid making the clinical situation worse with an unnecessary laparotomy.
- Chest – pneumonia, pleurisy and pulmonary embolism
- Cardiac – myocardial ischaemia or infarction
- Spinal conditions – osteomyelitis or acute disc prolapse
- Metabolic – diabetic ketoacidosis and porphyria
- Haematological – sickle cell crisis.

## MÜNCHHAUSEN SYNDROME

Some patients fabricate a history of abdominal pain to obtain a hospital admission or at least an opiate injection in a casualty department. The patients often come to hospital alone and have a number of abdominal scars from previous surgery. The diagnosis is made by exclusion and can be difficult. Careful examination with distraction of the patient's attention to overcome the voluntary guarding and tenderness is important. The diagnosis is also suspected if all other aspects of the examination and investigations are normal.

---

**CRIB BOX – ACUTE ABDOMEN**

Acute abdominal pain of <7 days duration, excluding trauma. **ABDOMINAL PAIN IS EITHER COLICKY OR CONTINUOUS**

**Pathology**

- Inflammation (local or generalized peritonitis)
- Obstruction
- Haemorrhage
- Infarction

**Diagnose on:**

- History – character, onset, site, radiation, relieving factors
- Examination – inspection, palpation, percussion, auscultation
- Investigations – urinalysis; blood tests; radiology (CXR and supine AXR)

**Treatment**

- Obstruction – simple obstruction can be treated conservatively. **Beware strangulation**
- Peritonitis – conservative treatment for cholecystitis, pancreatitis and sigmoid diverticulitis only. Surgery for generalized peritonitis **after** resuscitation

**Pathology outside the abdomen**

- Abdominal wall
- Medical
- Münchhausen

# chapter 25

# THE APPENDIX

## ACUTE APPENDICITIS

This is the commonest abdominal emergency (Figure 25.1) with an overall mortality rate of around 1%. Death results from generalized peritonitis and occurs most commonly in the very young and elderly. The majority of patients are aged 10–30 years and in this group the mortality is negligible.

Appendicitis is almost exclusively a disease of the Western world, depending not on any racial, climatic or geographical factors but presumably being related to diet

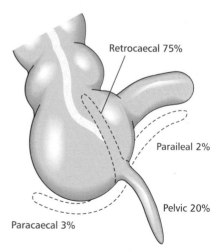

**Figure 25.1** Inflamed appendix at operation

or lifestyle. Thus the disease is rare amongst native inhabitants of undeveloped countries but immigrants become susceptible upon adopting Western habits.

### PATHOLOGY

**Obstruction to the lumen of the appendix** is the root cause of appendicitis but other factors must also be considered:

- **Structure** – lymphoid tissue is abundant in the wall of the appendix, forming follicles in the mucosa and submucosa. Swelling of this lymphoid tissue in response to viral or bacterial invasion can occlude the lumen and explains the variable seasonal incidence of appendicitis in children.
- **Contents** – at operation the appendix is often found to be obstructed by faecoliths and rarely by foreign bodies such as beads or teeth. Threadworm infestation is common in childhood.
- **Anatomy** – the position and length of the appendix is variable (Figure 25.2). A long kinked retrocaecal organ will be

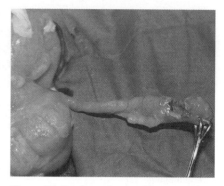

Retrocaecal 75%

Paraileal 2%

Pelvic 20%

Paracaecal 3%

**Figure 25.2** Appendix positions

more prone to blockage than a short straight one and anatomical differences probably account for a familial predisposition to develop appendicitis. In infancy the appendix is short and conical with a wide mouth whereas in later life the lumen tends to obliterate – thus appendicitis is rare at the extremes of life.

Two clinical types of appendicitis are recognized:

- **Congestive** appendicitis has no clear mechanical obstructive element. Inflammation arises either in the mucosa or submucosal lymphoid tissue and probably is initiated by ingested organisms. The resulting oedema and congestion undoubtedly produces an element of obstruction to the lumen of the appendix and subsequent colonization by enterobacteria leads to suppuration. This process occurs slowly over a period of days.
- **Obstructive** appendicitis is usually caused by a faecolith obstructing the lumen. Rare causes include parasitic worms, foreign bodies, carcinoma of the caecum or carcinoid tumours of the appendix. The rise in intraluminal pressure produced by the obstruction causes vascular stasis, resulting in ischaemia of the wall, bacterial invasion and eventual gangrene and perforation. This process occurs rapidly over a period of hours.

## DISEASE PROCESS

The natural course of appendicitis, as with inflammation elsewhere, can be derived from basic pathological principles.

- **Resolution** may be complete but more commonly there is a degree of damage with fibrosis or scarring. This renders the appendix prone to further attacks of obstruction and inflammation – recurrent appendicitis. Resolution is more likely to occur in congestive appendicitis.
- An **appendix abscess** results from the attempts of the body to wall off and isolate inflammation. The appendix lies bathed in pus within a cavity formed by adhesions, omentum, bowel and parietal peritoneum. The abscess usually takes several days to form but earlier than this an appendix mass may be felt in the right iliac fossa. The mass is composed of oedematous bowel and omentum surrounding the inflamed organ.
- **Gangrene and perforation** most often occurs in obstructive appendicitis and is due to distension of the wall and thrombosis of its arterial supply. Perforation may lead to diffuse peritonitis or, alternatively, abscess formation, depending upon the speed of onset and the efficacy of local defence mechanisms. **Generalized peritonitis is most common in the young and old** in whom the powers of localization of infection are reduced and the diagnosis difficult or delayed.
- Rarely, an obstructed appendix remains sterile and distends with mucus to form a **mucocele** which is felt as a smooth painless mobile lump in the right iliac fossa.

**Natural course of appendicitis**

**Appendicitis**
- → Complete resolution
- → Resolution with fibrosis
- → Suppuration → Abscess
- → Gangrene → Perforation

## DIAGNOSIS

The diagnosis of appendicitis rests entirely on the history (Figure 25.3) and clinical examination. Blood tests are usually unhelpful and a white count may be normal and misleading.

### History

Pain is the most constant feature and **initially is situated in the peri-umbilical region**. At first it may be colicky if the appendix is obstructed but this is eventually superseded by the more usual dull constant pain characteristic of inflammation. The time scale of the pain may give some indication of the type of appendicitis – either congestive or obstructive. In the former, the condition develops over many days and there may be a history of sore throat or flu-like illness, especially in children.

The onset of obstructive appendicitis is much more rapid, the patient usually presenting within 24 hours. As inflammation spreads from the appendix to involve the parietal peritoneum in **the right iliac fossa, the pain shifts to this area**. This feature is not invariable and depends on the anatomical position of the appendix; if it is retrocaecal or pelvic there may be no right iliac fossa pain, the patient complaining instead of flank tenderness in the former case or suprapubic discomfort in the latter. In the rare situation of malrotation or situs inversus, the pain will shift to the area closest to the appendix. Anorexia, nausea and vomiting follow the onset of pain.

### Examination

There is usually a fever and a pronounced 'alimentary' foetor oris with furring of the tongue (Figure 25.4). **Movement is painful because of the inflammation so the patient lies still**, but occasionally a patient may present early with appendicular colic and roll around in spasms of pain. The right leg may be flexed due to irritation of the psoas muscle which crosses the right iliac fossa posteriorly. **Palpation** reveals tenderness and guarding in

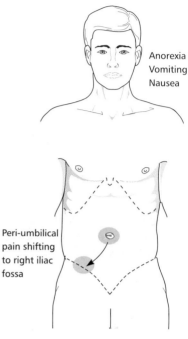

Anorexia
Vomiting
Nausea

Peri-umbilical pain shifting to right iliac fossa

**Figure 25.3** Appendicitis – history

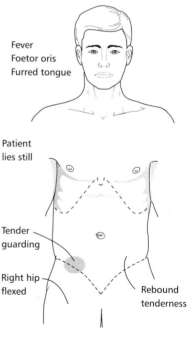

Fever
Foetor oris
Furred tongue

Patient lies still

Tender guarding

Right hip flexed

Rebound tenderness

Tender PR in pelvic appendicitis

**Figure 25.4** Appendicitis – examination

the right iliac fossa over **McBurney's point** – but only if this is the position of the appendix. A retrocaecal appendix may produce loin tenderness and in the case of a pelvic position, tenderness may only be elicited on rectal or vaginal examination. If the history is long a mass may be felt. Rebound tenderness is a sign of spreading peritoneal inflammation. Flexion and extension of the hip may be painful due to movement of the psoas muscle in the right iliac fossa. An inflamed appendix in the pelvis can be accompanied by diarrhoea or dysuria due to irritation of the rectum or bladder.

## TREATMENT

The treatment of appendicitis is **appendicectomy**. There should be as little delay as possible before surgery since the very presence of tenderness, guarding and fever mean that the patient has spreading peritonitis. However, if the patient is moribund with generalized peritonitis and dehydration, resuscitation with intravenous fluids and antibiotics must take precedence over immediate operation.

If there is a palpable appendix mass but the patient is well with no signs of toxicity or peritoneal irritation, the inflammation has been adequately isolated and immediate appendicectomy is unnecessary and difficult (see **Appendix mass**, page 333).

The operation is commonly done through a muscle-splitting 'grid-iron' incision at **McBurney's point – one-third of the distance between the anterior superior iliac spine and the umbilicus** (Figure 25.5). The procedure is usually simple but can be extremely difficult, particularly if the appendix is very long and retrocaecal. The experienced surgeon can often predict the position of the appendix from the preoperative clinical signs. When the patient is anaesthetized and before the incision is made, a mass is often palpable. This is of no consequence since the decision to operate was made on the grounds of toxicity and peritonitis – indications that the intra-abdominal defence mechanisms have failed to isolate the inflammation. If there is any doubt about the diagnosis and particularly in elderly patients who may have other pathology, it is usual to explore the abdomen through a formal laparotomy incision such as a midline or right paramedian. **Wound infection is very common after appendicectomy and the incidence is reduced with the use of perioperative antibiotics.**

Laparoscopic appendicectomy can also be performed with ports at the umbilicus,

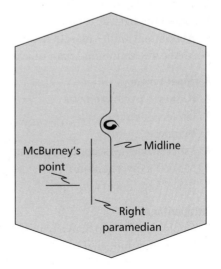

**Figure 25.5** Incisions for appendicectomy

lower midline and right iliac fossa. This method has the advantages of a better cosmetic result and earlier return to full activity.

## POST-OPERATIVE COMPLICATIONS

Appendicectomy is perceived by the public to be a simple operation for a relatively trivial condition and consequently any post-operative complications are often looked upon as a failing of the surgeon or his team. It is important therefore that early in the treatment process, patients and relatives are made aware of the potential complications of appendicitis and surgery:

- **General complications** such as pneumonia, atelectasis, DVT and thromboembolism.
- **Wound infection** is extremely common.
- **Pelvic abscess** or other intra-abdominal collections may occur.
- **Prolonged paralytic ileus** is common after removal of a particularly dirty appendix.
- **Faecal fistula** can develop between the appendix stump and the wound.
- **Adhesive obstruction** can develop months or years after appendicectomy.

## DIFFERENTIAL DIAGNOSIS OF APPENDICITIS

Acute appendicitis can be the easiest or the most difficult of diagnoses to make. In considering the differential diagnoses it is useful to list possible causes of pain arising outside the abdomen, in the retroperitoneal space or within the peritoneum.

### Outside the abdomen
- Chest – right basal pneumonia and pleurisy
- CNS – collapse of 11th and 12th thoracic vertebrae, shingles
- Inguinal – hernia, torsion of undescended testis
- Abdominal wall – muscle strain, Spigelian hernia
- Medical – abdominal pain of crises such as porphyria, sickle cell, diabetes.

### Retroperitoneal
- Kidney – pyelonephritis
- Ureter – ureteric colic
- Bladder – cystitis
- Psoas abscess – secondary to osteomyelitis of spine
- Meckel's diverticulum
- Iliac artery aneurysm.

### Intraperitoneal
- Cholecystitis – particularly in the elderly
- Perforated duodenal ulcer
- Ileum – Crohn's, Meckel's, intussusception
- Caecum – carcinoma, caecal diverticulitis

- Pelvis – salpingitis, ectopic pregnancy, ruptured follicle, torsion of cyst
- Mesenteric adenitis – common in children with sore throats and associated with adenitis palpable in the neck, axillae and groins.

> Such a plethora of possible diagnoses means that in every case of suspected appendicitis searching enquiries must be made regarding menstrual history, previous illness, chest disease, gynaecological and urological symptoms. Full examination of the chest, abdomen, pelvis and rectum must be undertaken and the urine examined. Laparoscopy is indicated where doubt remains.

## APPENDIX MASS AND APPENDIX ABSCESS

The distinction between an appendix mass and abscess is largely chronological and is best appreciated by examining the natural history of the condition:
- If acute appendicitis progresses rapidly to gangrene and perforation, the resulting clinical picture is one of diffusing or diffuse peritonitis and the patient requires urgent surgery.
- Conversely, if the inflammation has a more insidious onset the appendix is likely to become surrounded by greater omentum, oedematous caecum and small intestine.

Thus it is not uncommon for a patient to present with a history of pain over many days and on examination for there to be a palpable inflammatory mass in the right iliac fossa. The general health is good and although the mass is tender, there are no signs of peritonism such as rebound pain and guarding.
- Having once formed, the inflammatory mass will then resolve, or suppurate to form an abscess.
- An abscess must be drained surgically or else discharge spontaneously through the anterior abdominal wall, or into the caecum, small bowel, rectum or peritoneal cavity. If an abscess discharges into the bowel, resolution of the mass and fever coincide with a bout of foul diarrhoea.

### TREATMENT

- Treatment of an appendix mass is conservative.
- The patient is confined to bed on a light diet and the pulse and temperature carefully monitored (Figure 25.6).
- The mass is examined daily and the border outlined in ink on the skin.
- Antibiotics are usually given.
- The majority of masses resolve over a period of days.
- A rising pulse rate, swinging fever and increase in size of the mass indicate abscess formation.
- An abscess is drained via a retroperitoneal incision situated laterally to McBurney's point and usually no attempt is made to locate and remove the appendix unless it is easily accessible.

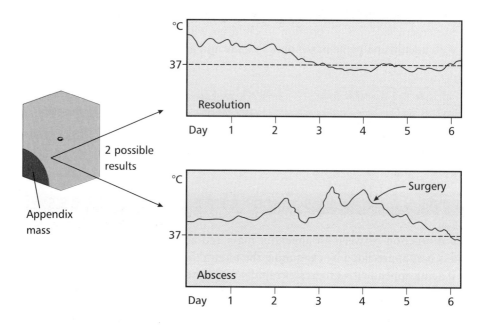

**Figure 25.6** Appendix mass with temperature charts

- Following resolution of an appendix mass or abscess it is generally advisable to let the inflammation settle completely and then to perform an appendicectomy to prevent further problems. The interval allowed between resolution and operation is usually 3 months – so-called '**interval appendicectomy**'.

## APPENDICITIS IN THE YOUNG AND AGED

- In infants under 3 years the incidence of perforation and peritonitis is greater than in adults, possibly because the greater omentum is short and underdeveloped and does not assist as readily in isolating inflammation.
- Diagnosis is difficult since a complete history is unavailable and usually the clinical picture is one of a miserable toxic child who resents examination of any kind. Abdominal signs can be impossible to elicit in an infant who is squirming and crying.
- Elderly patients tend to disregard symptoms until they are very unwell; consequently, they often present late with peritonitis or signs of low small bowel obstruction.

When doubt exists in both the very young and the very old, there should be no hesitation in establishing a diagnosis either by open operation or laparoscopy.

## APPENDICITIS IN PREGNANCY

- The appendix is displaced upwards and laterally by the enlarging uterus and with appendicitis the site of tenderness and guarding likewise follows suit.
- Pyelitis occurs frequently in pregnancy and the diagnosis of appendicitis can be delayed if the symptoms resemble renal tract infection.
- If the urine is clear and appendicitis is likely, it should be treated appropriately.
- Peritonitis following perforation of the appendix is associated with a high risk of abortion or premature labour.
- Miscarriage is most likely to occur in the first trimester.

## THE 'GRUMBLING APPENDIX'

This term is often used to describe a condition usually seen in older children or teenagers, many of whom have emotional problems. It is characterized by repeated attacks of right iliac fossa pain, of variable nature and degree and which are not accompanied by fever or other signs of inflammation. Exhaustive investigation usually fails to find an obvious cause and in any case of real doubt appendicectomy is advocated, using either the standard grid-iron incision or the laparoscope. The appendix is removed and a careful search made for abnormalities in the terminal ileum, caecum, pelvic organs in women or the presence of a Meckel's diverticulum. Often everything is normal but the patients continue to complain of pain.

## TUMOURS OF THE APPENDIX

- **Carcinoid tumour** is the most common neoplasm although it is found only in about 1 in 400 appendices removed at operation. It forms a discrete **yellow** nodule in the tip of the appendix or, more rarely, in the base. Derived from the **Kulchitsky** cells of the intestinal glands, the cells have an affinity for silver stains (argentaffinomas). The majority are benign, but, rarely, carcinoid tumours are malignant and metastasize to the mesenteric nodes and liver. **Carcinoid syndrome is caused by secretion of serotonin from liver metastases** and is characterized by flushing, diarrhoea and a pulmonary systolic murmur.
- **Carcinoma** of the appendix is very rare as a primary condition. Carcinoma of the caecum can invade the appendix, causing obstructive appendicitis. It is treated as for any adenocarcinoma of the large bowel.

**CRIB BOX – APPENDIX**

**Commonest abdominal emergency** – mortality 1% from peritonitis; disease of Western world

**Two types**

- Congestive – slow onset
- Obstructive – rapid onset

**Diagnose on:**

- History – central pain shifting to right iliac fossa
- Examination – RIF tenderness, guarding and rebound pain

**Treatment**

- Appendicectomy when fit for surgery (i.e. not moribund and dehydrated)
- McBurney's point incision (1/3 between anterior superior iliac spine and umbilicus) or using laparoscope
- Post-operative complications – general (chest, DVT), wound infection, pelvic abscess, ileus, faecal fistula, adhesions

**Differential diagnosis** – outside abdomen, retroperitoneal, intraperitoneal (especially gynaecological and mesenteric adenitis in children)

**Appendix mass** – treat conservatively (interval appendicectomy)

**Appendix abscess** – drain (interval appendicectomy)

**Young and old** – rare, dangerous and difficult to diagnose

**Tumours very rare** – carcinoid and adenocarcinoma

chapter 26

# THE OESOPHAGUS

## ANATOMY

The oesophagus is a muscular tube 25 cm in length which extends from cricopharyngeus in the neck (level C6) and passes through the posterior mediastinum to pierce the diaphragm (T10) and join the cardia of the stomach in the abdomen (T11). **The mucosa is non-keratizing squamous epithelium.** The submucosa contains numerous glands and an extensive network of lymphatics. The muscular layer consists of an outer longitudinal layer and an inner circular layer and is composed of skeletal muscle in the upper third, smooth muscle in the lower third, with a transitional middle third. Only the intra-abdominal oesophagus has a serosa. The oesophagus contains a plexus of nerves to co-ordinate peristalsis and propel food to the stomach. Oesophageal pH is normally 5–7 unless there is reflux of gastric contents.

## CONGENITAL ABNORMALITIES

The commonest (1 in 3000) congenital abnormality of the oesophagus is **oesophageal atresia** which is commonly associated with tracheo-oesophageal fistula. Half are associated with other congenital anomalies.

Other congenital conditions of the oesophagus include oesophageal duplication, duplication cysts, oesophageal webs and stenosis.

## DYSPHAGIA

Difficulty in swallowing is termed dysphagia and is **the most common symptom of oesophageal disease.** Swallowing is initiated either voluntarily or involuntarily by reflex action after dilatation of the pharyngeal muscles. It depends on the synchronized combined action of the pharyngeal and oesophageal muscles under neural control. Passage of food from the pharynx to the stomach relies on a wave of peristalsis initiated by the pharyngeal muscles or by upper oesophageal distension and depends on the neural plexus present in the oesophagus. Thus dysphagia may occur due to:

**Neuromuscular disease**
- Motor neurone disease
- Myasthenia gravis

- Cerebrovascular accident affecting the 9th, 10th, or 12th cranial nerves
- Achalasia
- Chagas' disease
- Diffuse spasm
- Diabetic autonomic neuropathy.

### Obstruction
- Foreign body
- Benign stricture (peptic, caustic)
- Tumour
- External compression (mediastinal mass).

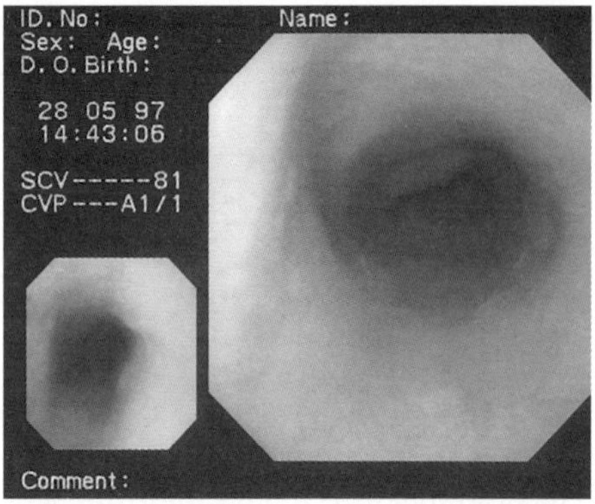

**Figure 26.1** Endoscopic view of oesophagus

### Non-compliance
- Scleroderma
- Other rheumatic diseases.

> In every case of dysphagia it is imperative that malignancy is excluded before attributing the symptom to another cause. This is done with an endoscopy (Figure 26.1) or barium swallow.

## ACHALASIA OF THE OESOPHAGUS (CARDIOSPASM)

Achalasia is a condition characterized **by absent peristalsis and failure of the lower oesophageal sphincter to relax.** The notable pathological change is absence of ganglion cells in the oesophageal muscles. The aetiology is unknown but abnormalities of the vagus nerve and its dorsal nucleus, viral infection, autoimmune disease and vitamin deficiency have been implicated.

### Symptoms
The condition develops slowly over many years. As food and liquid accumulate in the oesophagus, dilation takes place and dysphagia and regurgitation become the predominant symptoms. Regurgitation may not take place until some time after a meal. Patients occasionally learn to eat food and then wash it through with copious amounts of fluid or find that eating and drinking is facilitated by standing. Accumulation of food and liquid in the oesophagus can lead to aspiration and recurrent chest infection, bronchiectasis and lung abscess.

### Diagnosis
Diagnosis is confirmed with a barium swallow showing a dilated oesophagus which tapers at the lower oesophagus (**'bird's beak'**) to a non-peristaltic segment (Figure 26.2). Endoscopy is necessary to confirm absence of a stenosing tumour or other mechanical cause of dysphagia. Oesophageal manometry can be per-

formed to simultaneously measure intraluminal pressures throughout the length of the oesophagus. In achalasia there is a lack of peristaltic activity and a high resting pressure. Carcinoma complicates 3% of cases.

### Treatment

Initially treatment is by **endoscopic balloon dilatation** of the lower sphincter. Surgery is reserved for failure of dilation, perforation after dilation and children. The operation of **Heller's cardiomyotomy** involves dividing the muscles of the distal oesophagus and cardia, and may be performed in conjunction with an anti-reflux procedure.

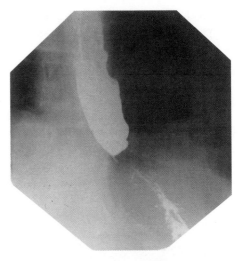

**Figure 26.2** Barium swallow in achalasia showing 'bird's beak'

## CHAGAS' DISEASE

In South America infection with *Trypanosoma cruzi* leads to destruction of the ganglion cells and mega-oesophagus. Chagas' disease also affects cardiac muscle (causing heart failure and cardiac rupture) and the rest of the gastrointestinal tract.

## SECONDARY OESOPHAGEAL MOTILITY DISORDERS

**Systemic sclerosis (scleroderma)** commonly presents with, or is complicated by, dysphagia due to the oesophagus becoming stiff and non-compliant. Reflux often complicates the condition. There is a characteristic appearance on barium swallow of a dilated oesophagus with aperistalsis, but unlike achalasia there is free flow of contrast into the stomach and often reflux the other way. Other connective tissue diseases such as **rheumatoid arthritis** and **systemic lupus erythematosis** can be complicated by this problem. Management is difficult, but usually most symptoms are controlled by decreasing acid reflux with medical therapy ($H_2$ blockers or proton pump inhibitors).

## GASTRO-OESOPHAGEAL REFLUX

This is a common condition caused by the reflux of gastric acid and enzymes into the oesophagus; it is also known as **reflux oesophagitis**.

### Pathogenesis

The aetiology is multifactorial but is predominantly due to **failure of the lower oesophageal sphincter**. This is not an anatomical sphincter but comprises several mechanisms:

- The lower oesophageal muscle tone
- The cardiac angle
- The crura of the diaphragm
- The folds of mucosa at the oesophagogastric junction
- The increased pressure on the intraperitoneal oesophagus.

An incompetent lower sphincter will allow gastric contents to reflux into the oesophagus in certain circumstances, e.g. when lying flat; when the stomach is full; when there is increased intra-abdominal pressure (obesity, pregnancy). Reflux of acid and enzymes produces mucosal damage and inflammation which can lead to:

- Bleeding – causing anaemia or occasionally haematemesis
- Ulceration – causing fibrotic strictures.

> If reflux irritates the mucosa for a sufficiently long period of time it changes from squamous to columnar epithelium – a condition named **Barrett's oesophagus**. The new epithelium may be junctional, gastric or intestinal in type and can be diagnosed only on endoscopy. **Such epithelium has an increased risk of malignant transformation.**

### Symptoms

Typically there is chest pain (often described as heartburn), regurgitation and dysphagia. Commonly there is pain on or after swallowing hot, spicy or acidic food and drink. **Symptoms are related to posture so that they are more prominent on lying down, bending or stooping and after eating or drinking large quantities.** Other symptoms may reflect the complications of reflux such as dysphagia from strictures, bleeding from ulcers and respiratory complaints from aspiration of refluxed material.

### Investigations

Investigations include ambulatory pH monitoring (which allows measurements of intraluminal pH for 24 hours or more as reflux may only occur at night or after meals), barium swallow and endoscopy.

### Medical management

This includes weight reduction, cessation of smoking and alcohol intake, and avoidance of foods and drinks that cause symptoms. Meals should be small and regular and should not be taken before sleep. The head of the bed should be raised, or the patient sleeps sitting up. Antacids and alginates can be used to protect the mucosa. Oesophageal and gastric motility and clearance can be improved with drugs such as metoclopramide and cisapride; acid production in the stomach is reduced by $H_2$ blockers (ranitidine), or proton pump inhibitors (omeprazole).

### Surgical management

If conservative and medical treatments fail, or patients are unwilling to undergo prolonged medical treatment, there are a number of **surgical options. These**

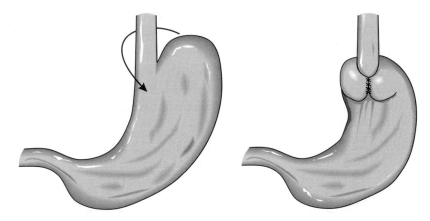

**Figure 26.3** Nissen fundoplication

operations aim to create a good segment of intra-abdominal oesophagus with a valve mechanism at the distal oesophagus to prevent reflux. The commonest procedure is the **Nissen fundoplication** (Figure 26.3) in which the fundus of the stomach is wrapped around the distal intraperitoneal oesophagus and sutured to itself, usually around a bougie to ensure that the wrap is neither too loose (rendering the operation ineffective), nor too tight (causing dysphagia). It can be performed through the abdomen (commonly) or chest, but has become rare with the advent of effective antacid therapy. The use of less invasive laparoscopic techniques is making the operation more popular.

### Strictures
Arising as a result of ulceration, these can usually be treated with endoscopic balloon dilatation although occasionally operative patch repair must be undertaken, usually with an anti-reflux procedure.

### Barretts's oesophagus
Should be kept under endoscopic surveillance and if the risk of malignant change (length of diseased oesophagus, length of time present, dysplasia on biopsy) is high, then surgical intervention is undertaken.

## NON-REFLUX OESOPHAGITIS

Other causes of oesophagitis include ingestion of caustic or corrosive agents such as acid, bleach, detergents and boiling water. Depending on the strength and time of exposure, the amount of tissue damage varies and, if significant, produces either a perforation or scarring and stricture. Infective causes include *Candida* and herpes virus, especially in the immunocompromised. Drugs (non-steroidal anti-inflammatory drugs), radiation (therapeutic or accidental) and a number of specific disorders such as Crohn's disease and Behçet's disease also cause oesophagitis and strictures.

## HIATUS HERNIA

Herniation of the stomach through the diaphragmatic hiatus is relatively common. It is a cause of reflux oesophagitis, although not all hiatus herniae are associated with reflux. There are three variants (Figure 26.4):

- Axial or sliding
- Para-oesophageal or rolling
- Mixed.

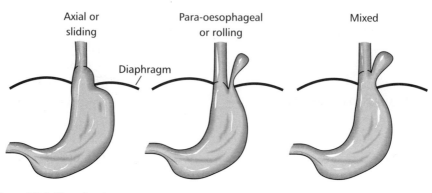

**Figure 26.4** Hiatus herniae

The axial variety is the commonest type and occurs when the distal oesophagus and proximal stomach slide through the hiatus, causing failure of the lower oesophageal sphincter mechanism. The para-oesophageal type, where the fundus of the stomach herniates through the hiatus alongside the oesophagus, is prone to incarceration, infarction and perforation. In the mixed type a large para-oesophageal hernia causes the gastro-oesophageal junction to migrate through the hiatus.

### Management

Only hiatus herniae causing significant symptoms are considered for surgery, the most usual conservative measure being weight loss and medical treatment of any associated reflux oesophagitis. Types of operation include simple reduction of the hernia followed by repair of the defect, or a Nissen fundoplication.

## OESOPHAGEAL TUMOURS

Benign oesophageal tumours are rare. The most common are leiomyomas in the distal oesophagus. Benign polyps such as squamous papillomas and adenomas may be found incidentally during upper gastrointestinal endoscopy.

Malignant tumours are:

### Carcinomas

- Squamous cell carcinomas (95%)
- Adenocarcinomas (lower third) (2%)
- Adenoid cystic carcinoma
- Mucoepidermoid carcinoma
- Bronchial (direct spread)
- Melanoma
- Carcinoid tumours.

## Sarcomas
- Leiomyosarcoma, Rhabdomyosarcoma.

## Others
- Lymphomas.

### Pathology
Squamous carcinoma of the oesophagus is **relatively common** world-wide and has a poor prognosis. It most commonly occurs in China, Iran and the Transkei. Proven aetiological factors include smoking, excess alcohol (especially spirits), poorly preserved foods, human papilloma virus infection, oesophageal reflux, Barrett's oesophagus and achalasia. The tumours can be polypoid, stenosing or ulcerating, and direct spread to adjacent organs occurs early (as the oesophagus lacks a serosa for most of its length). **Survival is related to the stage of the disease, depth of invasion and length of the primary tumour.**

### Clinical features
Oesophageal carcinoma **usually presents with dysphagia,** initially for solids (e.g. meat) and eventually liquids. Physical examination is usually normal unless there has been extensive distant nodal metastasis or weight loss from poor nutrition.

### Investigations
Barium swallow and endoscopy are the most important diagnostic investigations. Barium swallow shows a **characteristic shouldered stenosing lesion** (Figure 26.5). Endoscopy allows a tissue diagnosis (Figure 26.6). Staging investigations (CT

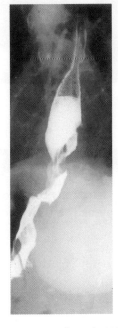

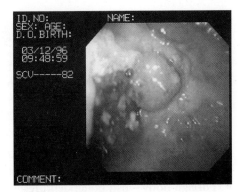

**Figure 26.5** Barium swallow of carcinoma of oesophagus

**Figure 26.6** Endoscopic view of carcinoma of oesophagus

scan, MRI) are needed to assess the suitability of the tumour for surgical excision. Most are not resectable due to direct spread into surrounding mediastinal structures (bronchus; diaphragm; aorta) or metastases. The fitness of the patient to undergo major surgery must also be determined with special attention paid to cardiovascular, respiratory and nutritional status. The final test of resectability is the operation itself.

### Management

- **Surgery** – there are a number of different approaches to oesophageal tumours depending on their site. Most are approached through the abdomen and thorax but total oesophagectomy also requires exploration and mobilization in the neck. The tumour is examined and, if free from invasion into adjacent organs, is removed. The resected oesophagus is replaced with either mobilized stomach or colon. Surgical bypass with stomach or a palliative resection may be attempted but these are associated with high perioperative mortality and morbidity. **All oesophageal surgery of this type has the potential complications of anastomotic leakage and stenosis.** Leaks are difficult to manage and are usually fatal.

- **Radiotherapy** – occasionally provides very long-term remission and is used for inoperable tumours or as first line treatment in the unfit.

- **Stenting** – when the tumour is inoperable dysphagia can be relieved by endoscopic insertion of an intraluminal wire-mesh tube (**stent**) to hold the malignant obstruction open (Figure 26.7). This allows ingestion of soft food and fluids. Other palliative treatment includes laser phototherapy to burn a lumen through the obstructing carcinoma.

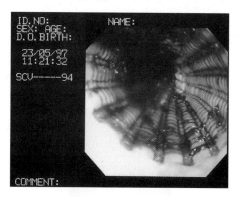

**Figure 26.7** Oesophageal stent

## OESOPHAGEAL PERFORATION

Although uncommon, oesophageal perforation is a dangerous condition which, when untreated, is fatal, and even when managed optimally has significant morbidity and mortality.

The causes are:
- **Iatrogenic** – endoscopy and related procedures; oesophageal surgery; radiotherapy; instrumentation (e.g. chest drain insertion)
- **Penetrating injury** – stab injury (mostly cervical); gun shot
- **Foreign body** – fish bone; dentures; needles
- **Boerhaave's syndrome** – prolonged or violent vomiting
- **Pathological** – tumour; peptic ulceration.

## Clinical features

These are **severe chest pain, tachycardia and fever.** Other features may include haematemesis if the cervical or distal oesophagus is involved, hoarseness of voice if cervical, supraclavicular swelling, surgical emphysema (crepitus of the skin), shortness of breath (pneumothorax), pleural effusion, upper abdominal tenderness and other signs of abdominal perforation. Septic shock is common.

## Investigations

Diagnosis is usually made with a plain chest x-ray showing surgical emphysema, widening of the mediastinum, pleural effusion, pneumothorax and air under the diaphragm if intra-abdominal. A Gastrografin swallow can be used to confirm the diagnosis.

## Management

Management consists of resuscitation, broad spectrum antibiotics, nasogastric drainage, drainage of the pleural cavity if an effusion is present and parenteral nutrition. Most perforations will require surgical repair.

## PHARYNGEAL POUCH AND OTHER OESOPHAGEAL DIVERTICULA

Long-term upper oesophageal dysfunction may be the cause of a pharyngeal diverticulum (**Zenker's diverticulum**) – an out-pouching of the pharyngeal mucosa just above the cricopharyngeus muscle posteriorly (Figures 26.8, 26.9). These can reach a large size and present as a lump in the neck, often on the left side. Other clinical features include regurgitation, halitosis, hoarseness, chronic

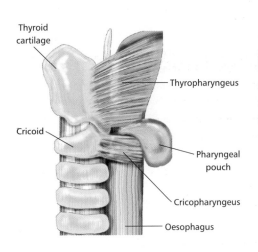

Figure 26.8 Pharyngeal pouch

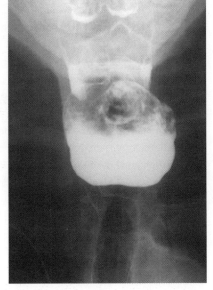

Figure 26.9 X-ray of pharyngeal pouch

cough, and recurrent chest infection due to aspiration. Bleeding, perforation, and the development of neoplasia are all rarer.

Barium swallow is the investigation of choice. Treatment ranges from cricopharyngeal myotomy, diverticulopexy, diverticulectomy and, in the frail, the septum between the diverticulum and the pharynx can be divided endoscopically (**Dohlman's procedure**).

Other diverticula are rarely found throughout the remaining length of the oesophagus and are causes of dysphagia and regurgitation. At the lower oesophagus these are thought to resemble pharyngeal pouch in aetiology. Diverticula in the mid-oesophagus are rare and result from traction of other structures in the mediastinum, usually lymph nodes.

## OESOPHAGEAL BLEEDING

The most common causes of bleeding from the oesophagus are oesophageal varices and **Mallory–Weiss** tears, which are longitudinal tears in the distal oesophagus or proximal stomach that arise as a result of prolonged or violent vomiting. The amount of bleeding varies, but occasionally can be torrential. Diagnosis is confirmed by endoscopy and usually the bleeding is self-limiting. The tear can be injected endoscopically or can be treated by surgical repair.

Other causes of bleeding include oesophagitis of any cause, tumours, perforation and diverticula.

---

**CRIB BOX – OESOPHAGUS**

- The oesophagus is lined by **non-keratinizing squamous epithelium**. Remember Barrett's oesophagus
- The most common symptom is **dysphagia**
- **Cancer must be excluded** before any other diagnosis is made
- **Reflux oesophagitis** is common and usually **treated medically**
- **Hiatus hernia** – sliding; rolling; mixed. Many are **symptomless**
- **Oesophageal cancer** – usually **squamous** and **often inoperable**. Palliation involves **radiotherapy and stenting**
- **Oesophageal perforation is usually iatrogenic**
- **Oesophageal bleeding** – varices; Mallory–Weiss tears; oesophagitis; tumours

# chapter 27

# DISEASES OF THE STOMACH AND DUODENUM

The commonest disease of the stomach and duodenum is peptic ulceration, which affects up to 10% of all men and many women in Britain. Ulceration occurs when the aggressive factors of hydrochloric acid and pepsin overcome the natural protective factors of mucosal integrity, mucus and bicarbonates. *Helicobacter pylori* infection is now known to be involved in the vast majority of gastritis and duodenal ulcers.

## GASTRIC SECRETION

The gastric glands contain parietal cells that produce hydrochloric acid, cells that secrete pepsin, and cells that secrete mucus. Mucus-secreting cells are also found in the cardia and pyloric mucosa where the secretion is weakly alkaline. Acid-producing glands occupy more than two-thirds of the stomach (body); the cardia and pyloric antrum are devoid of acid-secreting cells (Figure 27.1).

Resting acid secretion is 15% of maximum. Acid secretion in response to food is increased by:

- **Vagal reflex** – the first or **cephalic phase** of gastric secretion occurring in response to the smell, sight or taste of food
- **Gastrin secretion** – the second and most important **humoral phase** in which the hormone gastrin is released from the pyloric antrum when it is in contact with food. Gastrin circulates in the blood and stimulates acid production.

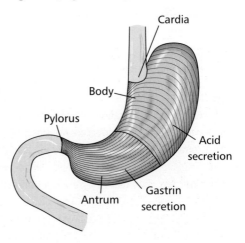

**Figure 27.1** Anatomy of the stomach

## *HELICOBACTER PYLORI*

*Helicobacter pylori* is a recently discovered micro-aerophilic bacillus that infects the stomach. It is found world wide, the risk of infection being greatest in developing countries.

The method of spread is unclear but is probably oro-faecal.

Apart from those who develop chronic peptic ulcer, most infected individuals remain well.

The two most important associated diseases are peptic ulcer and gastroduodenitis.

The organism is also implicated in the development of gastric cancer and lymphoma.

## H. PYLORI IN CHRONIC GASTRITIS AND NON-ULCER DYSPEPSIA (NUD)

*H. pylori* is the commonest cause of gastritis world wide.

The relationship between gastritis and dyspepsia is far from clear.

There is no convincing evidence that eradication of *H. pylori* improves symptoms in NUD.

Inflammation does, however, resolve with eradication of *H. pylori*.

Infection usually involves the **gastric antrum**, but in severe cases a **pangastritis** may occur.

With time, **glandular atrophy** may occur and **intestinal metaplasia** develops.

This sequence is thought to be important in the development of **gastric cancer**.

## H. PYLORI IN PEPTIC ULCERATION

*H. pylori* is present in >80% of adults with gastric ulcers and 95% of those with duodenal ulcers. Physiological changes cause marked hyperaemia and release of inflammatory cytokines. Changes in gastric acidity are inconsistent.

Eradication of *H. pylori* reduces the relapse rate of duodenal ulcer from 80% to less than 10%.

There is a similar reduction in gastric ulcer relapse.

The long-term complications of haemorrhage and perforation are reduced.

## H. PYLORI AND GASTRIC NEOPLASIA

Most patients with gastric adenocarcinoma have evidence of current or previous infection. However, both gastric cancer and infection with *H. pylori* are epidemiologically linked with increasing age and low socioeconomic status, so the relative importance of infection is difficult to ascertain.

Data from prospective studies indicate a three- to sixfold increase in the rate of gastric cancer. **The WHO has classified *H. pylori* as a definite carcinogen.**

*H. pylori* has also been linked with tumours of mucosa-associated lymphoid tissue (**MALT**).

These lymphomas have been shown in some instances to regress after eradication of *H. pylori*.

### Diagnosis and eradication

Tests for *H. pylori* include serology and $^{13}C$ urea breath tests, but the gold standard remains endoscopic mucosal biopsies and culture. A rapid urease test may be performed at the time of biopsy. The organism is resistant to single antibiotics and currently **the most effective regimen (>95% eradication) includes a proton pump inhibitor with two antibiotics.**

# PEPTIC ULCER

Peptic (Greek *peptein*: to digest) ulceration occurs in the presence of acid digestive juice at five sites:

1 Oesophagus – reflux
2 Stomach
3 Duodenum
4 Meckel's diverticulum – ectopic gastric mucosa
5 Gastrojejunal stoma – following gastric surgery.

Duodenal ulcer (DU) is five times more frequent than gastric ulcer (GU), but has been declining since the 1950s. It is seen commonly in all social groups and 80% occur in men. The most important aetiological factor is *H. pylori* (see above). The vast majority of ulcers are treated medically by reducing acid secretion and eradicating *H. pylori*.

### Aetiology
- *Helicobacter pylori*
- Smoking
- Aspirin, NSAIDs, steroids
- Alcohol
- Zollinger–Ellison syndrome – a rare non-β-cell tumour of the pancreas producing a hormone resembling **gastrin** (gastrinoma). The resulting continuous secretion of large volumes of gastric juice high in acid content gives rise to multiple duodenal and jejunal ulcers. It may occur as part of a MEN-1 syndrome. The tumours are often malignant and treatment is excision if possible or gastrectomy.
- Stress – nervous factors, presumably mediated through the vagus, may lead to hypersecretion of acid. Exacerbations of an ulcer are frequently associated with periods of anxiety and mental stress. Hospitalized patients, particularly those in ITU or having suffered burns, are predisposed to so-called stress ulcers (**Curling's ulcer**).

### Acid status
- **Most patients with DU have high acid output**; *H. pylori* antral gastritis causes high serum gastrin levels and therefore high acid production.
- **Most patients with GU have normal or low acid output**; severe *H. pylori* pangastritis causes reduced acid secretion.

### Pathology
Chronic peptic ulcers penetrate through the mucosal basement membrane into the muscle layer or beyond and **heal with scarring.**

Acute ulcers are simply mucosal erosions that heal rapidly by regrowth of mucosal cells without scarring (e.g. acute erosive gastritis).

- **Gastric ulcer** – most chronic GUs occur in the mid-part of the lesser curve. **Ulcers elsewhere in the stomach should be suspected of malignancy.** The ulcer penetrates the muscle coat of the stomach wall to a variable depth and may eventually involve structures such as the pancreas and liver. **Acute erosive gastritis** produces extensive superficial mucosal ulcers with associated hyperaemia and purpura; it may cause massive bleeding. The cause is often aspirin or NSAIDs taken to cure a hangover on top of alcohol-induced gastritis. It also occurs in severe illness such as septicaemia or uraemia.

- **Duodenal ulcer** – nearly always occur within 2–3 cm of the pylorus. The ulcer is usually solitary, lying on the anterior or posterior wall. **Anterior ulcers perforate to produce peritonitis. Posterior ulcers penetrate the gastroduodenal artery behind the duodenum and cause bleeding.**

### Symptoms and signs

It is not possible to distinguish accurately the symptoms of gastric and duodenal ulcer. Symptoms may be similar to those of gall stones, hiatus hernia, pancreatitis and myocardial ischaemia. However, there are a few truisms worth remembering:

- The classic DU patient is a strapping, overweight, middle-aged man. The classic GU patient is a wizened elderly lady who lives alone.
- Peptic ulcer pain is often intermittent and episodic, felt in the epigastrium or just below the xiphisternum and may radiate through to the back.
- Duodenal ulcer pain is usually relieved by food whereas gastric ulcer pain is exacerbated. Patients are said to **feed a DU and starve a GU**. Weight loss is minimal in DU, but may be a feature of GU and should alert the physician to the possibility of malignancy.
- Examination may or may not show epigastric tenderness.

### Investigations

**Fibreoptic endoscopy** is the investigation of choice (Figure 27.2) and has superseded radiological investigation with a barium meal. Ulcers may be visualized, localized, brushed and biopsied and the mucosa assessed for the presence of *H. pylori*. Bleeding ulcers may be treated endoscopically (see below). All gastric ulcers should be biopsied for evidence of malignancy. A test for *H. pylori* should be taken in all diagnosed cases.

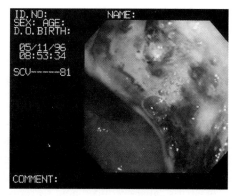

**Figure 27.2** Endoscopic view of an ulcer

### Treatment of peptic ulcer

- **Medical** More than 80% of ulcers will heal with a conventional course of an $H_2$ antagonist for 4–6 weeks. A further 10% will heal with more powerful proton-pump inhibitors (omeprazole or lansoprazole). Relapse rates remain high (80%) with this conventional treatment, but *H. pylori* eradication has revolutionized the management of peptic ulcer disease and reduced the relapse rate to

5–10%. Most regimens use a proton-pump inhibitor and two antibiotics (e.g. lansoprazole 30 mg twice daily with clarithromycin 250 mg and metronidazole 400 mg twice daily) for 1–2 weeks.

Sucralfate improves mucosal protection and is a useful agent, particularly in the management of stress ulcers and in patients in the ITU.

- **Endoscopic**  Bleeding is the most important complication of peptic ulcer disease. Certain endoscopic signs 'stigmata of bleeding' are helpful to determine the risk of bleeding – the visible vessel, red spots, fresh clot. A bleeding ulcer may be treated endoscopically to reduce the transfusion rate, length of hospital stay, operation rate, **but not overall mortality** which remains at 5–10%. Various modes of treatment are available and in skilled hands all are equally effective:
  - Injection with adrenaline ± sclerosing agent
  - Heat probe or bipolar electrocoagulation
  - Laser photocoagulation.

Endoscopy with therapy should be available within 24 hours of presentation of upper gastrointestinal bleeding, and most hospitals have treatment protocols with on-call endoscopists for this purpose.

- **Surgical**  Indications for surgical treatment of peptic ulcer are:

1 **Failure of medical treatment to relieve symptoms.** This is now most unusual.
2 **Complications.** Uncontrolled haemorrhage necessitates emergency surgery. Perforation and stenosis usually warrant an operation.
3 **Malignancy.** A non-healing gastric ulcer with or without suspicious histology should be excised and frank malignancy should be treated surgically after appropriate assessment for operability (see below).

## OPERATIONS FOR PEPTIC ULCERATION

### Gastric ulcer

Billroth I partial gastrectomy is the operation of choice for gastric ulcer (see Figure 27.3). This is essentially a plastic operation to remove the ulcer and the ulcer-bear-

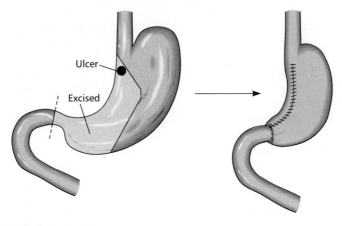

Ulcer

Excised

**Figure 27.3** Billroth I gastrectomy

ing area of the lesser curve and then to fashion a new functional stomach. There is no primary intention to reduce acid output since this is normal or low in gastric ulceration; it will, of course, happen anyway since the majority of the antrum (gastrin production) and a proportion of the body (acid production) is excised.

### Duodenal ulcer

The primary intention of duodenal ulcer surgery is to reduce acid secretion. This can be achieved by vagotomy or gastrectomy.

- **Vagotomy** – eliminates the cephalic phase of acid secretion (Figure 27.4). In this operation the vagal nerves are identified at the gastro-oesophageal junction. If they are divided at this level (**truncal vagotomy**) the stomach loses its capacity to produce acid, but it will also lose motility and a drainage procedure will be necessary – either a pyloroplasty or gastrojejunostomy. However, if the vagal supply to the pylorus is preserved whilst the vagal supply to the body of the stomach is divided, the stomach will retain its ability to empty and a drainage procedure is not required. This is the operation of **highly selective vagotomy**. Vagotomy can be performed laparoscopically.

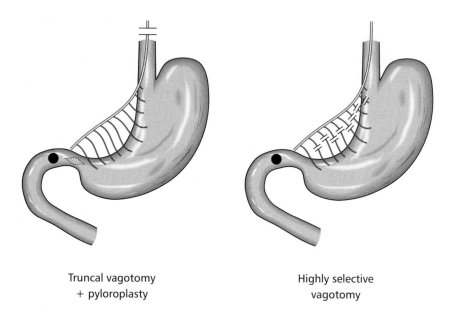

| Truncal vagotomy | Highly selective |
| + pyloroplasty | vagotomy |

**Figure 27.4** Truncal and highly selective vagotomy

- **Gastrectomy** – eliminates the humoral phase of acid secretion (antrum). The Billroth II or Polya gastrectomy involves a two-thirds gastric resection and restoration with a gastrojejunostomy (see Figure 27.5). Removing a portion of the gastric body also reduces acid secretion by reducing the total parietal cell mass.

Gastrectomy for duodenal ulcer is probably now indicated only in the Zollinger–Ellison syndrome or as an emergency procedure for bleeding.

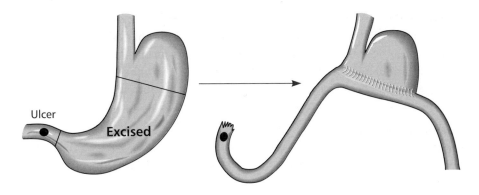

**Figure 27.5** Polya gastrectomy

## SPECIFIC COMPLICATIONS OF SURGERY

- Post-vagotomy diarrhoea – seen in truncal vagotomy because of vagal denervation of most of the gut. Not seen in patients who have undergone highly selective vagotomy.
- Dumping syndrome – fainting and giddiness within half an hour of eating. Possibly caused by hypovolaemia due to the osmotic effect of food entering the jejunum rapidly. 'Late' dumping occurs at around 2 hours due to hypoglycaemia from rebound hyperinsulinaemia following a period of high sugar levels caused by rapid absorption.
- Anastomotic or stomal ulceration – seen most commonly on the jejunal side of a gastrojejunal anastomosis.
- Bilious vomiting – following gastrojejunostomy bile may acccumulate in the stomach, giving rise to bouts of green bilious vomiting.
- Malabsorption – deficient absorption of iron, vitamin B12 and calcium may occur, particularly after gastrectomy.

## COMPLICATIONS OF CHRONIC PEPTIC ULCER

There are five complications of chronic peptic ulcer:

1 Perforation
2 Penetration
3 Haemorrhage
4 Stenosis (pyloric stenosis; hour-glass stomach)
5 Maligancy (gastric ulcer).

### Perforation
Perforation of peptic ulcer is usually a sudden event leading to diffuse peritonitis. Less often, a small leak through a tiny perforation is walled off by omentum and nearby viscera, resulting in localized peritonitis and sometimes a subphrenic abscess.

Duodenal ulcers perforate much more often than gastric ulcers and men are more commonly affected than women. The perforation that causes diffuse peritonitis lies on the anterior wall of the duodenum or stomach. Posterior ulcers burrow into the pancreas or, in the case of a gastric ulcer, into the liver, lesser sac and pancreas. Often there is a long history of dyspepsia before the perforation, but many occur without any previous history.

**Symptoms and signs:**
- Pain which is sudden and excruciating
- Generalized peritonitis, causing 'board-like rigidity' of the abdomen
- Referred pain may be felt in the shoulder due to irritation of the diaphragm
- Shock and collapse
- The patient lies still, for every movement causes pain.

**Diagnosis:**
- The history and physical signs usually make the diagnosis easy.
- An erect chest x-ray may show air under the diaphragm (Figure 27.6).
- The differential diagnosis includes any cause of generalized peritonitis, cholecystitis, pancreatitis, myocardial infarct, pneumothorax and dissecting aneurysm.

**Treatment:**
- Intravenous fluid resuscitation for shock
- Analgesia for pain
- Antibiotics
- Surgery – via laparotomy or laparoscopy the peritoneal cavity is thoroughly washed out and the perforation oversewn (Figure 27.7).

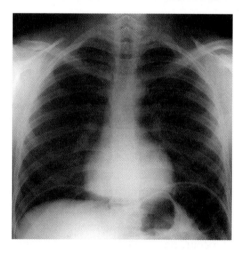

**Figure 27.6** Erect chest x-ray with free gas under the diaphragm

Medical therapy is instituted following repair of the perforation.

An appreciable number of perforated gastric ulcers are malignant, so there is a strong case for immediate partial gastrectomy to be performed for perforated gastric ulcer. If it is to be only oversewn a biopsy must be taken first.

Patients may be too ill for any operation, particularly if the diag-

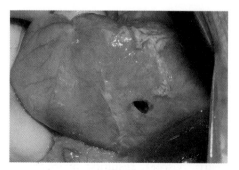

**Figure 27.7** Perforated peptic ulcer at surgery

nosis has been long delayed; conservative treatment is nasogastric suction, intravenous fluids and antibiotics.

### Penetration

Sometimes a duodenal or gastric ulcer may extend into the pancreas, liver or other neighbouring viscera. Invasion of the pancreas is suggested by the change in the character of the pain, which becomes more constant and often radiates to the back. It may be difficult clinically to distinguish carcinoma of the stomach from a benign ulcer, but the diagnosis can always be made from endoscopic biopsy. In gastrectomy for gastric ulcer the base of the ulcer may often have to be left on the pancreas, but this causes no complications. The most important complication of penetration is haemorrhage.

### Haemorrhage

Haemorrhage from a duodenal or gastric ulcer may present as haematemesis or melaena or sometimes both. There are many causes of bleeding from the upper GI tract. The approximate order of frequency is:

- Peptic ulcer – 90%
- Oesophageal varices – portal hypertension
- Drugs – aspirin; NSAIDs; steroids – acute erosive gastritis
- Tumours of the stomach – benign and malignant
- Blood dyscrasias – haemophilia, thrombocytopenia and the reticuloses
- Toxaemia and septicaemia – stress ulcer, especially following uraemia and burns
- Vessel-wall defects – von Willebrand's disease and pseudoxanthoma elasticum
- Mallory–Weiss syndrome – haematemesis due to a tear at the cardia produced by violent vomiting.

**Investigation and treatment of haemorrhage** Following a detailed history and examination, the patient must be resuscitated:
- Oxygen by mask
- Intravenous fluid and **blood replacement**
- CVP monitoring if necessary
- Urinary catheter to monitor renal function.

Most bleeding stops spontaneously. Once the patient is stable, **endoscopy is performed** (Figure 27.8) for diagnosis and treatment, e.g. injection sclerotherapy.

**Indications for surgery:**
- Failure of medical treatment – often due to massive haemorrhage, making it impossible to visualize a bleeding vessel

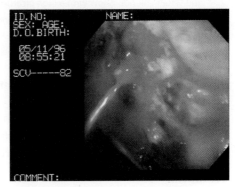

**Figure 27.8** Endoscopic view of bleeding gastric ulcer

- Re-bleeding following initial successful medical treatment
- Simultaneous perforation
- Malignant gastric ulcer
- In elderly patients, possibly because of sclerotic vessels, bleeding is less likely to stop spontaneously or respond to sclerotherapy, and surgery should be considered earlier.

For gastric ulcers a partial gastrectomy is done. A bleeding vessel in a duodenal ulcer may be under-run by a suture and recurrence prevented by vagotomy or post-operative medical treatment.

### Pyloric stenosis

Pyloric stenosis is caused by:
- Fibrosis and narrowing secondary to duodenal ulceration
- Carcinoma of the antrum
- Hypertrophic pyloric stenosis occurs in babies, but rarely in adults.

### Clinical features:
- Vomiting is the cardinal sign of pyloric stenosis. The vomitus is large in amount, forceful (projectile), and contains undigested food – often the contents of meals eaten days before are recognized.
- A long history of dyspepsia is common. Starvation causes a rapid loss of weight.
- Visible gastric peristalsis may be seen when the stomach is full. Waves of peristalsis pass from left to right across the epigastrium.
- A mass may be felt in cases of carcinoma and in babies with hypertrophic pyloric stenosis.
- Splashing may be elicited by sudden pressure over the distended stomach (succussion splash).
- Dehydration occurs with persistent vomiting.

### Investigations:

- Electrolytes – the patient loses water and HCl, resulting in **hypochloraemic alkalosis,** i.e. the serum chloride is low with a high bicarbonate and in late cases an inappropriate acid urine is excreted. These findings are pathognomonic. The level of ionized calcium falls in alkalosis, so tetany may occur.

- Barium meal – shows gastric dilatation with food residue and outlet obstruction.
- Endoscopy – often impossible until the stomach has been washed out. Reveals antral carcinoma or a stenosed pylorus.
- Ultrasound scan – in babies a hypertrophied pyloric 'tumour' is seen.

### Treatment:
- Dehydration and electrolyte imbalance are corrected with normal saline.
- Stomach washouts are performed to clear old food debris.

- Endoscopic balloon dilatation can be used for benign strictures.
- The usual surgical procedure is a drainage operation to bypass the duodenum (gastrojejunostomy), often combined with a vagotomy.
- Partial gastrectomy is performed for carcinoma of the stomach.
- Ramstedt's pyloromyotomy is performed for infantile hypertrophic pyloric stenosis.

### Hour-glass constriction of the stomach

Stenosis of the mid-part of the stomach is almost entirely confined to women; it is very rare nowadays. An ulcer in the middle of the lesser curve may cause fibrosis and scarring, dividing the stomach into two sacs. Rarely, the cause is carcinoma. The symptoms and signs are those of pyloric stenosis. Hour-glass constriction is treated by partial gastrectomy.

## CARCINOMA OF THE STOMACH

Carcinoma of the stomach is relatively common – about 8000 people die of it in England and Wales every year. It is one of the few cancers that seem to be declining in incidence, especially in North America. Men are more often affected than women at an age usually between 40 and 70 years. Carcinoma of the stomach is associated more commonly with blood group A. It is relatively rare in Jews and Asians and common in Japan. **World wide it is most common in lower socioeconomic groups and it now seems clear that there is a causal connection between _H. pylori_, atrophic gastritis, low acid secretion, and gastric cancer.** Pernicious anaemia sufferers (atrophic gastritis; achlorhydria) also have a high incidence of carcinoma of the stomach. It is thought that 1% of benign gastric ulcers become malignant.

### Pathology

The regions of the stomach affected by carcinoma are mainly the pyloric antrum (50%), lesser curve (25%) and cardia (10%). Carcinoma of the stomach (Figure 27.9) may present as a malignant ulcer with rolled everted edges, a proliferating polypoid mass or a thickening that may be localized or may diffusely involve the whole stomach ('**leather-bottle stomach**').

Histology shows an adenocarcinoma of varying degrees of differentiation. Rarely, squamous carcinoma is seen at the cardia.

Spread is by:

- Lymph nodes – along the lesser and greater curves and eventually to those around the coeliac axis. Nodes

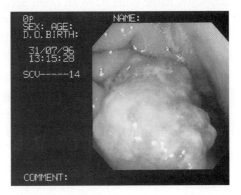

**Figure 27.9** Endoscopic view of carcinoma of the stomach

in the porta hepatis cause jaundice from pressure on the hepatic ducts. At a late stage, there may be spread to the left supraclavicular lymph nodes (**Troisier's sign or Virchow's node**).

- Portal vein spread gives rise to metastases in the liver, lungs and elsewhere.
- Trans-coelomic implantation of cancer cells throughout the peritoneum produces ascites. Occasionally cancer cells grow in the ovaries, producing large cysts or solid tumours – (Krukenberg tumours).
- Lastly, carcinoma of the stomach may directly invade surrounding structures, such as the pancreas and transverse colon. A gastrocolic fistula may be produced with distressing vomiting of faeces.

## Symptoms

The onset of carcinoma of the stomach is often insidious, with increasing weakness, anaemia, loss of energy, loss of weight and anorexia. Symptoms referable to the stomach include:

- Dyspepsia
- Pain – due to posterior invasion of the pancreas
- Dysphagia – due to obstructing tumour at the cardia
- Vomiting – due to antral obstruction causing pyloric stenosis
- Jaundice – due to liver metastasis or bile duct obstruction
- Abdominal distension – due to ascites
- Perforation (peritonitis) and severe haemorrhage are common.

## Physical signs

These depend on the mode of presentation, but include epigastric mass, ascites, jaundice, visible peristalsis with succussion splash, and supraclavicular glands. Rarely, a malignant nodule is felt at the umbilicus (**Sister Joseph's nodule**).

## Diagnosis

Any patient who has suspicious symptoms should be investigated. **Dyspepsia beginning after the age of 40 years is suspicious**, especially where the history is brief. Because stomach cancer has such a poor prognosis when diagnosed late, it is important that dyspeptic symptoms are taken seriously and investigated expeditiously. Most units have an open access diagnostic endoscopy service for such patients. Endoscopy with biopsy confirms the diagnosis and can be used as a screening procedure (Japan) to pick up early gastric cancer.

## Treatment

Surgical excision is presently the first line treatment. Preoperative assessment should include CT scanning and, in some cases, laparoscopy to assess operability.

- **Curative surgery** – radical gastrectomy to include all loco-regional lymph nodes, omentum, tail of pancreas and spleen improves long-term survival compared with less extensive surgery.
- **Palliative surgery** – at laparotomy many patients are incurable because of secondary deposits in the liver, spread through the peritoneum or penetration into viscera which cannot be removed. Palliation in the form of partial gastrectomy or gastrojejunostomy can prevent bleeding and gastric outlet obstruction.

- **Adjuvant therapy** – trials of adjuvant chemotherapy and/or radiotherapy are in progress.

> The long-term results of surgery for carcinoma of the stomach have previously been poor, perhaps only 10% of those who have a resection surviving for more than 5 years. The prognosis appears to be greatly improved by early diagnosis and radical surgery – a concept introduced by Japanese surgeons.

## OTHER TUMOURS OF THE STOMACH AND DUODENUM

Benign gastric tumours are rare. Adenomata occur as single or multiple polyps. Leiomyomas are liable to ulceration and haemorrhage; occasionally they become malignant. Neurofibromas and neurogenic sarcomas rarely occur in the stomach. Sarcomas are very rare; usually lymphosarcoma or leiomyosarcoma. Adenoma and adenocarcinoma rarely occur in the duodenum.

## FOREIGN BODIES IN THE STOMACH

Most foreign bodies are swallowed by children and many must never be noticed. The objects swallowed are of infinite variety, including whistles, nails, pins and dentures. Psychiatric patients and prisoners commonly swallow foreign bodies. If hair is swallowed over a period of years a hairball (**trichobezoar**) may form in the stomach, giving rise to a large mass in the shape of the stomach. Usually foreign bodies cause no symptoms, because the vast majority pass spontaneously. Warning symptoms are pain and vomiting; very rarely perforation may occur.

If a foreign body passes the cardia it is also likely to pass through the pylorus and eventually the rectum. The only foreign bodies that require removal are sharp objects likely to cause perforation and very large bodies such as spoons which can never pass through the pylorus.

As long as there are no symptoms and the shape of the object and its size suggest that it will pass, no treatment is required. Infrequent x-rays monitor progress through the gut. If the object remains in the stomach after several days it should be removed by endoscopy or open operation.

## ACUTE DILATATION OF THE STOMACH

Acute dilatation of the stomach used to be a common complication of abdominal operations, but it is rare nowadays because of the nasogastric tube and intravenous fluid replacement. It may follow any operation, abdominal trauma, or immobilization. The cause is not known, but at post mortem (this condition used to be highly fatal) not only is the stomach dilated, but also the duodenum up to the third part, suggesting some degree of duodenal ileus from pressure of the mesenteric vessels. Dilatation of the stomach causes severe discomfort in the epigastrium, distension and vomiting of large volumes of brown offensive fluid. Once vomiting starts, there is grave danger of inhalation of vomit and cardiac arrest. If the condition is suspected, the stomach should be emptied and kept empty by continuous nasogastric aspiration, and i.v. fluid replacement started.

---

### CRIB BOX – STOMACH AND DUODENUM

#### Physiology

- The body secretes acid; the antrum secretes gastrin
- Two phases of acid production – cephalic/vagal and humoral/gastrin

*Helicobacter pylori* – implicated in chronic gastritis, NUD, peptic ulcer and cancer

#### Peptic ulcer

- Oesophagus, stomach, duodenum, Meckel's, and stomal
- Acute – superficial gastric erosions
- Chronic – deep, heal with scarring
- Treatment – medical triple therapy, i.e. proton-pump blocker and two antibiotics
- Indications for surgery – failure of medical treatment and/or complications
- Complications – perforation, penetration, haemorrhage, scarring (stenosis), malignancy (GU)

Remember the biochemistry of pyloric stenosis

#### Carcinoma of stomach

- Reducing in incidence
- *H. pylori* responsible for atrophic gastritis which in turn is responsible for malignant change??
- Treat with radical surgery for best results

# chapter 28

# THE BILIARY AND PORTAL SYSTEMS

Gall stone disease is a common cause of hospital admissions in Western society. It is increasing in developing countries where diet is becoming more westernized.

## THE GALL BLADDER

### GALL STONES (CHOLELITHIASIS)

#### Aetiology
Gall stones are found in **20% of the population in old age. Women account for 80% of patients** – classically 'fair, fat, female, fertile and forty'. Gall stones are caused by a combination of three factors – **metabolic, stasis and infection.**

- Metabolic
  Bile is 97% water containing small amounts of:
  - Bile salts (detergents)
  - Bile pigment (breakdown products of haemoglobin; bilirubin, biliverdin)
  - Fatty acids and cholesterol.
  The gall bladder concentrates the bile up to tenfold and the poorly soluble fats are kept in solution by the **detergent action of the bile salts**. This balance is upset if the concentration of solutes increases, or the concentration of bile salts diminishes. Thus **bile pigment stones** are found in the presence of **haemolytic anaemias** or diseases that result in excessive haemolysis, e.g. spherocytosis; malaria. The **concentration of bile salts is reduced in liver disease, and disease or excision of the terminal ileum** which is the site of **bile salt resorption from the gut** (enterohepatic circulation). Supersaturation of bile with cholesterol will result in crystal formation.

- Stasis
  Minor congenital anatomical anomalies of the gall bladder or bile ducts are very common (up to 10%) and predispose to bile stasis. **The very presence of stones means that stasis must be present** since otherwise they would pass into the gut while still in particulate form. Progesterone relaxes smooth muscle and no doubt contributes to stasis and stone formation in multiparous women.

- Infection
  Many **bacteria deconjugate bilirubin** which will then combine with calcium to form **insoluble calcium bilirubinate**. Gut bacteria reach the gall bladder via the portal bloodstream and lymphatics.

## Types of stone
There are three types of gall stone (Figure 28.1):

1 **Mixed – 80%**; calcium bilirubinate and cholesterol; usually associated with infection; nearly always multiple and faceted.
2 **Cholesterol – 10%**; often solitary (cholesterol 'solitaire') and may become very large. On section they have a crystalline interior.
3 **Pigment – 10%**; (calcium bilirubinate) is seen typically in haemolytic disease; soft, black, crumbly and multiple.

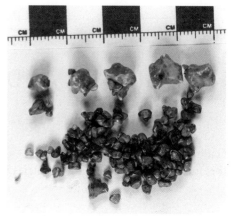

**Figure 28.1** Gall stones

About 10% of all gall stones contain enough calcium for them to be radio-opaque.

## Clinicopathological features of gall stones
**The majority of gall stones produce no symptoms**; 10% of patients will develop symptoms in the first 5 years after incidental diagnosis and only 20% by 20 years (Figure 28.2). Asymptomatic gall stones discovered during routine examination should be left alone. It is estimated that 30% of gall stones will pass spontaneously.

Gall stones cause problems by their presence:
- In the gall bladder
- In the bile ducts.

### In the gall bladder
Stones in the gall bladder (cholelithiasis) are usually asymptomatic.
- **Flatulent dyspepsia** – often cited as a symptom. Dysfunction of the gall bladder is presumed to cause poor fat digestion with resulting flatulence. However, fullness after meals, heartburn, dyspepsia and bloating are symptoms that can similarly be applied to diverticular disease, irritable bowel syndrome and hiatus hernia. Cholecystectomy in patients with flatulent dyspepsia is likely to result in recurrent

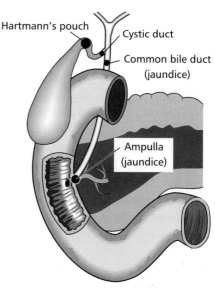

**Figure 28.2** Sites of gall stone obstruction

symptoms in 30% of these patients. It is therefore essential to exclude other causes of flatulent dyspepsia before embarking on cholecystectomy ('**Saint's triad' – hiatus hernia, diverticular disease and gall stones occurring in the same patient**).

- **Biliary colic** – this typical symptom is caused by a stone lodging in Hartmann's pouch or passing through the cystic duct. **Pain is felt in the upper abdomen, radiating around to the right subscapular region and up the back; it is so severe that the victim often believes he/she will die.** Rolling around in agony and vomiting is common. The attack seldom lasts more than a few hours and pain disappears as rapidly as it started once the stone falls back into the body of the gall bladder or passes into the common bile duct. Colic often occurs at night when the supine position in bed allows stones to gravitate to the neck of the gall bladder. Constitutional disturbance is slight, but biliary colic can progress to **acute cholecystitis or empyema**. Rarely, an obstructed gall bladder remains sterile and a mucocele forms.

- **Acute cholecystitis** – the disease process is similar to acute appendicitis save for the lower incidence of gangrene and perforation. Resolution is the usual outcome but severe life-threatening complications such as biliary peritonitis are not uncommon.

> **Acute cholecystitis**
> → Resolution ± fibrosis
> → Suppuration/empyema
> → Gangrene/perforation
> → Chronic cholecystitis

Acute cholecystitis is characterized by **constant inflammatory pain maximal in the right hypochondrium**. The patient is febrile and unwell. Irritation of the diaphragm may give rise to shoulder tip pain while peritoneal irritation may cause the patient to catch their breath in pain if the gall bladder is palpated during inspiration – **Murphy's sign**.

- **Chronic cholecystitis** – Chronic low grade inflammation caused by gall stones, infected bile and stone impaction causes repeated attacks of subacute cholecystitis and colic. The gall bladder becomes scarred, contracted and non-functioning with a thickened fibrotic wall and loss of normal mucosal pattern. Cysts and sinuses may occur in the submucosa (**Rokitansky–Aschoff sinuses**), with abscess formation. Cholesterol impregnation of the inflamed mucosa may produce a red appearance with flecks of yellow – 'strawberry gall bladder'.

- **Gall stone ileus** – Erosion of a large gall stone through the gall bladder wall into the adherent duodenum occurs rarely. Patients present with intestinal obstruction due to the stone, which usually impacts in the terminal ileum. The classic plain x-ray shows dilated bowel with gas in the biliary tree. A laparotomy is required to remove the obstructing stone.

- **Carcinoma of the gall bladder** – This is a rare condition. There is a direct association between gall stones and carcinoma of the gall bladder and the risk correlates with the increasing size of the stone. If the tumour is confined to the mucosa, cholecystectomy is usually curative. Cholecystectomy and wedge resection of the liver may be indicated for more advanced disease. The risk of gall bladder cancer developing in association with gall stones is too low to justify prophylactic cholecystectomy.

**Table 28.1** Symptoms of gall stones

| In the gall bladder | In the bile ducts |
| --- | --- |
| Asymptomatic | Asymptomatic |
| Flatulent dyspepsia | Cholangitis |
| Biliary colic | Jaundice |
| Acute cholecystitis | Pancreatitis |
| Mucocele | |
| Empyema | |
| Gall stone ileus | |
| Carcinoma | |

### In the bile ducts

Stones in the common bile duct (choledocholithiasis) may be asymptomatic and pass harmlessly through the sphincter of Oddi to be expelled in the faeces. Symptoms are caused by infection and obstruction.

- **Cholangitis** – This is a serious infective inflammation of the biliary tree which ascends into the liver. Caused usually by obstructing stones, thick inspissated bile (sludge) or stricture of the common bile duct; rarely by parasitic infection (*Clonorchis* – common in the Far East) and tumour (cholangio-carcinoma and periampullary carcinoma). The patient is unwell and toxic with an alarmingly high swinging **temperature**, a **tender painful liver** and **jaundice** (**Charcot's intermittent fever**).

  Urgent drainage of the biliary tree is required to prevent liver failure.

- **Jaundice** – Stones impacted in the common bile duct will cause obstructive jaundice. Differentiating between obstructive jaundice due to stones or malignancy in the ampulla or head of pancreas is a common clinical problem. Stones are often associated with previous biliary pain whereas **malignant obstruction is usually painless**. Also, the gall bladder distends and is palpable in malignancy whereas the fibrotic gall bladder harbouring stones will not distend (see **Courvoisier's law**).

- **Pancreatitis** – Impaction at the sphincter may cause obstruction of the pancreatic duct and pancreatitis.

### Investigation of gall bladder and biliary tree

History and examination are the first steps, then urine examination for bilirubin and urobilinogen; blood for liver function tests; and imaging of the biliary tree.

- **Ultrasound scanning** – Ultrasound (Figure 28.3) is the safest and most cost-effective method of diagnosing stones in the gall bladder and biliary tree. Acute cholecystitis can be diagnosed with extreme accuracy. Common bile duct (CBD) stones are less easily detected when located behind the duodenum but a dilated CBD is easily imaged and measured (normal <7 mm diameter). The presence of a raised bilirubin, alkaline phosphatase and a dilated CBD suggests stones. Mobile machines can be used for outpatient diagnosis.

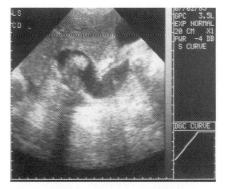

**Figure 28.3** Ultrasound scan of gall stones

- **Endoscopic retrograde cholangiopancreatography (ERCP)** – Under light sedation an endoscope is swallowed and passed into the duodenum to visualize and cannulate the ampulla of Vater. Injection of contrast medium produces x-ray images of the biliary tree and pancreatic ducts (Figure 28.4). This procedure is invasive but has the advantage of being **diagnostic and therapeutic** – stones can be grasped and removed from the bile ducts; sphincterotomy performed to allow passage of stones and free flow of bile; tumours biopsied or stented.

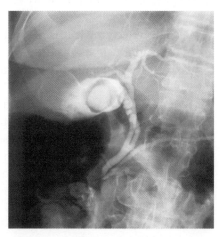

**Figure 28.4** ERCP showing gall stones in gall bladder

- **Percutaneous transhepatic cholangiography (PTC)** – Used in the diagnosis and treatment/palliation of obstructive jaundice. Using local anaesthetic, a fine needle is passed directly into the liver substance until a dilated biliary radical is entered. Injection of contrast details the intra- and extrahepatic biliary system (Figure 28.5). Stents or drains can be inserted percutaneously. A combination of ERCP and PTC may be required to deal with difficult bile duct strictures or tumours.

- **Radioisotope scan** – Technetium-labelled aminodiacetic acid derivatives (HIDA) are excreted rapidly from the blood and concentrated by the liver. Dynamic imaging of the biliary system is obtained and an assessment of hepato-enteric flow (e.g. after hepatico-jejunostomy) can be made.

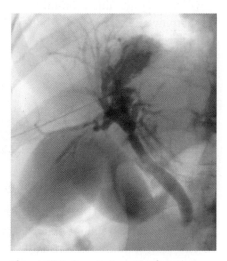

**Figure 28.5** Percutaneous transhepatic cholangiography (PTC) showing lower CBD obstruction

## Treatment of gall stones

Asymptomatic gall stones require no treatment.

- **Non-surgical treatments** have been used with limited success. Such techniques are only suitable in poor-risk patients as the stone recurrence rate is high, for example:
  - **Dissolution therapy** – oral chenodeoxycholic acid or similar dissolution agents may be used to dissolve gall stones. Stones may recur in 50% of patients on completion of treatment.
  - **Extracorporeal shock-wave lithotripsy (ESWL)** – can be used for solitary radiolucent stones less than 2 cm in diameter. Passage of the stone fragments may produce colic.
- **Surgical treatment** is normally employed unless there are medical contraindications.
  - **Cholecystectomy** is feasible and often easier during the first 3–4 days of an acute attack. If early surgery is not possible, acute attacks are treated with analgesics and antibiotics and surgery planned after resolution.

The **aim of cholecystectomy** is to define and expose the structures in **Calot's triangle** (cystic duct, CBD and liver), to ligate the cystic duct and artery and to remove the diseased gall bladder and stones therein **without injury to the common bile duct**. Both 'open' and laparoscopic methods are employed.

- **Open cholecystectomy** – Conventional surgery via Kocher's, transverse or midline incision is still practised and may be required when a laparoscopic procedure is converted to open surgery. **'Mini' cholecystectomy** via a small 5 cm transverse incision over the gall bladder is advocated by some surgeons and gives similar results to laparoscopic surgery. **Peroperative cholangiography** is done routinely in open cholecystectomy by injecting dye into the biliary tree via the cystic duct, on-table radiology providing information on biliary anatomy and stones in the bile ducts.
- **Laparoscopic cholecystectomy** – The operation (Figure 28.6) is essentially the same as open cholecystectomy but performed after producing a $CO_2$ pneumoperitoneum. Placement of four trocars provide access for a camera probe and instruments and negates the need for a formal incision, thus allowing rapid post-operative recovery to full mobility. The patient must be warned that technical difficulties may necessitate conversion to an open operation.

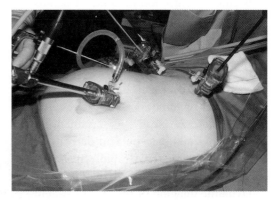

**Figure 28.6** Laparoscopic cholecystectomy ports

### Specific complications of laparoscopic cholecystectomy

#### Intraoperative
- Hypercapnia
- Trocar injuries to bowel, aortoiliac vessels and abdominal wall vessels
- Diathermy injuries
- Bile duct injuries

#### Early post-operative
- Haemorrhage
- Wound infection
- Bile peritonitis

#### Late
- Bile duct strictures, jaundice
- Intra-abdominal abscesses due to dropped stones
- Retained stones in CBD
- Incisional hernia

Injury of the bile duct was initially reported as more than 1% during laparoscopic cholecystectomy. With increasing experience the bile duct injury rate has reduced to about 0.3% of all cases performed in the UK. Missed stones in the common bile duct may remain silent and pass spontaneously or give rise to symptoms.

### Treatment of common bile duct stones

Stones in the common bile duct are found in approximately 10% of patients with gall bladder stones and may give rise to jaundice and ascending cholangitis if bile flow is obstructed. **The aim of treatment is to relieve jaundice and to clear the ducts of stones.**

- **Preoperative methods:** Diagnostic ERCP and sphincterotomy.
  - Stone clearance with Dormia basket or balloons;
  - Insertion of stent for decompression and relief of jaundice.
- **Operative methods:**
  - Open surgery with cholecystectomy and exploration of common bile duct (ECBD);
  - Laparoscopic cholecystectomy and choledochotomy using choledochoscope to remove common bile duct stones.

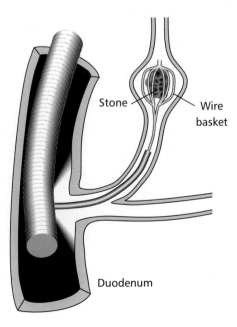

**Figure 28.7** ERCP and stone retrieval

- Post-operative methods:
  - for residual stones detected after routine cholecystectomy
  - ERCP and sphincterotomy
  - Reoperation and ECBD.

## JAUNDICE

- The normal level of bilirubin in the serum is 5–17 μmol.
- Above 30 μmol jaundice is apparent with yellowness of the sclera and skin.
- **Bilirubin** derives from the breakdown products of **haemoglobin** and reaches the liver as unconjugated bilirubin which is insoluble in water (Figure 28.8).
- In the liver it is conjugated with glucuronic acid to become water-soluble and enters the duodenum in the bile.
- In the gut bacterial action breaks it down to stercobilin which is excreted in the faeces and is responsible for their brown colour.
- A small amount is converted to urobilinogen which is reabsorbed from the gut and excreted in the urine.

Thus jaundice occurs with:

- **Excess bilirubin production** (haemolysis)
- **Incomplete conjugation** (liver disease)
- **Inefficient excretion** (biliary obstruction).

**Types of jaundice**

Jaundice is classified as:
- Pre-hepatic (haemolysis)
- Hepatic (hepatocellular)
- Post-hepatic (obstructive)

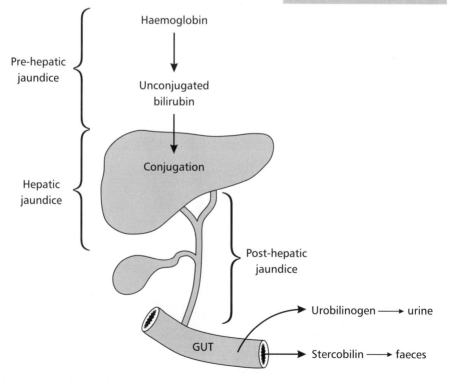

**Figure 28.8** Pathways of bilirubin metabolism

### Diagnosis

The history may suggest exposure to infectious hepatitis, previous transfusion, drugs, liver toxins, Weil's disease. Pain suggests a stone. Painless jaundice with a palpable gall bladder suggests pancreatic carcinoma (see **Courvoisier's law**).

Deciding which type of jaundice a patient has is made easier if some simple clues are used:

- Absence of bilirubin in the urine (**acholuric jaundice**) suggests unconjugated hyperbilirubinaemia and therefore a pre-hepatic cause.
- If the urine contains urobilinogen, the jaundice is unlikely to be post-hepatic (obstructive).
- **Pale or white stools** are diagnostic of obstructive jaundice (do a rectal examination).
- Bile salts escaping retrogradely into the bloodstream in **obstructive jaundice cause intolerable itching** and their presence in the urine produces frothing (detergent action).

**Table 28.2** Biochemical diagnosis of jaundice

|  | Pre-hepatic | Hepatic | Post-hepatic |
| --- | --- | --- | --- |
| Blood |  |  |  |
| Bilirubin | + | +++ | +++ |
| Alkaline phosphatase | N | ++ | +++ |
| Urine |  |  |  |
| Bilirubin | 0 | + | + |
| Urobilinogen | +++ | N | 0 |

N, normal; 0, zero.

### Causes of jaundice

**Pre-hepatic** (haemolytic) jaundice is caused by:
- Spherocytosis
- Pernicious anaemia
- Transfusion reaction
- Haematoma resorption.

**Hepatic** (hepatocellular) jaundice is caused by:
- Cirrhosis
- Viral hepatitis
- Weil's disease
- Poisons and drugs
- Liver tumours.

**Post-hepatic** (obstructive) jaundice is caused by:
- Obstruction in the lumen – gall stones; *Clonorchis*; blood clots
- Obstruction in the wall – atresia; strictures; tumours of bile duct
- Extrinsic compression – carcinoma of head of pancreas; carcinoma of ampulla of Vater; pancreatitis; secondary nodes around porta hepatis.

There remain many cases in which the distinction between hepatic and obstructive jaundice can only be made by ERCP or percutaneous transhepatic cholangiography.

> **IMPORTANT LESSON**
> Obstructive jaundice prevents adequate absorption of fat-soluble vitamin K which is essential for the production of clotting factors.

# THE LIVER

A normal liver is not usually palpable below the costal margin except in thin adults and children. The abnormal liver enlarges below the costal margin and moves with respiration; it may have a smooth or irregular edge and is dull to percussion. Enlargement of the liver may be due to:

- **Congenital abnormalities** – Reidel's lobe, polycystic liver
- **Acquired conditions** – traumatic; infective; parasitic; malignancy; cirrhosis; engorgement, e.g. cardiac failure, Budd–Chiari syndrome.

## TRAUMA

The liver is well protected by the rib cage but is vulnerable to stabbing, gunshot wounds and high velocity road accidents; there may be associated fractures of the ribs and injuries to other intra-abdominal organs and the diaphragm. The clinical features are those of shock and peritonism due to intraperitoneal bleeding.

Major liver injury may require formal laparotomy with a thoracoabdominal incision. The liver is sutured or packed to achieve haemostasis. The patient is then transferred to a specialized liver unit if major resection is anticipated.

## ABSCESSES

Infection reaches the liver by three different routes:

1 Ascending cholangitis – gut organisms
2 Via the hepatic artery – septicaemia producing multiple pyaemic abscesses
3 Via the portal vein – amoebic abscess and hydatid cyst, rarely portal pyaemia from appendicitis or other peritoneal sepsis.

### Amoebic abscess
This is seen in tropical countries as a complication of amoebic dysentery. Spread of *Entamoeba histolytica* to the liver occurs following penetration of the portal vein tributaries in the gut. A large abscess develops, usually in the right lobe of the liver. It is filled with pus that has been described as 'chocolate syrup' or 'anchovy sauce'. Treatment may require a long course of metronidazole followed by diloxanide to eradicate infection in the gut. Needle aspiration of the abscess may be necessary.

## Hydatid cyst

Hydatid disease is due to *Taenia echinococcus*, a tapeworm infesting the gut of **dogs**. Eggs are passed in the dog's faeces and usually complete their life cycle in their intermediate host, the **sheep**. Man may take the place of the sheep, and thus the disease is common in **sheep-rearing countries** like Australia, Greece and Turkey. The eggs are digested in the gut, and the parasite passes up the portal vein to the liver, where a cyst is formed with a dense fibrous capsule, the germinal layer producing daughter cysts. Symptoms are due to a space-occupying lesion which may press on the bile ducts, become infected or, rarely, rupture.

Treatment consists of medication with mebendazole or albendazole. Persistent cysts can be treated by laparoscopy and aspiration, injecting hypertonic saline to kill the daughter cysts. If open surgery is required, care must be taken to prevent spillage of intact cysts within the abdominal cavity.

## PORTAL HYPERTENSION

The normal portal venous pressure is $120-140$ mmH$_2$O when measured on the operating table. Portal hypertension is defined as a portal pressure of over 300 mmH$_2$O at surgery, and is caused by an obstruction to portal blood flow (Figure 28.9). Such an obstruction can occur in three sites:

1 Hepatic veins – Budd–Chiari syndrome
2 Intrahepatic – cirrhosis, tumours
3 Portal vein – thrombosis, malignant obstruction.

The site of obstruction is intrahepatic in about 80% of cases and by far the **commonest cause is cirrhosis** restricting flow in the intralobular tributaries of the hepatic veins. Obstruction of the portal vein by tumour or portal vein thrombosis is the commonest extrahepatic lesion.

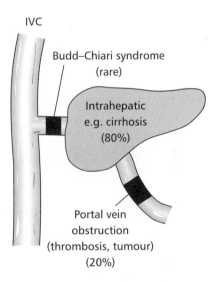

**Figure 28.9** Sites of portal blood flow obstruction

## Clinical features

The clinical problems are caused simply by the **high pressure within the portal venous system**. Thus portal hypertension opens abnormal venous collaterals (shunts) into the systemic bloodstream; these same collaterals may bleed; the blood they carry contains ammoniacal digestive toxins which affect the nervous system; hydrostatically produced oedema fluid may collect in the peritoneum as ascites; the spleen swells and enlarges. There are four major signs:

1 **Portal-systemic anastomotic shunting** – lower oesophageal and upper gastric varices which bleed, caput medusae (radiating veins) at umbilicus, haemorrhoids in anal canal.
2 **Splenomegaly and hypersplenism** – reduction in red and white cells and platelets.
3 **Portal-systemic encephalopathy** – a protein load (often blood) in the gut increases ammonia production with attendant intoxication (flapping hand tremor, mental confusion, stupor and coma).
4 **Ascites** – associated with a low serum albumin and secondary hyperaldosteronism.

Unremitting jaundice is a sign of terminal liver failure.

### Treatment of variceal haemorrhage
- Bleeding from oesophageal varices may be torrential and is life-threatening (30% mortality at first episode).
- Emergency control of bleeding is achieved by endoscopy and injection with a sclerosing agent (sclerotherapy).
- Occasionally oral insertion of a Sengstaken tube (Figure 28.10) is needed – inflating the balloons holds the tube in position and compresses the varices to arrest haemorrhage; the third and fourth lumen are used to aspirate blood from the stomach and oesophagus.

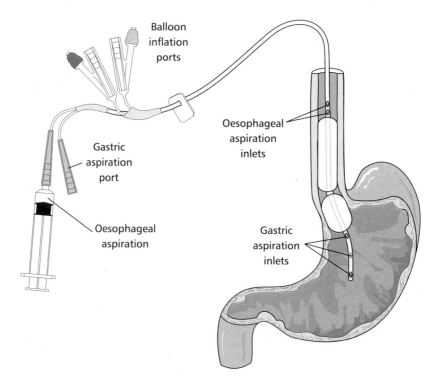

**Figure 28.10** Sengstaken tube

- Medical treatment includes vasopressin and somatostatin to reduce portal pressure and flow.
- Complete oesophageal transection and reanastomosis just above the cardia of the stomach using a stapling gun interrupts the oesophageal venous shunts and may be necessary in otherwise uncontrollable bleeding.
- Long-term control employs endoscopic sclerotherapy or banding.

When direct obliteration of oesophageal varices fails, it is possible to **decrease the portal venous pressure** by increasing the portal-systemic shunting in a controlled fashion. This is rarely required and carries considerable mortality and morbidity (hepatic coma). It can be achieved by:

- **Transjugular intrahepatic portasystemic shunt (TIPS)** – transjugular vein insertion of a stent between the hepatic vein and the portal system
- **Open porta-caval shunt** – anastomosis of the portal vein to the inferior vena cava; or the splenic vein to the left renal vein.

Liver transplantation is the final option.

## TUMOURS OF THE LIVER

### Benign
- Cavernous haemangiomas
- Adenomas

### Primary malignant tumours
1. **Primary hepatocellular carcinoma** (hepatoma) is the commonest malignant primary tumour of the liver. Although rare in the Western world, it accounts for 30% of all cancer deaths in many parts of Asia and Africa. Patients have a high incidence of cirrhosis and exposure to the hepatitis B virus. In addition, various mould toxins such as aflatoxin are found in the food in areas of high incidence.

2. **Cholangiocarcinoma** is much rarer than hepatocellular carcinoma and is less often associated with cirrhosis. It arises from the intrahepatic ducts, and may be associated with *Clonorchis* infestation.
- Diagnosis of primary liver cancer depends on ultrasonography, scanning, angiography and fine needle biopsy.
- Serum **alpha-fetoprotein** is raised in approximately 70% of patients with hepatocellular carcinoma and is **used as a tumour marker.**
- Primary liver tumours are rapidly fatal and the only hope of **cure is by hepatic resection or transplantation.**
- Palliative treatment involves the use of systemic chemotherapy, hepatic artery ligation and embolization.
- Jaundice in cholangiocarcinoma is relieved by insertion of stents.

### Secondary malignant tumours

The liver is one of the commonest sites of metastatic cancer, particularly lung, breast, colorectal, stomach, pancreas, oesophagus and melanoma. **Secondary liver tumours are far more common than primary growths, and of all cases of fatal cancer the liver is involved in 30%.** Secondary tumours are usually multiple and when on the liver surface characteristically have a central depression due to necrosis. The usual cause of death in patients with hepatic metastases is liver failure from destruction of normal tissue and obstruction of the biliary tree.

Solitary and multiple deposits within the liver can be removed using several methods, including cryotherapy and hepatic resection. The greater part of the blood supply of both primary and secondary liver tumours comes from the hepatic artery rather than the portal vein. Infusion of the hepatic artery delivers chemotherapy directly to the tumour and has been used to achieve palliation.

## THE PANCREAS

The exocrine glands of the pancreas secrete amylase, lipase and trypsin into the duodenum. The most common disease encountered in this organ is pancreatitis, but it should be noted that acute pancreatitis and chronic or relapsing pancreatitis are two quite different conditions, despite the similarity of their names. They will be discussed separately here.

### ACUTE PANCREATITIS

The cause of this condition is unknown, but it is often associated with gall stones (up to 60%) or alcohol abuse. The most plausible explanation for acute pancreatitis is that a small gall stone blocks the ampulla of Vater, thus preventing the free outflow of pancreatic juice and possibly permitting the reflux of bile or infected material into the pancreatic ducts.

**Causes of acute pancreatitis**

- Gall stones (60%)
- Alcohol abuse
- Surgery (ERCP)
- Viral (mumps)
- Hyperparathyroidism

Pancreatitis is seen, very rarely, complicating mumps and even more rarely in hyperparathyroidism. Occasionally it complicates operations in the vicinity of bile ducts (e.g. ERCP), trauma, and hypothermia.

### Symptoms and signs

- In simplistic terms the symptoms and signs of pancreatitis result from autodigestion of the gland and intraperitoneal leak of digestive pancreatic enzymes.
- The latter produce a peritoneal chemical 'burn' which may be small or extensive depending on the severity of the pancreatitis.
- Since the peritoneum has the same surface area as the skin, the potential injury is huge.

By extending the analogy to skin burns, the clinical picture of pancreatitis is better understood.

Local effects:
- **Pain** – severe epigastric pain which radiates through to the back
- **Peritonitis** – with accompanying signs and paralytic ileus
- **Fluid loss** – water, protein, electrolytes, blood
- **Tissue damage** – may be minimal (a small burn) or gross with necrosis of the entire pancreas and surrounding organs.

Systemic effects:
- **Shock** – often profound; due to fluid loss within the peritoneum and extracellular space
- **Cyanosis and hypoxia** – pancreatitis impedes gaseous exchange in the lungs (reason unclear); respiratory movement is reduced due to pain
- **Hypocalcaemia** – unique to pancreatitis; retroperitoneal fat is broken down to soap (saponification) which absorbs large amounts of calcium. Resulting hypocalcaemia may cause tetany (**Chvostek's sign** – facial nerve sensitivity; and **Trousseau's sign** – carpal spasm after applying a blood pressure cuff).

Special signs:
- **Grey Turner's sign** – discoloration of the flanks indicative of severe disease
- **Sentinel loop** – plain x-ray may show a distended 'sentinel' loop of jejunum overlying the pancreatic area; flecks of calcification may be present from previous attacks
- **Diabetes** – occurs early in severe cases or as a late sequel. Due to destruction of β-cells.

### Diagnosis
- A history of gall stones or alcohol abuse in a shocked ill patient with epigastric pain and signs of peritonitis is the usual presentation.
- **Serum amylase is raised 5–10 times normal and is diagnostic.**
- Abdominal ultrasound shows free fluid, a 'bright' oedematous pancreas and gall stones, if present.

### Treatment
When the diagnosis of acute pancreatitis has been established, treatment should be expectant and supportive:
- Intravenous fluid replacement to treat shock; CVP monitoring to gauge hydration; urinary catheter to monitor renal function; blood transfusion if necessary.
- Oxygen by mask with blood gas analysis and $P_{O_2}$ monitoring. Intubation and mechanical ventilation may be needed.
- Adequate analgesia.
- Serum calcium needs monitoring; hypocalcaemia is corrected by intravenous infusion.
- Intravenous parenteral nutrition is commonly required.

If the diagnosis is doubtful or conservative measures fail, laparoscopy is advised with **peritoneal lavage**. The peritoneal effusion is blood-stained and the omentum shows signs of fat necrosis with chalky patches indicating saponification. In the presence of gall stones and depending on the patient's condition, laparoscopic cholecystectomy or open cholecystectomy may be performed. Some centres advocate ERCP with sphincterotomy and clearance of bile duct stones but there is a risk that pancreatitis may be aggravated by this manoeuvre. In severe cases the whole of the pancreas may necrose and become a haemorrhagic mass with abscess formation. This can be removed surgically (**necrosectomy**) but there is a high mortality.

Rarely, a **pancreatic pseudo-cyst** forms as a collection of pancreatic fluid contained within the lesser sac. It should be suspected when the patient continues to complain of pain and the serum amylase remains elevated. A firm rounded swelling in the epigastrium may be felt and the cyst can be visualized using ultrasound scanning.

### Prognosis

In most patients acute pancreatitis runs a benign course and recovery occurs within a week; if gall stones are the cause, routine cholecystectomy is then planned to prevent further attacks. However, in about 10–20% the disease is overwhelmingly severe and death occurs despite many weeks of ITU treatment and surgical intervention. Prognostic indicators of severity are shown in the box:

- Age >55
- High white count
- Anaemia
- High blood glucose
- Severe hypoxia
- Low serum calcium

## CHRONIC RELAPSING PANCREATITIS

This disease has a geographical distribution, being more common in the USA and France than the UK. It is generally seen in men rather than women and about a third of patients are alcoholics. A number become drug addicts because of intractable pain.

### Symptoms and signs

- Recurrent attacks of epigastric pain radiating through to the back.
- The pain may be so severe that the patient will rest a hot water bottle on his/her back to soothe it – the resulting discoloration of the skin is known as *erythema ab igne.*
- Each attack is associated with varying degrees of ileus, and the repeated damage to the pancreas results eventually in **steatorrhoea and diabetes**.
- Serum amylase rises in each attack, and may remain elevated between attacks in the absence of symptoms.
- Radiographs of the abdomen may show a stippled calcification of the pancreas and stones in the pancreatic ducts.
- Gall stones may or may not be present.
- ERCP shows multiple strictures of the pancreatic ducts with stones and dilated radicals forming 'lakes' of contrast.

## Treatment

- Acute or chronic episodes should be treated as for acute pancreatitis.
- Cholecystectomy and clearance of the bile duct is required for choledocholithiasis.
- Stones in the pancreatic duct may be cleared by a distal pancreatectomy and anastomosis to a loop of jejunum.
- In patients with persistent and debilitating pain, pylorus-preserving total pancreatectomy is now the treatment of choice.

## CARCINOMA OF THE PANCREAS

- The incidence of carcinoma is rising.
- It usually occurs after 50 years of age and is more common in men – 2:1.
- About 75% occur in the ampulla and head of the pancreas.
- Tumours of the lower end of the bile duct are often confused with peri-ampullary carcinomas.
- Spread of tumour is usually to the lymphatic glands along the upper border of the pancreas and around the superior mesenteric vessels.
- Venous and perineural spread is common.
- Peritoneal spread eventually causes ascites.

> **Courvoisier's law**
> If in the presence of jaundice the gall bladder is palpable, then the jaundice is unlikely to be due to stones.

## Symptoms and signs

- **Jaundice** due to malignant obstruction of the bile duct, dyspepsia, loss of weight and a **palpable gall bladder** are the most frequent findings.
- Obstruction to the pancreatic duct may cause **steatorrhoea** and sometimes chronic pancreatitis or pancreatic cysts.
- **Diabetes** can be a presenting feature.
- Tumours of the **distal part of the body and tail of the pancreas produce few symptoms** and often present late with distant metastases or peritoneal carcinomatosis. Jaundice in such patients indicates metastatic disease in the liver. The first symptoms of such tumours may be the presence of non-specific thrombophlebitis migrans, malaise, anorexia and weight loss.

## Diagnosis

- ERCP shows a 'rat tail' stricture at the lower end of the common bile duct. Brushings for cytology confirm the diagnosis.
- Ultrasound or CT scanning shows a mass which can be needled for FNAC.

## Treatment

Treatment is primarily surgical.

> In jaundiced patients **vitamin K is required to correct the prothrombin time** preoperatively; fresh frozen plasma may also be needed. An additional problem in jaundiced patients is **renal failure (hepatorenal syndrome)** associated with surgical intervention of any sort, including ERCP. It is prevented by good hydration and osmotic diuretics (mannitol) to maintain urine output.

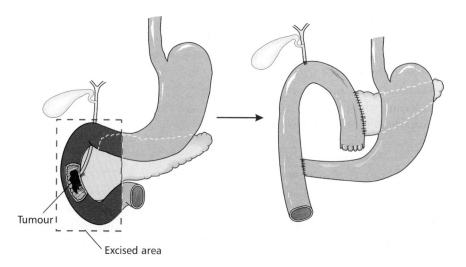

**Figure 28.11** Pancreatico-duodenectomy

- **Curative** – early tumours of the ampulla and lower common bile duct which do not involve the portal vein (determined by angiography or scanning) are suitable for resection. **Pylorus-preserving pancreatico-duodenectomy** (Figure 28.11) is now the procedure of choice and has a lower mortality than Whipple's procedure first described in 1935. Patients with carcinomas of the head and body of the pancreas have a significantly low survival rate, very few surviving beyond 5 years.
- **Palliative** – most patients at laparotomy are only suitable for palliative surgery to prevent or relieve jaundice; achieved by anastomosing a loop of jejunum to the gall bladder to drain the bile (**cholecysto-jejunostomy**) (Figure 28.12). If inoperability is determined before laparotomy, biliary obstruction can be relieved **endoscopically by inserting a stent** into the common bile duct.

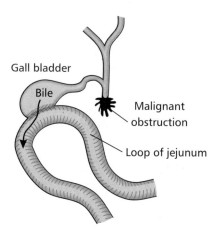

**Figure 28.12** Cholecysto-jejunostomy

Palliation also includes pain relief – this can be achieved by destruction of the coeliac ganglia using alcohol injection.

Carcinoma of the pancreas is a rapidly fatal disease with few patients surviving more than 1 year.

## PANCREATIC CYSTS

- The commonest cyst of the pancreas is **the pseudo-cyst, encountered as a sequela of pancreatitis.**
- Any part of the pancreas may be involved but the body is the usual site.

- It may also follow trauma to the gland by a crushing injury or sharp blow which transects the body of the pancreas against the vertebral column.
- A cyst may fill the lesser sac or lie in the mesocolon.
- Cysts contain pancreatic fluid and sloughs of pancreas which can be difficult to aspirate.

> **Management of pseudo-cysts**
>
> - Expectant → resolution
> - Active → percutaneous drainage
>   - → surgical cysto-gastrostomy

### Treatment

No action is taken for 6 weeks as the cyst may resolve spontaneously or proceed to develop a firm capsule. Percutaneous drainage may aid resolution but failing this permanent drainage may be achieved by anastomosing the cyst to the posterior aspect of the stomach (**cysto-gastrostomy**). This procedure can be performed laparoscopically or by open surgery.

Other rare causes of pancreatic cyst are hydatid disease and fibrocystic disease.

## TRAUMA

The pancreas is well protected and is not often traumatized. Occasionally crushing injuries will transect it across the vertebral column. Stab wounds and gunshot wounds are common in some countries. Laparotomy is indicated if pancreatitis occurs and partial pancreatectomy may be required. Pancreatic fistula is a common complication.

## THE SPLEEN

Splenectomy may be required for splenic injuries and in certain blood diseases. In order to preserve immunological integrity, a traumatized spleen is repaired and preserved whenever possible.

## TRAUMA

- The normal spleen is protected by overlying ribs.
- If the spleen is enlarged (malaria; glandular fever) it is much more easily damaged.
- Penetrating injuries and blunt trauma (especially if a rib is fractured) may cause rupture.
- The spleen may also undergo **delayed rupture** – there is an initial silent period of 7–14 days following injury and then haemorrhage suddenly occurs, perhaps while the patient is at rest; the original injury presumably causes a subscapular haematoma which later bursts.

### Symptoms and signs

- Pain and tenderness occur in the left upper abdomen.
- Radiation of **pain to the left shoulder tip** is caused by diaphragmatic irritation by blood.

- Tenderness on the left side increases and is followed by generalized rigidity.
- The patient is restless, pale, shocked and sweating.
- X-rays may show a diffuse haziness and absence of a splenic shadow.

### Treatment
- Shock and blood loss are treated by immediate blood transfusion.
- Laparoscopy allows small splenic tears to be treated with a haemostatic dressing.
- Uncontrolled bleeding warrants conversion to open laparotomy with splenectomy.

## SPLENOMEGALY

In many tropical countries enlargement of the spleen is endemic. It may be due to malaria or to other parasites. If the organ is so big that it displaces the other abdominal organs and raises the diaphragm, it may be removed for mechanical reasons. The operation (Figure 28.13) can be very difficult because of vascular adhesions. Prolonged ileus may follow from decompression of the peritoneal cavity, with attendant collapse of the left lower lobe of lung due to disturbance of the diaphragm.

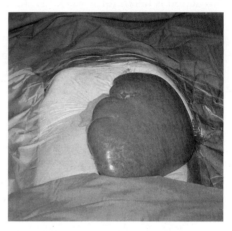

**Figure 28.13** Splenomegaly at operation

**Splenectomy** is occasionally indicated for the treatment of some haematological conditions:
- Haemolytic anaemia
- Thrombocytopenic purpura
- Hypersplenism.

**The spleen is part of the immune defence system.** Splenectomy patients require **active immunization against pneumococcal, meningococcal and** *Haemophilus influenzae* **type b (Hib) infection.** Long-term penicillin is essential in children and recommended in adults. A 'Medic-alert' card is also available (Figure 28.14).

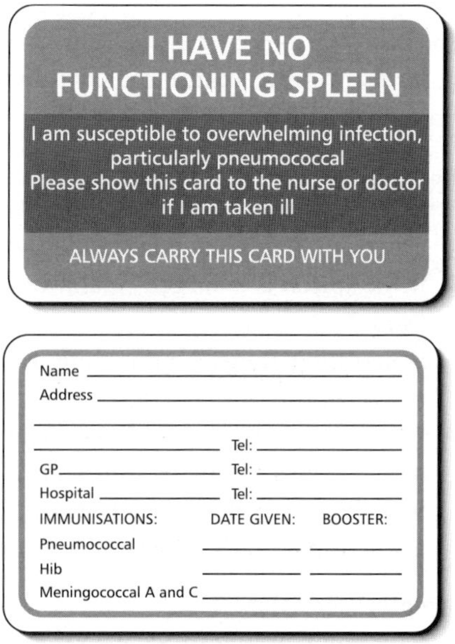

**I HAVE NO FUNCTIONING SPLEEN**

I am susceptible to overwhelming infection, particularly pneumococcal
Please show this card to the nurse or doctor if I am taken ill

ALWAYS CARRY THIS CARD WITH YOU

Name _____
Address _____
_____ Tel: _____
GP_____ Tel: _____
Hospital _____ Tel: _____
IMMUNISATIONS:        DATE GIVEN:        BOOSTER:
Pneumococcal        _____
Hib        _____
Meningococcal A and C _____

**Figure 28.14** 'Medic-alert' card: (a) front; (b) back

## CRIB BOX – BILIARY AND PORTAL SYSTEMS

### Gall stones

- Causes – metabolic, stasis, infection
- Types - pigment, cholesterol, mixed
- Majority are asymptomatic – remember **Saint's triad**
- Cause symptoms (80% women) – in the gall bladder; in the bile ducts
- Treatment – mainly surgical; open, mini or laparoscopic cholecystectomy. Stones in bile ducts removed by surgery or ERCP and sphincterotomy

### Jaundice

- Pre-hepatic (haemolytic); hepatic (hepatocellular); post-hepatic (obstructive)
- Surgery mainly concerned with obstruction to bile duct; in the lumen, in the wall, extrinsic compression
- Obstructive type causes itching, pale (white) stools, dark urine

### Portal hypertension

- Obstruction to portal venous flow in – portal vein; liver; hepatic veins
- Cirrhosis is commonest
- Produces – haemorrhage, splenomegaly, encephalopathy, ascites
- Bleeding from oesophageal varices is a medical emergency – Sengstaken tube; sclerotherapy; oesophageal transection; portal-systemic shunt

### Liver tumours

- Benign – haemangioma; adenoma
- Malignant – primary hepatocellular (common in Asia, Africa); cholangiocarcinoma; secondary metastatic (commonest overall)

### Pancreatitis

- Acute – gall stones; alcohol abuse; surgery; viral. Treatment supportive followed by cholecystectomy if stones present. Remember calcium drops
- Chronic relapsing – alcohol abuse

### Carcinoma of pancreas

- Common and increasing. Often presents with obstructive jaundice
- Remember Courvoisier's law
- Treatment usually surgical palliation of jaundice and pain control. Pancreatectomy possible but long-term survival poor

**Surgery and jaundice** – remember clotting disorder (vitamin K) and hepatorenal syndrome

**Splenectomy** – remember the immunological consequences

# chapter 29

# THE SMALL INTESTINE

## ABSORPTION

The small intestine is the main site for digestion and absorption of foodstuffs, i.e. carbohydrates, fats and proteins. It is largely completed in the jejunum and upper ileum but **bile salts** and **vitamin B12** are absorbed in the **terminal ileum**. Hence, disease or excision of the terminal ileum may lead to:

- Gall stones (disruption of the **enterohepatic circulation of bile salts**)
- Deconjugation of bile salts in the colon (causing diarrhoea)
- Malabsorption of vitamin B12 (leading eventually to pernicious anaemia).

Abnormalities of the upper small bowel (coeliac disease; Whipple's disease; diverticula) cause malabsorption syndromes which come under the care of medical gastroenterologists.

## IMAGING THE SMALL INTESTINE

- **Plain abdominal film** – shows abnormalities such as bowel dilatation, fluid levels (erect film), free gas or fluid, and even gas in the biliary tree.
- **Barium meal and follow-through** – the patient drinks a barium solution, the course of which is followed through the stomach, duodenum and small intestine with serial films taken over several hours (Figure 29.1).
- **Small bowel enema** – an oral tube passed to the duodenojejunal junction is used to instil contrast into the small intestine which is then followed on serial x-rays through to the caecum and beyond. This study allows more precise definition of small bowel mucosal abnormalities.
- **Endoscopy** – visualizes the oesophagus, stomach, duodenum and upper jejunum. Biopsies of the duodenal mucosa will confirm coeliac disease and other malabsorption disorders.
- **Selective angiography** – superior mesenteric artery angiograms may identify obscure sites of haemorrhage, e.g. small bowel ulcers, Meckel's diverticulum, angiodysplasia. Isotope-labelled red cells can also

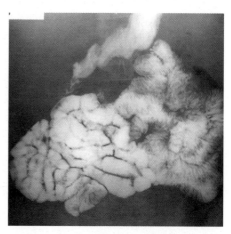

**Figure 29.1** Barium follow-through

be used but both methods depend on an adequate rate of blood loss at the time of the investigation.

- **Isotopic scanning** – shows foci of inflammation such as Crohn's disease.

## SMALL BOWEL OBSTRUCTION

This is a common surgical problem (see also Chapter 24). Causes of **mechanical obstruction** are numerous and can be classified usefully into those outside the bowel, in the wall or in the lumen, e.g.:

- **Lesions outside the bowel wall** – hernia; adhesions; volvulus
- **Lesions in the bowel wall** – Crohn's; tumour; atresia; intussusception
- **Lesions in the lumen** – bolus obstruction; gall stone ileus; meconium ileus.

Hernia and adhesions are by far the most common causes of mechanical obstruction.

**Functional obstruction** (adynamic, paralytic) is equally important:

- Peritonitis (calor, rubor, dolor, tumour and loss of function)
- Post-operative paralytic ileus
- Ischaemia
- Electrolyte imbalance (including metabolic causes, e.g. diabetic ketoacidosis)
- Retroperitoneal haematoma
- Pancreatitis
- Prolonged bed rest
- Malignant infiltration
- Long-standing mechanical obstruction.

### Pathology

**Mechanical obstruction**

The small intestine distal to the site of mechanical obstruction is empty and collapsed. Proximal to the obstruction, waves of forcible peristalsis produce intense symptoms of **midgut colic**. If the obstruction is not relieved the proximal intestine eventually distends, peristalsis ceases, and **the colic stops**. The patient is pain free but remains obstructed. If the distension is gross, blood flow in the bowel wall is compromised due to compression and the resulting **ischaemia** produces **continuous midgut pain**. If further neglected, the ischaemic bowel **perforates to produce generalized peritonitis**. Thus, depending at which stage a patient presents, pain may be colicky, absent, continuous, or peritonitic. Some causes of mechanical obstruction are frequently complicated by **strangulation** of the bowel; notably hernia, volvulus and intussusception.

**Functional obstruction**

The whole small intestine is distended with absent or ineffectual peristalsis. Pain is either absent or continuous (ischaemia; peritonitis) depending on the underlying pathology. Vomiting, dehydration, distension and absolute constipation are prominent features. Bowel sounds are absent or 'tinkling' due to fluid pouring from one distended loop of bowel into another under the effects of gravity or body movement.

## Management of obstruction

Clearly, the management of small bowel obstruction will differ according to the aetiology but all patients will need a 'drip and suck' regimen:

- Nil by mouth
- Nasogastric suction – to alleviate vomiting
- Intravenous fluid replacement – daily requirements **plus** nasogastric losses.

> Any evidence of small bowel **strangulation** or **peritonitis** is an indication for immediate surgery following adequate resuscitation.

Apart from adhesions (see below), most mechanical obstruction requires surgical intervention. Functional obstruction resolves with conservative treatment once the precipitating cause is treated.

## ADHESIONS

> Normal resolution of the inflammatory process following intra-abdominal surgery, sepsis or injury produces fibrous tissue. As a result, viscera which are usually separated can become united by fibrous **adhesions** or bands. Ordinarily this causes no problems but adhesions can result in obstruction due to compression, torsion or narrowing of the small bowel.

- Minor abdominal procedures may produce dense adhesions, whereas multiple major abdominal operations might produce few.
- Talc undoubtedly was a cause of extensive adhesions in the past, and the use of talc-free operating gloves has removed this risk.
- Excessive handling of the small intestine probably provokes excessive adhesion formation, a theory substantiated by the finding that there is less than expected adhesion formation following minimally invasive procedures.
- Adhesions may occur following an intra-abdominal septic episode, e.g. diverticulitis, acute cholecystitis, salpingitis.
- All patients who have had abdominal surgery remain at risk of developing intestinal obstruction due to adhesions.

## Clinical features

- The majority of patients never develop symptoms.
- Repeated abdominal surgery becomes increasingly difficult due to further adhesion formation at each operation.
- Patients with symptomatic adhesions present with:
  - Repeated episodes of colic which resolve spontaneously
  - Small bowel obstruction which resolves
  - Small bowel obstruction requiring surgery.

## Management

Most adhesive obstruction resolves on a conservative regimen of 'drip and suck', recovery being heralded by reduced nasogastric aspirate, passage of flatus and return of normal bowel sounds. Failure of the obstruction to resolve despite several days of conservative treatment is an indication for surgery. Early surgery is avoided, except where strangulation or ischaemia is suspected, because of the risk of subsequent increase in the density of adhesions.

## VOLVULUS

Volvulus may involve any abdominal viscus on a long mesentery, e.g. volvulus neonatorum; sigmoid volvulus; gastric volvulus; caecal volvulus. As well as causing obstruction, there is a significant chance of **strangulation due to occlusion of the twisted mesenteric vessels**.

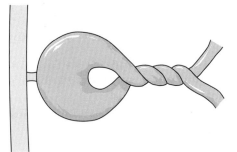

**Figure 29.2** Volvulus

- **Small bowel volvulus** – usually occurs as the result of adhesion formation with the **gut rotating around a single dense band** (Figure 29.2). Because of the risk of strangulation, early operation is recommended to release the band and untwist the rotated gut.
- **Complex volvulus** – involving small bowel and colon, is seen in the underdeveloped world, but is rare in the West.

## INTUSSUSCEPTION

This is mainly a problem in infants under 2 years old (see Chapter 22) but is seen in adults secondary to **mucosal polyps** (Peutz–Jeghers syndrome) and tumours (lipoma; leiomyoma). An intussusception (Figure 29.3) tends to progress distally with the apex or caput remaining constant as more and more bowel and mesentery is invaginated behind it. Stretching, compression and **occlusion of the mesenteric vessels** eventually leads to strangulation.

- Presentation in adults is with small bowel obstruction.
- In adults surgery is necessary to reduce the intussusception and excise the causative lesion (polyp, etc.).
- The ileocolic intussusception of infancy is most often reduced hydrostatically with a barium enema without the need for surgery.

Apex

**Figure 29.3** Intussusception

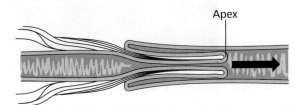

## POST-OPERATIVE PARALYTIC ILEUS

Following any abdominal operation, there is a delay in return of effective peristalsis (ileus). The delay may vary from a few hours, e.g. after a cholecystectomy, to 3–4 days after a hemicolectomy. Patients must be treated for intestinal obstruction with a 'drip and suck' regimen. The return of peristalsis is heralded by:
- Passage of flatus
- Return of bowel sounds
- Reduction in nasogastric aspirate
- Soft, concave abdomen on palpation.

Occasionally ileus may be prolonged and a cause for this should be sought:
- Blood biochemistry derangement (often due to poorly managed intravenous fluid replacement)
- Intra-abdominal sepsis (leaking anastomosis; abscess formation)
- Adhesions
- Internal hernia
- Bowel ischaemia
- Pancreatitis.

Diagnosing the reason for prolonged post-operative ileus is difficult and requires skill and experience. Ultrasound scanning may show an abscess or fluid collection. A careful water-soluble contrast study might identify an anastomotic leakage or a mechanical obstruction. Sometimes a diagnostic laparotomy is needed.

Intravenous feeding may be necessary with a prolonged ileus.

## INTRALUMINAL CAUSES OF OBSTRUCTION

Intraluminal obstruction has unusual causes and is **rare**.
- **Gall stone ileus** – a large gall stone passes through a cholecysto-duodenal fistula to lodge in the distal ileum. The stone is usually radiolucent, but plain x-ray findings of **dilated loops of small intestine and gas within the biliary tree** are diagnostic (Figure 29.4). The treatment is to remove the gall stone surgically from the ileum; usually no attempt is made to interfere with the gall bladder which has decompressed itself through the fistula into the duodenum.
- **Pith balls** – from fruit will sometimes obstruct the small intestine (particularly after gastrectomy) and need to be removed.

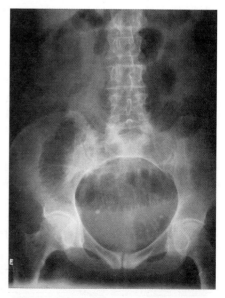

**Figure 29.4** Gall stone ileus — note dilated small bowel and gas in biliary tree

- Trichobezoar – young women and girls with long hair have been described as chewing their hair to produce an obstructing mass in the small intestine.
- 'Mules' – illicit carriage of drugs, wrapped in condoms and swallowed, produce no shadow on abdominal x-rays, but may cause bolus obstruction.

## INFLAMMATION OF THE SMALL BOWEL

There are predominantly two diseases that need to be considered under this heading – **Crohn's disease and tuberculosis.**

### CROHN'S DISEASE

Crohn's disease is an inflammatory disorder which may affect the gastrointestinal tract from the **mouth to the anus**. The aetiology is unknown, but it is characterized by **non-caseating granulomas** affecting the **full thickness** of the bowel wall.

- Patients with small bowel Crohn's usually present aged between 20 and 55 years.
- **Chronic diarrhoea, abdominal pain and weight loss** are caused by **ileitis** and **stricture formation** which can affect jejunum or ileum, although **typically the terminal ileum** is involved.
- Fissure formation and sepsis outside the lumen of the bowel, coupled with **fistulae** to other loops of intestine, the skin and bladder may complicate the disease. The majority of patients run a chronic course, which eventually requires surgical intervention. However, there are a **minority who become acutely toxic,** and require intensive in-patient medical therapy or emergency surgery. The acute presentation may include toxic megacolon, not unlike the equivalent in ulcerative colitis.

In the chronic disease, evidence of anaemia and hypoalbuminaemia are usually found. Indices of inflammation, such as ESR and C-reactive protein, are raised. A mass may be palpable in the right iliac fossa, and there may be evidence of subacute intestinal obstruction.

### Diagnosis

The diagnosis is based on suspicion. Raised **inflammatory indices, a barium follow-through** or small bowel enema showing stricture formation alternating with normal bowel (**skip lesions**) and fissures or fistulae support the diagnosis (Figure 29.5). A biopsy of an accessible lesion might show granuloma formation. An **iridium scan** indicates the extent of involvement of the small intestine.

### Management

The main treatment is medical.
- Steroids are used and can be administered orally, intravenously or rectally.
- Azathioprine, cyclosporin and thalidomide have been shown to be useful adjunctive therapy.

- A mesalazine derivative (Pentasa) has been shown to be effective in sustaining remission.
- The acutely ill should be supported with intravenous feeding and steroids until fit for surgery.

**Operative intervention** is eventually required in 75% of patients with Crohn's disease.

> - **Failure of medical treatment** to control the symptoms **and/or complications** necessitates resection or bypassing of diseased bowel.

- As the disease is chronic, further resections may be required, so attempts to conserve small bowel length are a priority.
- Multiple **stricturoplasties** may be performed. In this procedure the narrowed segments are opened but not resected, and then sutured in such a way as to widen the lumen.

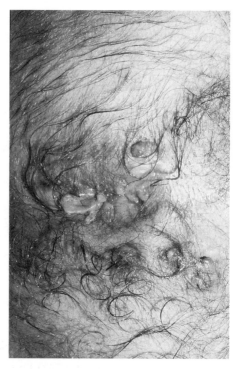

**Figure 29.5** Small bowel Crohn's presenting as perineal fistula

## TUBERCULOSIS

This disease is reappearing in the Western world, partly through immigration but also indigenously.

**Primary intestinal TB** is acquired by drinking infected milk (*Mycobacterium bovis*). **Secondary intestinal TB** is caused by infection with *Mycobacterium tuberculosis* and is secondary to pulmonary disease.

- The distal ileum is usually affected and may either be fibrotic or ulcerative.
- The patient may complain of abdominal pain, weight loss and **night sweats**.
- A mass or ascites may be present on abdominal palpation.
- Uncomplicated disease is treated with antituberculous drugs.
- If complicated by haemorrhage, perforation or obstruction, emergency resection is also required.

## ISCHAEMIA

Three main causes of ischaemic small bowel need to be considered:

1 Ischaemia due to small bowel **strangulation**
2 **Thrombosis** or **arterial embolus** of the superior mesenteric artery

3 **Atherosclerosis** of the superior mesenteric artery.

Strangulation has been discussed elsewhere (Chapter 23).

- An arterial embolus or thrombosis may produce acute ischaemia of the jejunum and ileum, leading to massive infarction and fatal perforation. The patient is severely shocked with gas visible within the bowel wall on abdominal x-ray. There are no specific clinical or diagnostic tests. Surgery reveals loops of black, atonic small bowel.
- Rarely, atherosclerotic narrowing or occlusion of the superior mesenteric artery results in chronic small bowel ischaemia with weight loss and pain after eating – **mesenteric angina.**

## SHORT GUT SYNDROME

This may follow massive resections of small intestine for ischaemia or even occasionally multiple resections for Crohn's disease.

- If **2 metres** of small intestine remains the patient can maintain his/her weight on enteral nutrition.
- Lengths of **less than 1 metre** will require permanent home parenteral nutrition.
- Ileal resections are less well tolerated than jejunal resections due to the inability to absorb bile salts and vitamin B12.

Immediately after a massive resection, absorption is greatly reduced. However, within weeks a **process of adaptation** occurs, whereby the residual small intestine dilates and the absorptive surface of the villi enlarge. Most patients will need intestinal sedative drugs such as codeine phosphate or loperamide for the remainder of their lives.

Other complications of short gut syndrome are:

- Gastric hypersecretion
- Kidney stone and gall stone formation
- Metabolic bone disease.

Ingenious techniques have been described to lengthen the absorptive capacity of the remaining small intestine. A further option now available is small bowel transplantation.

## TUMOURS

Unlike the colon, malignant tumours of the small intestine are rare. The mucosa of the small intestine is rich in immunoglobulins, which may act to protect against mitotic change.

**Benign tumours** include:

- Adenomatous polyps
- Leiomyoma
- Lipoma

- Angioma
- Multiple polyposis of the **Peutz–Jeghers syndrome**. This latter condition is associated with pigmentation of the lips and buccal mucosa.

**Malignant tumours** include:
- Lymphoma
- Adenocarcinoma
- Carcinoid.

## LYMPHOMA

Lymphoma in the small intestine produces large bulky lesions which may bleed, obstruct or perforate. It may be a rare complication of coeliac disease.

The diagnosis is usually made by a combination of endoscopic biopsies and barium studies. Wide **resection** is performed at laparotomy, and subsequent **chemotherapy or radiotherapy** offers a 5-year survival of 50%. Downgrading of a lymphoma can be attempted using preoperative chemotherapy or radiotherapy.

## ADENOCARCINOMA

Primary adenocarcinoma occurs rarely in the small intestine. It presents with obstructive symptoms, haemorrhage or hepatic metastases. Barium follow-through should demonstrate the lesion, but often it is an unexpected finding at laparotomy for obstruction. Patients with long-standing Crohn's are at increased risk.

## CARCINOID

Carcinoid tumours are **neuroendocrine APUD tumours** which arise from enterochromaffin cells in the crypts of Lieberkühn. They can arise anywhere within the gastrointestinal tract, but half are found within the appendix and most of the remainder in the small intestine.
- Appendix – carcinoid tumours in the appendix are usually a chance finding at appendicectomy and they rarely metastasize.
- Small intestine – carcinoid tumours in the small bowel may enlarge to cause obstruction and may later metastasize to the liver.
- When there are significant **hepatic metastases** from carcinoid, a variety of catecholamines are secreted, including **serotonin**.
- This may cause the **carcinoid syndrome**, which presents with **transient cutaneous flushing, diarrhoea, asthma and tricuspid insufficiency and pulmonary stenosis**.

The diagnosis of carcinoid syndrome is made by measuring a metabolite of serotonin – **5-hydroxy-indole acetic acid (5-HIAA)** – in the urine.

**Management**
- Small bowel lesions should be resected.

- Hepatic metastases grow very slowly and **hepatic lobectomy or liver transplantation** can be offered to the patient.
- **Octreotide, a somatostatin analogue,** has been useful in the control of symptoms from the carcinoid syndrome.

---

**CRIB BOX – SMALL INTESTINE**

- The terminal ileum absorbs **bile salts** and **vitamin B12**
- Imaging with plain films, Ba meal and FT, small bowel enema, endoscopy, angiogram, isotope scan
- **Obstruction is common** – adhesions, hernia, ileus, volvulus, Crohn's, TB
- Obstruction can be complicated by **ischaemia** and/or **strangulation**
- Hernia, volvulus and intussusception are most likely to strangulate
- Prolonged post-operative ileus is most often due to poor fluid and electrolyte management
- Appreciate that Crohn's involves the **full thickness** of the bowel which is why it causes fistulae (compare it with ulcerative colitis which affects mucosa only)
- Tumours are **benign** or **malignant** and both are rare

# chapter 30

# DISEASES OF THE COLON

## ANATOMY

The colon (Figure 30.1) is considered in two parts:

- The right colon extends from the ileocaecal valve to two-thirds of the way across the transverse colon, embryologically derived from the midgut and receiving its blood supply from the superior mesenteric artery via the ileocolic, right colic and middle colic arteries.
- The left colon deriving from the hindgut nominally ends at the rectosigmoid junction at the level of the sacral promontory. It derives its blood supply from the inferior mesenteric artery.

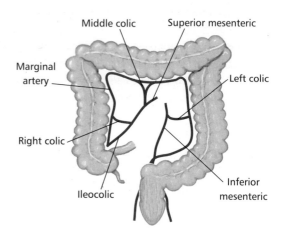

**Figure 30.1** The anatomy of the colon with schematic of blood supply

The colon also has a marginal artery running along its mesenteric border which derives supply from all the major colonic vessels.

> The colon can be distinguished from the small bowel at laparotomy and laparoscopy by the presence of the taenia coli (three longitudinal stripes of muscle) on the colon.

## PHYSIOLOGY

The colon absorbs water and electrolytes and then acts as a reservoir for the remaining faecal material. The 1000–2000 ml/day of ileal effluent is reduced to 100–150 ml of stool. Between one and three times a day the colon contracts along its whole length to stimulate defaecation (mass action).

## SIGNS AND SYMPTOMS OF COLONIC DISEASE

- **Pain** – visceral pain from the gut is not well localized in the absence of somatic stimulation from parietal peritoneal inflammation. The **right colon is midgut** in its origin and pain arising from it is usually **peri-umbilical**. **Left colonic pain is hindgut** pain and felt in the **lower abdomen** (suprapubic).
- **Bleeding** – unlike bleeding arising from anorectal pathology, blood from the colon tends to be a darker red in colour and is often mixed in with the stool.
- **Change in bowel habit** – the most significant change in bowel habit is one that persists; an arbitrary duration of 2 weeks is a reasonable guide to divide significant from insignificant changes. There are only a few variations on a theme which may feature on their own or in combination – increased, decreased or variable stool frequency; firmer, looser or variable stool consistency.

Some patients find it both difficult and embarrassing to describe these symptoms although some patients are so obsessed that they will talk about little else.

## EXAMINATION AND INVESTIGATION OF COLONIC DISEASE

The colon can be investigated by double contrast barium enema or colonoscopy (Figure 30.2). Although a colonoscopy is the test of choice it may not be practical for the examination of many patients in a busy hospital (see below). No examination of the colon is complete without a digital rectal examination and if a bar-

ium enema is to be performed a rigid or flexible sigmoidoscopy is mandatory. The role of faecal occult blood tests is unclear although recent reports suggest their importance in screening; however, the colonoscopic workload that a national screening programme would generate is prohibitive at present.

### Colonoscopy
This is the most effective investigation as it not only permits diagnosis but allows biopsy and polypectomy as well. The drawbacks are that it is a sedated procedure requiring a half day admission, it needs a trained colonoscopist who is usually a gastroenterologist or a colorectal surgeon with service commitments other than investigations and has a perforation rate of approximately 1 in

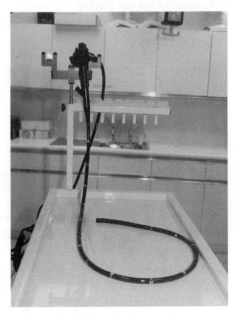

**Figure 30.2** A colonoscope

2000 procedures. If there is an annular carcinoma then the proximal colon may not be visualized.

### Barium enema

This is a very useful investigation but does not permit any therapy in adults. As it is a procedure performed by radiologists it does not impinge on the workload of gastroenterologists or colorectal surgeons. The drawbacks are that it does not permit biopsy or therapy, it may miss small mucosal lesions especially in the presence of diverticular disease, it has a significant impact on the workload of radiologists and it involves radiation exposure for the patient.

### CT scanning

CT scanning can be useful in investigation of masses associated with the colon when double contrast enema or colonoscopy cannot demonstrate the cause. Developmental work is in progress to use spiral CT scanning and advanced computer techniques to image the colon.

### Plain abdominal radiology

This is of little use except in the emergency situation where it can be of some help. In obstruction the level can sometimes be seen on plain radiographs. In patients with acute exacerbations of inflammatory bowel disease the diameter of the colon measured on a plain abdominal film is an important index of toxic megacolon.

### Transit studies

These are of limited use in determining whether a patient has slow transit constipation. Radio-opaque markers are swallowed and after they have reached the caecum the transit time is checked by serial (daily) plain radiographs.

### $^{99m}$Tc-labelled red cell studies

$^{99m}$Tc-labelled red cell studies can be of use in identifying the source of obscure colonic bleeding.

## COLONIC SURGERY

For elective surgery the bowel is emptied of faecal residue using laxatives such as sodium picosulphate (Picolax®, Nordic).

> Bowel preparation and preoperative starvation can lead to marked dehydration and therefore intravenous preoperative hydration during the bowel preparation is advisable.

For emergency surgery no bowel preparation can be given but if the lesion is in the left side of the colon, on-table lavage can be performed during the operation to permit safe anastomosis and thus avoid a colostomy.

> Only if the patient is unfit for a major emergency surgery should lesser procedures be considered, such as a defunctioning colostomy or a resection with end colostomy and closure of the distal limb (Hartmann's procedure).

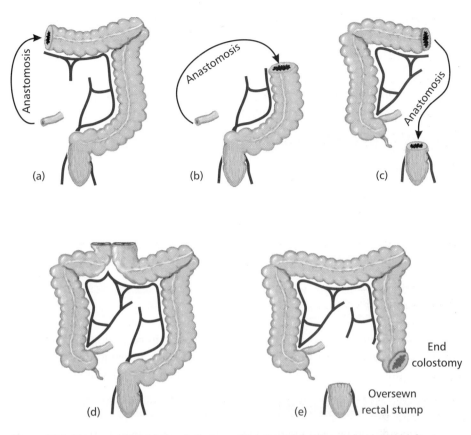

**Figure 30.3** Diagrams of (a) right hemicolectomy; (b) extended right hemicolectomy; (c) left hemicolectomy; (d) transverse loop colostomy; and (e) Hartmann's procedure.

## Resection

The extent of the resection (Figure 30.3) depends on the major arterial supply of the colon and also the marginal artery (a good blood supply is essential for anastomotic healing). In malignant disease the arterial basis of the resection is also important as this defines the lines of lymphatic drainage. The anastomosis is fashioned either with sutures or with stapling devices (Figure 30.4).

## Defunctioning

Defunctioning, either with a loop or an end colostomy, diverts faeces away from the site of distal colonic pathology or an anastomosis. The whole colon can be defunctioned with an ileostomy.

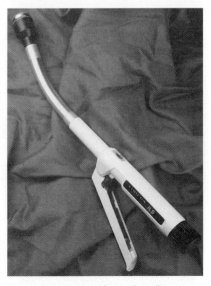

**Figure 30.4** An intraluminal stapling gun

### Decompression

This can be achieved with a caecostomy; however, this stoma is difficult for the patient to manage post-operatively.

### Bypass

In some circumstances (such as an inoperable obstructing carcinoma) a bypass procedure may be helpful in palliating the obstructive symptoms.

## COLONIC OBSTRUCTION

This is a serious condition requiring surgery after resuscitation and rehydration. If the ileocaecal valve is incompetent, then bowel contents can accumulate also in the small bowel, giving a mixed picture of small and large bowel obstruction (**open loop obstruction**). If the ileocaecal valve is competent, the picture will be one of large bowel distension only (**closed loop obstruction**); a dangerous dilatation of the caecum with caecal perforation can follow.

> In a closed loop large bowel obstruction, tenderness over the caecum is an indication for immediate surgery.

In a patient presenting with a history and plain abdominal radiographs suggesting a distal colonic obstruction, it is essential to exclude a pseudo-obstruction by demonstrating a mechanical obstruction with an unprepared barium enema.

## COLONIC CARCINOMA

This section should be read in combination with the section on carcinoma of the rectum which describes the Dukes' classification.

> Colorectal carcinoma is now the second commonest carcinoma in England and Wales.

Rectal carcinoma differs from colonic carcinoma only in its treatment.

### Pathology

Colonic carcinoma (Figures 30.5, 30.6) is an adenocarcinoma of varying degrees of differentiation which metastasizes to the pericolonic lymph nodes and to the liver.

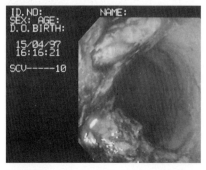

**Figure 30.5** Endoscopic view of carcinoma of colon

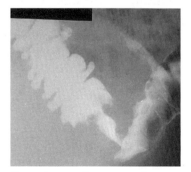

**Figure 30.6** Barium enema of an 'apple core' lesion

The classical staging uses Dukes' classification (see Chapter 31):

- A – not penetrating the bowel wall (muscularis propria) and no nodal spread
- B – penetrating the muscularis propria and no nodal spread
- C – nodal disease regardless of the local stage.

The importance of a staging is that it should have prognostic significance: the 5-year survival for Dukes' A is usually given as >90%, B 65–70% and C <20%. Survival is more usefully given in life tables (actuarial tables) – see Figure 30.7.

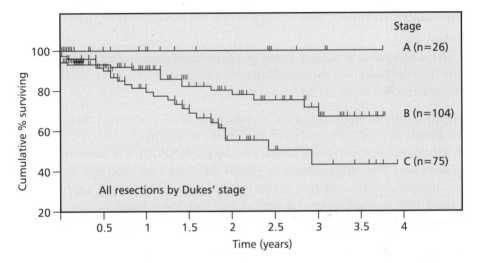

**Figure 30.7** Life table of survival by Dukes' stage

## Symptoms

Rectal bleeding from the colon is usually dark and often mixed in with the stool – it is a symptom to be taken seriously.

Other symptoms include a sustained change in bowel habit, mucous discharge and midgut or hindgut colic caused by progressive obstruction. Late disease can lead to weight loss, vesicocolic fistula, colovaginal fistula, jaundice (liver metastasis) and ascites (peritoneal seeding).

## Signs

Abdominal examination may reveal a mass in late cases. In most cases there are rarely any physical signs.

## Treatment

### Surgery

The treatment is primarily surgical. Most tumours are treated by major resection after preoperative bowel preparation – right hemicolectomy, extended right hemicolectomy or left hemicolectomy, depending on the position in the colon. In cases of malignant large bowel obstruction the procedure is complicated by faecal loading of the colon which predisposes to anastomotic failure. A right hemicolectomy or an extended right hemicolectomy is reasonably safe as the ileocolic anastomosis has a low leak rate if correctly performed. For obstructing tumours of the left colon, on-table colonic lavage (i.e. intraoperative) can be performed to clean the colon and permit primary colo-colonic anastomosis.

### Adjuvant therapy

Radiotherapy is of little proven benefit in tumours above the pelvis due to poor localization and higher side-effects (mainly small bowel damage). For cancers with nodal involvement, post-operative adjuvant chemotherapy can be helpful.

### Follow-up

There is no nationally accepted plan of follow-up to detect recurrent or new cancers. Regular colonoscopic surveillance or measurement of tumour markers (carcinoembryonic antigen – CEA) are options.

**Family history** is important in colorectal cancer as it is estimated that up to 5% are genetic in origin. There are two recognized syndromes:

- **Hereditary non-polyposis colorectal cancer (HNPCC)** is a dominant defect associated with other cancers in groups that have been described by **Lynch** – colorectal, uterine, gastric, urothelial and ovarian cancers. Twenty-five per cent have multiple colorectal cancers but with few adenomas. The condition should be suspected if there are three relatives over more than one generation with cancer, one of whom has presented under the age of 55 years.
- **Familial adenomatous polyposis** is a rare autosomal dominant condition with incomplete penetrance. It is characterized by the development of hundreds of colonic polyps. It is associated with upper gastrointestinal polyposis, desmoid tumours and retinal lesions. **Untreated, 100% of those with the mutation will die in early adult life from colorectal cancer.** In those in whom the diagnosis has been made, a prophylactic colectomy is performed and reconstructed with either an ileorectal anastomosis or, in younger patients, a restorative proctocolectomy. In those who have undergone a colectomy, there is a 5% risk of death from duodenal carcinoma.

## ADENOMA

See the section in diseases of the anus and rectum (Chapter 31). The most important fact about adenomas is that they must be considered to be premalignant.

## INFLAMMATORY BOWEL DISEASE

This name is given to a non-specific inflammation of the colon and rectum. There are two main diseases – **Crohn's colitis** and **ulcerative colitis**. The hypothesis that they are separate diseases is neither proved or disproved – they are either the same condition manifesting itself in different ways or two conditions which can only provoke certain responses in a single organ. The likely cause is an unknown trigger (or triggers) occurring in a genetically susceptible person which starts a self-perpetuating mucosal injury. It is thought that multiple genes are involved.

### Symptoms

Bloody diarrhoea is the main symptom; in more severe cases there is abdominal pain, weight loss, fever, anaemia, septicaemia, toxic dilatation, perforation and peritonitis. **Toxic dilatation or megacolon is a surgical emergency** – the patient is extremely toxic with a tender distended abdomen caused by an inflamed, thin-walled, grossly distended colon which has lost its protective mucosal barrier. Left untreated by colectomy, the colon will perforate to cause faecal peritonitis and death.

### Signs

In mild cases there may be no physical signs except on sigmoidoscopic examination where the rectum shows the signs of inflammation – contact bleeding, erythema, ulceration and mucopus. **Extracolonic manifestations include uveitis, iritis, ankylosing spondylitis, erythema nodosum and pyoderma gangrenosum.**

### Treatment

- **Medical** – aminosalicylates such as 5-aminosalicylic acid (5-ASA) and olsalazine, steroids (prednisolone, hydrocortisone and budesonide), immunomodulators (azathioprine, methotrexate, cyclosporin).
- **Surgical** – total colectomy and ileostomy with mucous fistula; panproctocolectomy with permanent ileostomy; restorative proctocolectomy (pouch procedure).

> The role of surgery in inflammatory bowel disease is to manage the complications or when medical management has failed. Surgery may be required as an emergency in fulminant colitis where the patient fails to respond to treatment or develops a toxic megacolon. Elective surgery is performed when the long-term debility of the illness is too great or when long-term complications such as dysplasia have occurred. Ten per cent of patients with colitis come to colectomy in the first year after diagnosis.

Surgical procedures in inflammatory bowel disease:

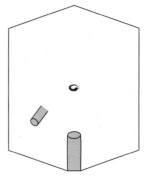

**Figure 30.8** Total colectomy, ileostomy and mucous fistula

1 **Total colectomy and ileostomy with mucous fistula** (Figure 30.8) – the emergency procedure for fulminant colitis is to excise the colon; the proximal end is brought out as an end ileostomy and the distal end out as a mucous fistula. This may, at a later date, be completed as option 2 or 3. An alternative is to close the rectal stump; however, this can be a potential source of sepsis if the suture line leaks.

2 **Panproctocolectomy with permanent ileostomy** (Figure 30.9) – this is the older elective surgical

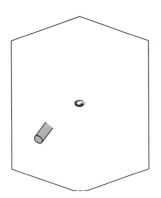

**Figure 30.9** Panproctocolectomy and permanent ileostomy

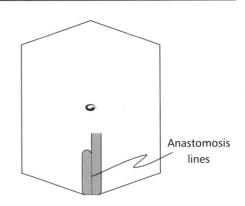

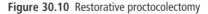

Anastomosis lines

**Figure 30.10** Restorative proctocolectomy

excised and the distal ileum brought out as an end ileostomy. The anal canal is excised, preserving the anal sphincters (intersphincteric proctectomy).

3 **Restorative proctocolectomy** (pouch procedure, Figure 30.10) – the colon and rectum are excised, a pouch is fashioned from the terminal ileum and anastomosed to the distal 1–2 cm of rectum with or without removing the mucosa from the remaining cuff of rectum. This may be done with a temporary defunctioning loop ileostomy (two-stage procedure). Once the pouch function has stabilized, 4–6 loose stools are passed per day. **The procedure has a 15% long-term pouch failure rate due to pelvic sepsis, fistula or pouchitis** (inflammation of the ileal pouch mucosa). This procedure is contraindicated in patients over 60, those with defective anal sphincters and those with Crohn's colitis.

## DIVERTICULAR DISEASE

This is a disease of older ages and can be found in approximately **50% of the population over 70 years of age.** Diverticular disease is thought to be diet related with inadequate stool bulk leading to high intraluminal pressure and subsequently an appearance of hypersegmentation prior to the formation of numerous false pulsion diverticula. Each **diverticulum is a herniation of mucosa** through the bowel wall at weak points where the muscularis propria is traversed by blood vessels. Inspissated pellets of faeces trapped within the diverticula may cause inflammation which presents like left-sided appendicitis – **diverticulitis.** Diverticular disease is often blamed by the patient for a variety of abdominal symptoms but it is usually an innocent bystander. There is no relationship between diverticular disease and colorectal cancer other than that they both occur in similar aged populations.

## Symptoms

The symptoms depend on which complications are present; usually asymptomatic. Women with vaginal fistula formation present to the gynaecologist with a faecal vaginal discharge. Fistulae into the bladder causes urinary tract infection and the classic symptom of pneumaturia.

## Signs

Signs depend on whether complications are present. There may be left iliac fossa tenderness and in severe cases signs of peritonitis. Barium enema (Figure 30.11) reveals a number of diverticula which fill with barium and this may obscure the mucosal detail in the sigmoid colon. In patients with rectal bleeding and a barium enema showing dense sigmoid diverticula, these appearances may obscure neoplastic lesions (adenoma or carcinoma) in up to 30%.

Colonoscopy (Figure 30.12) can reveal the mucosal detail but the presence of diverticular disease may prevent the passage of the colonoscope proximal to the sigmoid colon.

## Treatment

This depends on the complication that has arisen. It is reasonable to advise a patient with diverticular disease to attempt to adhere to a high fibre diet. For inflammation (diverticulitis), bed rest, intravenous fluids and antibiotics are usually enough. Other complications usually necessitate a colonic resection – often as an emergency procedure for spreading peritonitis. In cases of large bowel obstruction it can be impossible to assess at operation whether the pathology is due to diverticular disease or an inflammation secondary to a tumour.

The importance of diverticular disease is that it can lead to complications:

- Diverticulitis (inflammation)
- Perforation
- Pericolic abscess
- Colovaginal or colovesical fistula
- Stricturing
- Obstruction
- Rectal bleeding.

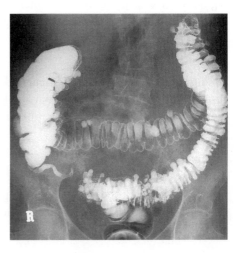

**Figure 30.11** Barium enema appearance of diverticular disease

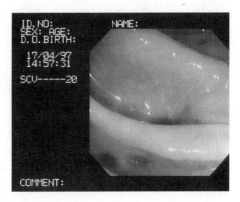

**Figure 30.12** Colonoscopic appearance of diverticular disease

whether the pathology is due to diverticular disease or an inflammation secondary to a tumour.

## VOLVULUS

This unusual cause of obstruction (approximately 5% of colonic obstruction in developed counties) is more common in people with chronic medical or psychiatric disorders. A long mesentery predisposes to a volvulus. Sigmoid volvulus occurs about the mesenteric axis and caecal volvulus around an axis across the ascending colon.

### Symptoms
Sigmoid volvulus presents with colicky lower abdominal pain, abdominal distension, constipation, nausea and vomiting. Caecal volvulus presents with vomiting and mid to lower abdominal pain.

### Signs
Both types of volvulus cause tympanic distension which may be sufficient to compromise respiration. In sigmoid volvulus the rectum is usually ballooned and empty. Plain abdominal radiographs show a hugely distended colon (sigmoid or caecum).

### Treatment
Caecal volvulus is best treated by right hemicolectomy. Sigmoid volvulus can be treated by sigmoidoscopic or colonoscopic decompression but this has a high incidence of recurrence. A sigmoid resection with primary anastomosis is the operation of choice.

## PSEUDO-OBSTRUCTION

Pseudo-obstruction occurs in patients with other medical conditions. It mimics large bowel obstruction but occurs in the absence of a mechanical blockage. An obstructing lesion must be excluded by an unprepared barium enema. Surgery is best avoided unless right iliac fossa tenderness suggests impending caecal perforation.

## PSEUDOMEMBRANOUS COLITIS

### Symptoms
There is pyrexia and diarrhoea, usually without bleeding or mucus, often occurring in patients who have had courses of antibiotics (particularly clindamycin).

### Signs
Sigmoidoscopy shows pseudomembranes which are filmy yellow-white areas partially attached to the mucosa. Confirmation can be made by biopsy (too slow for active management) or by demonstrating *Clostridium difficile* enterotoxin.

**Treatment**

Treatment consists of resuscitation and appropriate antibiotics (vancomycin and metronidazole).

# LESS COMMON COLONIC CAUSES OF RECTAL BLEEDING

> In a shocked patient bright red rectal bleeding may be coming from an upper gastrointestinal cause, such as a duodenal ulcer or oesophageal varices.

## ANGIODYSPLASIA

This is the most common vascular malformation of the colon, associated with aortic stenosis and chronic respiratory disorders. They are small, flat, bright red lesions more common in the right side of the colon, which tend to cause low grade intermittent bleeding.

## DIVERTICULAR DISEASE

Profuse bleeding can arise where a diverticulum passes through the colonic wall alongside the perforating vessels.

## ISCHAEMIC COLITIS

This usually occurs in atherosclerotic elderly patients and affects the left side of the colon. It is associated with ulceration, stricture formation and sometimes gangrene of the colon.

# IRRITABLE BOWEL SYNDROME

This name is given to a cluster of abdominal or gastrointestinal symptoms, the underlying cause of which is unclear. Some evidence suggests that this is related to an abnormality of smooth muscle both inside and outside the gastrointestinal tract.

This syndrome must only be diagnosed when organic pathology of the colon has been excluded.

> A diagnosis of irritable bowel syndrome must never be made in the presence of rectal bleeding unless the colon has been fully investigated to exclude carcinoma of the colon.

**Symptoms**

Symptoms include bloating, abdominal pain and variable bowel habit. Many of

## Treatment

**There is no role for surgery.** Medical management is aimed at reducing smooth muscle spasm in the colon – mebeverine or peppermint oil capsules may be of limited help.

---

**CRIB BOX – THE COLON**

**The colon** stores faeces and reabsorbs water. Disease can cause only a limited number of symptoms:

- Change of bowel habit
- Rectal bleeding
- Pain

**Colorectal cancer** is the second most common cancer in England and Wales. The premalignant stage (adenoma) can be successfully treated

**Inflammatory bowel disease** is treated medically initially – 10% of patients come to colectomy in the first year after diagnosis

- Q: What are the indications for surgery in inflammatory bowel disease?
- A: Failure of medical treatment or complications

**Diverticular disease** is very common in the over 60s – asymptomatic, diverticulitis, pericolic abscess, fistula, stricture, bleeding

**Irritable bowel syndrome** never ever causes rectal bleeding. It is not treated surgically

**LEARN DUKES' CLASSIFICATION**

# chapter 31

# DISEASES OF THE ANUS AND RECTUM

## ANATOMY OF ANUS

The anus (Figure 31.1) is the junction between the rectum and the perineal skin. It is lined in its upper part by colonic mucosa with visceral sensation and in its lower part by stratified squamous epithelium with somatic innervation.

There are two concentric sphincters; the internal sphincter is derived from gut muscle whereas the external sphincter is striated muscle and is in continuity with puborectalis.

The dentate line is a visible landmark just above the level of the epithelial transition zone. There are 6–10 vertical anal columns with horizontal folds (anal valves).

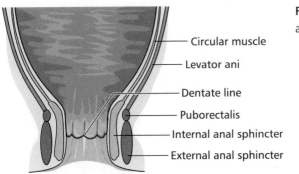

**Figure 31.1** Coronal section of anus

— Circular muscle

— Levator ani

— Dentate line

— Puborectalis

— Internal anal sphincter

— External anal sphincter

## SIGNS AND SYMPTOMS OF ANORECTAL DISEASE

- **Pain** – pain from the anal canal is due to **inflammation, tumour infiltration, perianal haematoma** or **anal sphincter spasm**. Rectal carcinoma is usually painless unless the anus or pelvic nerves are involved. **Haemorrhoids are usually painless** unless they are complicated by strangulation or thrombosis. Intense sharp (tearing) pain on defaecation is characteristic of an anal fissure.
- **Bleeding** – streaks of **bright red blood** seen only on the toilet paper after wiping are usually due to anal problems such as haemorrhoids or fissure.

Haemorrhoidal bleeding also splashes or sprays into the toilet pan or drips after defaecation. **Dark blood** or blood mixed with the faeces suggests a more proximal cause, such as a carcinoma or an adenoma.

- **Mucus** – 'slime' or moist discharge is due to haemorrhoids, rectal prolapse, rectal adenoma or adenocarcinoma.
- **Tenesmus** – an intense desire to defaecate but without results. It is caused by tumour filling the lower rectum or faecal impaction.
- **Pruritus** – perianal irritation is a common symptom in local anal lesions such as fistula, fissure or haemorrhoids. It can also occur with Crohn's disease or worm infestation. Pruritus most commonly occurs with perianal skin soiling in the absence of anal pathology.

## EXAMINATION AND INVESTIGATION OF ANORECTAL DISEASE

The patient should lie on his/her left side with the knees drawn up and buttocks on the edge of the couch (Figure 31.2).

> Careful and thorough examination is essential but if there is a lesion causing severe pain (such as a fissure) then an examination under anaesthetic should be considered.

Reassure the patient that he/she should not feel pain. If a rigid or flexible sigmoidoscopy is to be performed then the patient is warned of the discomfort that air insufflation will cause.

### Inspection
The buttocks are held apart and the skin inspected for:
- Perianal soiling
- Excoriation
- Skin tags
- Prolapsed haemorrhoids
- Fistulous openings
- Ulceration
- Fissure.

The patient is asked to push down to enable the examiner to look for:
- Rectal prolapse
- Perineal descent.

### Palpation
Palpation is carried out in the following areas:
- The anal canal for sphincter tone, induration and ulceration

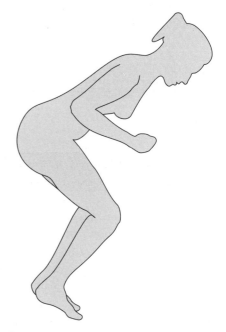

**Figure 31.2** Diagram of left lateral position

- The rectum for contents (faeces, blood)
- The mucosa for ulceration, tumour
- The prostate or cervix
- Extrarectal masses.

If digital examination is too painful, then this is abandoned and instrumentation is not performed; an examination under anaesthetic is likely to be needed.

### Proctoscopy
Haemorrhoids can be inspected and treated by injection sclerotherapy, band ligation, cryotherapy or infrared therapy. Other conditions of the anal canal, such as fibroepithelial anal polyps, can be seen.

### Sigmoidoscopy
The rectum and lower sigmoid can be inspected and biopsied but this examination takes practice. The examination can be performed with a rigid or a flexible sigmoidoscope. After a simple enema preparation, a flexible instrument can usually be passed to the region of the splenic flexure (50–60 cm).

### Imaging
A double contrast barium enema can image the whole colon but diverticular disease can mask mucosal lesions in the sigmoid. If a patient has diverticular disease and rectal bleeding, then a flexible sigmoidoscopy should be performed.

Endo-anal ultrasound is useful for determining sphincter defects, fistula tracks and for the local staging of anal and rectal cancers.

Magnetic resonance imaging gives high definition pictures.

The position of lesions in or around the anal canal are described as hours on a clock face with 12 o'clock anteriorly (as though the patient was in the lithotomy position). The depth of a lesion is reported in centimetres measured from the anal verge.

## HAEMORRHOIDS

Internal haemorrhoids (Figure 31.3) are thickenings of the fibromuscular tissue in the anal canal overlying the submucous venous plexus. Hypertrophy and fibrous scarring from repetitive trauma leads to them prolapsing through the anal sphincter. The causes are unclear but there is a familial tendency. Constipation, straining and pregnancy are contributory factors. There is a very occasional association between intra-abdominal tumours, portal hypertension and congestive cardiac failure. The internal haemorrhoids are found in the **3, 7 and 11 o'clock positions**. Perianal tags of skin are not haemorrhoids but patients often describe them as such. The

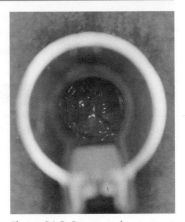

**Figure 31.3** Proctoscopic appearance of haemorrhoids

most common symptom is bleeding at defaecation – the blood is described as **bright red, separate from the stool, smeared on the toilet paper, or dripping into the pan.**

> Most patients attribute any anorectal symptom to an 'attack of piles'.

### Symptoms
- Bleeding
- Mucus
- Pruritus
- Discomfort.

### Staging
- **First degree** – never prolapse
- **Second degree** – prolapse and reduce (either spontaneously or with assistance)
- **Third degree** – never reduce.

### Investigation
The examination must include a sigmoidoscopy (either rigid or flexible).

> If there is any suspicion of a higher colorectal problem then full investigation with a barium enema or colonoscopy is mandatory.

### Treatment
- High fibre diet, topical ointments
- Chemical/physical treatments to cause submucosal fibrosis
  - Injection sclerotherapy (usually with 5% oily phenol)
  - Infrared therapy
  - Cryotherapy
  - Rubber band ligation (Barron's bands)
- Surgery – a haemorrhoidectomy is a very painful procedure and should be avoided unless the patient has severe symptoms.

## PERIANAL HAEMATOMA

This is often referred to as a **thrombosed external pile** but it is simply a tense thrombosis in one of the venous sacs of the external haemorrhoidal plexus. It presents acutely after straining as a tense, tender bluish swelling close to the anal margin.

### Treatment
- Early – drainage under local anaesthetic
- Late – left alone it will resolve over a few weeks to leave a small skin tag.

# ABSCESS AND FISTULA IN ANO

**A fistula is an abnormal track between two epithelial surfaces,** in this instance between the anal canal and the perianal skin (Figure 31.4). It is thought that an anal gland becomes blocked and leads to an abscess in the intersphincteric space. This infection can either stay localized and discharge back into the anal canal (intersphincteric abscess) or, more commonly, track elsewhere (perianal abscess, ischiorectal abscess or pelvic abscess). The resulting track forms a fistula and the nomenclature depends on its relationship to the sphincter mechanism. Both abscesses and fistulae may also run circumferentially around the anal canal (horseshoe abscess or fistula).

> Perianal abscesses (or more importantly ischiorectal abscesses) should be recognized quickly and drained as they can lead to the serious complication of bacterial synergistic gangrene.

**Types of abscess are:**
- Intersphincteric – an unusual cause of anal pain causing an intra-anal tender lump which may discharge back into the anal canal
- Submucous – tracks to anal verge

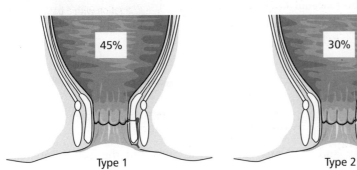
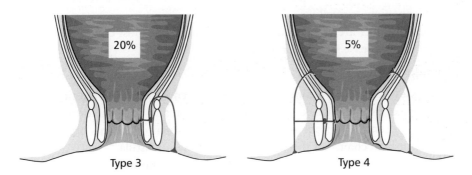

**Figure 31.4** Coronal sections of anal canal showing fistulous tracks: type 1, intersphincteric; type 2, trans-sphincteric; type 3, suprasphincteric; type 4, extrasphincteric

- Ischiorectal – often missed as it presents with pain, erythema and oedema in the skin between the anal canal and ischial tuberosity
- Pelvic – rare. Can arise from anal canal sepsis tracking above levator ani (associated with inflammatory bowel disease or tumour) but more commonly arising from intraperitoneal sepsis (appendicitis, pelvic inflammatory disease or post-surgery).

### Types of fistula are:

- Intersphincteric – 45%; running in the plane between the internal and external sphincters
- Trans-sphincteric – 30%; traversing the sphincters (most common with ischiorectal abscesses)
- Suprasphincteric – 20%; these run above the puborectalis and back down through levator ani
- Extrasphincteric – 5%; these communicate with the rectum above the anal canal.

### Goodsall's law

If the external opening of a fistula is behind a line drawn transversely across the anus, then, however complex the track, the internal opening is single and in the midline. If the external opening is in front of the line, then the track opens radially into the anal canal (Figure 31.5).

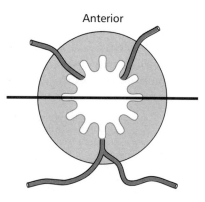

Anterior

**Figure 31.5** Goodsall's law

### Symptoms and signs

Abscesses present with pain and, later, swelling. Ischiorectal abscesses are frequently diagnosed late as they present with pain and little swelling until late on; usually induration and erythema between the anus and the ischial tuberosity rather than an acute, tender perianal swelling.

Fistulae present with either intermittent abscesses or with a recurrently discharging opening or swelling.

A small number are associated with other conditions, most commonly inflammatory bowel disease such as Crohn's or ulcerative colitis.

### Treatment

- Abscesses **need to be drained by an experienced surgeon**. At the time of the drainage a fistulous track should be looked for and if possible treated. Pus should be sent for microbiology – if gastrointestinal organisms are identified there is a high chance of this being associated with a fistula.
- The treatment of fistulae depends on their relationship to the anal sphincters; 75% can be treated by laying open the lower part of the internal or both sphincters without rendering the patient incontinent. **The treatment of the more complicated fistulae is highly specialized and may require multiple procedures.**

# FISSURE IN ANO

This is a common condition where there is a mucocutaneous ulcer or split in the anal canal (Figure 31.6), most commonly in the midline posteriorly, but sometimes anteriorly. It often occurs in women after childbirth. Rarely, they are multiple and superficial. Frequently in a chronic fissure a tag at the outer end is seen – a 'sentinel pile'.

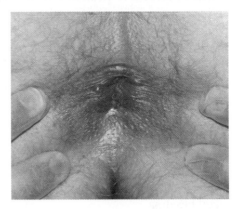

**Figure 31.6** Posterior fissure in ano

### Symptoms
There is pain and bleeding; usually pain on defaecation like 'broken glass' or 'a knife'.

### Signs
Inspection of the anal canal can often reveal the presence of a fissure. Palpation of the anal canal may be impossible because of extreme tenderness.

### Treatment
Acute fissures can be healed by twice daily application of glyceral trinitrate ointment 0.2% for six weeks. In chronic or unresponsive cases a lateral internal anal sphincterotomy can relieve the symptoms and lead on to healing. This operation is performed under a general anaesthetic where the lower border of the internal anal sphincter is divided through a tiny perianal incision. The older treatment is a forcible anal dilatation under a general anaesthetic but this leads to uncontrolled sphincter damage.

# PERIANAL WARTS

Warts (Figure 31.7), like elsewhere on the skin, are viral in origin. They are associated with warts on the digits and are also transmitted sexually.

### Symptoms
They may itch or cause difficulty cleaning the perianal skin, leading to soreness.

### Signs
They are usually multiple around the anal orifice but may also occur inside the anal canal. They may form plaque-like (condylomata acuminata) areas on the perianal skin.

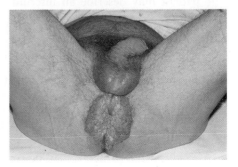

**Figure 31.7** Perianal warts

## Treatment

Perianal warts can respond well to topical chemical therapy but those inside the anal canal are inaccessible. Larger collections of warts and those inside the anal canal are best treated by scissor excision under a general anaesthetic. Histological examination of any excised warts is important as they can undergo a malignant change.

## FIBROEPITHELIAL ANAL POLYP

An epithelialized fibrous polyp arises from hypertrophy of the anal papillae at the level of the dentate line.

### Symptoms

There is a prolapsing polypoid lesion which may or may not be associated with rectal bleeding.

### Signs

A polypoid lesion may be visible at the anal margin. Palpation reveals a firm sometimes mobile lump within the anal canal, arising 2–3 cm from the anal verge.

### Treatment

If symptoms are severe enough then the polyp can be excised under a general anaesthetic.

## PROLAPSE OF RECTUM

Prolapse (Figure 31.8) is most common in elderly women but can occur at younger ages. A partially circumferential prolapse can be due to weak sphincters but a complete prolapse requires very lax pararectal tissues and indicates chronic straining. The prolapse may be reducible or it may strangulate.

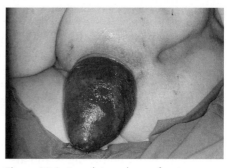

Figure 31.8 Complete prolapse of rectum

### Symptoms

The patient may describe an intermittent lump the size of a grape up to the size of a tennis ball.

### Signs

Nothing may be visible, in which case the patient should sit on a commode and strain for a few minutes. The prolapse may be the colour of normal rectal mucosa, engorged or dark and oedematous.

### Treatment

- A small partial prolapse may be treated by rubber band ligation or injection sclerotherapy.

- A large prolapse needs surgery:
  - Abdominal rectopexy (either open or laparoscopic) where the rectum is mobilized and fixed up to the sacrum
  - Anterior resection of the rectum
  - Delorme's procedure where the redundant mucosa is excised and the muscle layers plicated and reduced.

## CARCINOMA OF RECTUM

Colorectal carcinoma is now the second commonest carcinoma in England and Wales.

### Pathology

This is an adenocarcinoma of varying degrees of differentiation which metastasizes to the pericolonic lymph nodes and to the liver. There are often extranodal deposits in the mesorectum and these may be the source of local recurrences if surgical excision is incomplete.

The tumour may be seen to arise in a polyp, may be a firm-edged ulcer or an annular stricturing lesion. The macroscopic appearances are thought to progress with time and with this the stage and prognosis deteriorates. Early diagnosis is therefore important.

The classical staging uses Dukes' classification (Figure 31.9):

- A – not penetrating the bowel wall (muscularis propria) and no nodal spread
- B – penetrating the muscularis propria and no nodal spread
- C – nodal disease regardless of the local stage.

The importance of a staging is that it should have prognostic significance: the 5-year survival for Dukes' A is usually given as >90%, B 65–70% and C <20%.

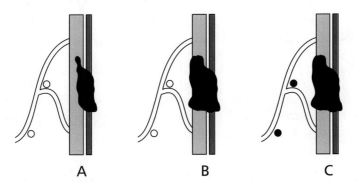

A        B        C

**Figure 31.9** Dukes' classification

## Symptoms

**Rectal bleeding is a common symptom and this is often incorrectly attributed to haemorrhoids.** Other symptoms include a sustained change in bowel habit, mucus discharge and sometimes dragging, dull pelvic pain. Late disease can lead to weight loss, vesicocolic fistula, jaundice, ascites and obstruction. Invasion of the sacral nerve plexus can cause severe pain.

## Signs

**Digital examination is vital;** 75% of rectal cancers are palpable on digital examination, and the tumour mobility can be assessed. Sigmoidoscopy and biopsy should be performed.

## Treatment

**Surgery** The treatment is primarily surgical. Most tumours are treated by major resection. If the tumour is above 7–8 cm from the anal verge, then an **anterior resection with reconstruction** (± temporary colostomy) is feasible but below this level the possible involvement of the pelvic floor muscles or the sphincters necessitates an **abdominoperineal resection** of the anus and rectum with a permanent colostomy (Figure 31.10). Pelvic dissection can compromise the pelvic nerves which in the male can lead to impotence or urinary dysfunction. To reduce the risk of local recurrence a total mesorectal excision is performed.

**Adjuvant therapy** Radiotherapy is of benefit in tumours penetrating the rectal wall. A short course of adjuvant radiotherapy (5 days in the immediate preoperative period) is as effective as a 4-week course of post-operative radiotherapy. For cancers with nodal involvement, post-operative adjuvant chemotherapy is helpful.

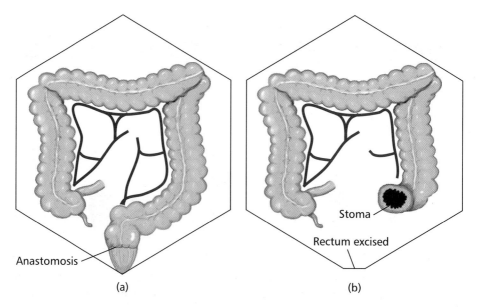

Anastomosis

Stoma

Rectum excised

(a)

(b)

**Figure 31.10** (a) Anterior resection of rectum. (b) Abdominoperineal excision of rectum

# ADENOMA

The most important fact about adenomas (Figure 31.11) is that they must be considered to be premalignant. They are classified into three histological types with increasing malignant potential: **tubular, tubulovillous and villous**. The malignant potential also increases with adenoma size. Histological grading of dysplasia is also important as many are mildly or moderately dysplastic; the severely dysplastic adenomas should be considered as carcinoma *in situ.*

### Symptoms

Rectal adenomas commonly cause rectal bleeding and sometimes a change in bowel habit (looseness) with mucus discharge.

### Signs

A low adenoma may be palpable on digital rectal examination, otherwise it may be seen on sigmoidoscopy.

### Treatment

This consists of colonoscopic snaring or endo-anal excision (operative resection via the anus).

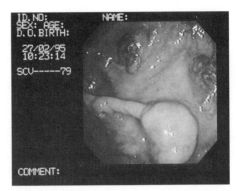

**Figure 31.11** Colorectal pedunculated adenoma

# INFLAMMATORY BOWEL DISEASE

For a description of ulcerative colitis and Crohn's colitis the reader is referred to Chapter 30 (Inflammatory bowel disease).

# IDIOPATHIC PROCTITIS

It is not clear whether this is a variant of ulcerative colitis or a separate entity although the histology is similar. **Thirty per cent of patients experience disease extension proximal to the rectum.**

### Symptoms

Symptoms are rectal bleeding, mucus discharge with or without change in bowel habit, and occasionally lower abdominal pain.

### Signs

Sigmoidoscopy shows an inflamed mucosa with granularity, contact bleeding and mucopus.

### Treatment

It is important to exclude infective or venereal proctitis, radiation proctitis or ischaemic proctitis. Traditionally steroid suppositories or enemas have been used but 5-aminosalicylic acid (5-ASA) suppositories are more effective.

## MALIGNANT DISEASE OF THE ANUS

This is a rare malignancy arising from the anal canal. It may be squamous or basiloid (cloacogenic – arising from the embryological cloaca). **The lymphatic drainage is to the inguinal nodes.** The carcinoma may arise from malignant change in perianal warts. Diagnosis depends on a biopsy, usually performed under a general anaesthetic.

### Symptoms
There is pruritus and severe pain.

### Signs
There is a perianal ulcer externally or a firm ulcerated mass in the anal canal.

### Treatment
The treatment is a combination of radiotherapy and chemotherapy, only resorting to surgery if this fails, at which point an abdominoperineal excision of the anus and rectum may be needed.

## PILONIDAL SINUS

This is a disease of the natal cleft rather than the anus and rectum. The microscopic appearance of a hair shows a series of barbs all pointing in one direction due to its construction from keratinized cells. Trapping of hair between the buttocks leads to it being driven into the skin by buttock movement and causing a chronic subcutaneous infection around a 'nest of hairs' (Figure 31.12). Typically it occurs in young men with dark coarse hair and in the armed forces is commonly termed 'jeep driver's bottom'. Pilonidal sinuses are also occasionally seen in the interdigital spaces of barbers' hands and the umbilicus.

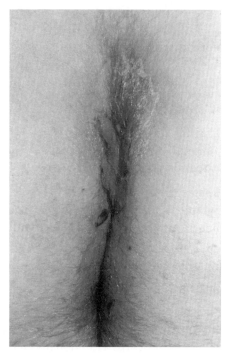

### Symptoms
Intermittent abscesses occur.

### Signs
If the area is inflamed, there is an abscess in or adjacent to the natal cleft. If it is not inflamed, there is one or more sinus openings around the natal cleft. The sinus can often be probed to reveal a track extending to other openings.

**Figure 31.12** Pilonidal sinus

## Treatment

The treatment is surgical. An abscess should be drained. Chronic sinuses are treated by a variety of techniques:

- Laying open
- Excision with packing, primary closure or Z-plasty
- Brushing of the track and chemical ablation.

## BACTERIAL SYNERGISTIC GANGRENE

This is a disease of the skin but most commonly arises from perianal sepsis, although it can arise from other sites (Figure 31.13). Synergism between anaerobic and aerobic organisms in subcutaneous tissues can cause a rapidly spreading cutaneous gangrene which, when treated inadequately, is fatal.

There is much confusion over the nomenclature (see Chapter 5) but two frequently used terms are:

- **Necrotizing fasciitis** – a rapidly spreading cutaneous gangrene which extends most rapidly in the subcutaneous panniculus carnosus muscle layers (corrugator cutis ani, dartos or platysma) although it can occur elsewhere. There is not usually involvement of tissues deep to the deep fascia. **In the scrotum this is known as Fournier's gangrene.**
- **Necrotizing cellulitis** – a more slowly spreading condition, often through the deep fascia into underlying muscle. It is more common in the immunocompromised (particularly in diabetics). This is sometimes described as **Melleney's gangrene**, particularly if it arises on the abdominal wall from intra-abdominal sepsis (or colorectal cancer).

## Symptoms

It often presents as general ill health and sepsis and is only later recognized to be arising from an ischiorectal abscess. Sometimes there is just cutaneous pain and localized tenderness.

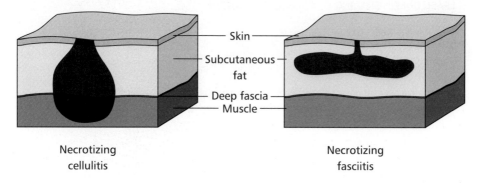

**Figure 31.13** Types of bacterial synergistic gangrene

### Signs

- Necrotizing fasciitis – a central area of necrosis is surrounded by apparently normal skin although this is widely undermined by a layer of thin, foul-smelling 'dishwater' pus and sometimes gas formation.
- Necrotizing cellulitis – an area of central gangrene surrounded by erythema and oedema.

### Treatment

Treatment consists of rapid and aggressive surgery to debride and drain the area in combination with broad spectrum antibiotics. If this arises from perianal sepsis, then it may be necessary to consider a defunctioning colostomy.

---

### CRIB BOX – ANUS AND RECTUM

**Haemorrhoids** – are painless unless third degree, prolapsed and thrombosed

**Pain** is caused by:

- Haematoma
- Fissure
- Abscess
- Fistula
- Carcinoma

Patients attribute **any** anal symptom to an attack of 'piles' (haemorrhoids)

**Diagnosis** requires digital rectal examination, proctoscopy and sigmoidoscopy

Any suggestion of **proximal disease** needs a barium enema or colonoscopy

**Patients over 45 with new symptoms** are assumed to have cancer until proved otherwise

**Perianal abscess** should be drained by an experienced surgeon

**Fistulae** can be complicated and require multiple procedures

### LEARN DUKES' GRADING OF COLORECTAL CANCER:

- A – in the wall
- B – through the wall
- C – nodal spread

Seventy-five per cent of rectal cancers are palpable on digital examination

# chapter 32

# DISEASES OF THE KIDNEY AND URETER

## CONGENITAL ABNORMALITIES

Developmental abnormalities of the kidney and ureter are relatively common and predispose in later life to **stasis** of urine, **infection** and **stone** formation. The commonest malformation is persistence of fetal lobulation; it is of no significance.

Other abnormalities are shown in Figure 32.1.

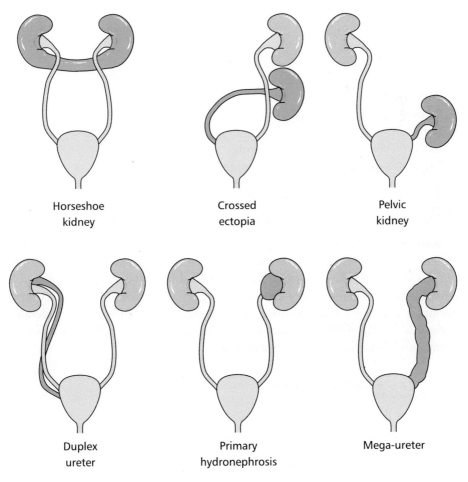

Horseshoe
kidney

Crossed
ectopia

Pelvic
kidney

Duplex
ureter

Primary
hydronephrosis

Mega-ureter

**Figure 32.1** Congenital abnormalities

## SYMPTOMS

The most common symptoms in disease of the urinary tract are **pain**, problems with **micturition** and **haematuria**.

### Pain
- **Fixed renal pain** is a dull ache in the loin – it usually denotes distension or inflammation of the kidney.
- **Ureteric colic** is extremely severe, intermittent in character and radiates from the loin to the groin, testicle or upper thigh. It is usually of such severity as to cause vomiting, sweating and restlessness. The pain is relieved with opiates and NSAIDs.
- **Bladder pain** is suprapubic – caused by distension or inflammation.
- **Strangury** is a painful and frequent desire to micturate frustrated by the passage of only a few drops of urine.
- **Dysuria** may mean difficulty or pain on micturition. The pain is usually described as burning.

### Micturition
Symptoms reflect bladder tone and function, and urinary flow through the urethra:
- Frequency – going too often
- Urgency – sudden need to void
- Hesitancy – difficulty starting
- Poor stream – thin with no power
- Straining – pushing to void urine
- Dribbling – leaking after voiding
- Incontinence – uncontrollable leaking
- Nocturia – disturbed sleep due to frequency
- Retention – inability to void.

### Haematuria
Blood in urine is always a very important sign of disease and demands full investigation. Routine 'dip-stick' testing of urine is a common source of detection. The volume of blood passed may vary from frank to microscopic haematuria. Bright red blood in urine indicates fresh bleeding. **Initial** haematuria, in which blood is passed at the beginning of micturition, suggests a urethral cause. **Terminal** haematuria suggests a vesical cause. The passage of clots indicates considerable haemorrhage. **Painful** haematuria suggests infection, inflammation or calculus. **Frank painless haematuria suggests tumour.**

## PHYSICAL EXAMINATION

The patient is examined for:
- Loss of weight, anaemia or uraemia
- Tenderness, loin masses, bladder distension, asymmetry of the loins
- Urethral discharge, genitalia abnormalities
- **Rectal examination** to palpate the **prostate gland**

- Vaginal examination for gynaecological problems
- A neurological cause of symptoms.

## INVESTIGATIONS

A wide range of tests are available for the investigation of urological disorders.

### Urine

Urine is routinely tested for protein, blood, sugar and pH. For microscopy, bacterial culture and antibiotic sensitivity (MC&S), specimens of urine free of urethral contaminants are taken either in midstream (MSU) or by catheter (CSU). Cytological examination on spun samples detects malignant cells.

### Blood

There has to be considerable kidney damage before evidence of renal failure becomes apparent. Plasma urea and creatinine are measures of renal function – both rise in renal failure with creatinine being more sensitive.

### Imaging of the urinary tract

- **Plain radiographs** – show the shape and size of the kidneys, the presence of calculi (90% of which are radio-opaque) and the psoas shadows which may be obscured in perinephric inflammation. Abnormalities of bone such as spina bifida, secondary deposits from carcinoma of prostate and osteoporosis from hyperparathyroidism may also be revealed.
- **Intravenous urography (IVU)** – the urinary tract is outlined following the intravenous injection of a contrast medium that is selectively excreted by the kidneys (Figure 32.2). Subsequent films show the anatomy of the urinary tract and are of use in assessing renal function – poor renal concentration correlates with poor renal function. The bladder may show pouches or diverticula, filling defects due to growths and enlargement of the prostate. The persistence of contrast medium in the bladder after micturition is a guide to incomplete emptying; residual urine is a common feature of enlargement of the prostate.
- **Retrograde urography** – sometimes indicated if no function is seen on the IVU or if more detail of a suspicious filling defect in the ureter, pelvis or calyces of the kidney is needed. Via a cytoscope one or both ureters are catheterized and contrast injected. Occasionally antegrade studies will help to determine the level of an obstruction – under ultrasound control, contrast can be injected directly into the renal pelvis using a fine needle.

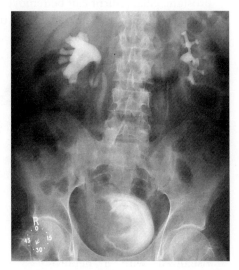

**Figure 32.2** IVU showing bladder tumour with right hydronephrosis due to ureteric obstruction

The bladder can be outlined by **cystography**, in which radio-opaque fluid is injected through a catheter – a micturating cystogram will demonstrate ureteric reflux and a cystometrogram simultaneously measures intravesical pressure during the investigation of bladder dysfunction. **Urethrography** demonstrates strictures or trauma to the urethra.

- **Arteriography** – outlines the arterial system of the kidneys. A catheter is passed via the femoral artery to the level of the renal arteries and contrast medium injected. The catheter can also be used to embolize tumours or bleeding points and for angioplasty of renal artery stenosis.

- **Ultrasound** – used extensively because it is quick, non-invasive and portable. It is particularly useful in differentiating between a solid tumour and a cyst and allows accurate percutaneous aspiration or biopsy. **Transrectal** ultrasound images the prostate and tumours within to guide biopsy needles.

- **CT and MRI** – particularly helpful in the diagnosis and staging of renal, suprarenal and pelvic tumours.

- **Radionuclide scans** – when given intravenously the passage of an isotope (e.g. DMSA; DTPA; MAG3) through the renal system can be monitored with a gamma camera producing a graph of uptake and excretion. The initial uptake is a function of blood flow to the kidney and the subsequent fall monitors excretion. Scans are used to measure relative renal parenchymal function of one kidney compared with the other ('split renal function'), vesicoureteric reflux, renal scarring, and renal filtration.

- **Endoscopy** – the mainstay of urological practice. Specialized endoscopes are available for retrograde inspection and treatment of conditions affecting the urethra, prostate, bladder and ureter. Through these endoscopes, catheters, diathermy electrodes, biopsy forceps, balloons, baskets, lasers and lithotripters can be passed (Figure 32.3). With a special form of cystoscope, a **resectoscope**, prostatic enlargement can be removed piecemeal via the urethra, an operation called trans-urethral resection of the prostate (**TURP**). Suitable bladder tumours may be removed in the same way – trans-urethral resection of bladder tumour (**TURBT**). Flexible fibreoptic cystoscopes passed with local anaesthetic allow inspection of the urethra, prostate and bladder in the clinic. Antegrade endoscopy requires percutaneous formation of a track into the renal pelvis under x-ray control. The renal pelvis can then be visualized with a nephroscope and stones removed or catheters passed.

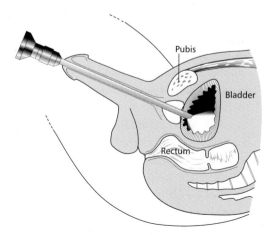

**Figure 32.3** Cystoscopy

# RENAL AND URETERIC INFECTIONS

## ACUTE PYELONEPHRITIS

Acute pyelonephritis is infection, inflammation and suppuration of the kidney parenchyma and renal pelvis. The most common predisposing factors in any urinary infection are **obstruction and stasis:**

- Enlarged prostate
- Stone
- Congenital abnormality of the renal tract
- Ureteric reflux
- Pregnancy.

The most common organisms in urinary tract infection are coliforms (*Escherichia coli, Klebsiella*), *Proteus* and *Pseudomonas*. The route of infection is usually ascending but infection may be blood-borne. In severe acute pyelonephritis the kidney is swollen and oedematous and the changes of acute inflammation extend into the parenchyma. Suppuration may occur and progress to a pyonephrosis or perinephric abscess.

### Symptoms and signs
- Fever
- Rigors
- Loin pain and tenderness
- Frequency and scalding dysuria
- Microscopy of the urine reveals pus cells, organisms and red blood cells.

### Treatment
- Intravenous antibiotics
- Ultrasound – to exclude an obstruction or dilatation of the ureters and pelvices
- IVU – may be indicated after the acute attack has subsided to uncover any predisposing cause such as a calculus, hydronephrosis or a congenital anomaly.

## PYONEPHROSIS

Invariably secondary to ureteric or pelvi-ureteric obstruction causing distension of the renal pelvis and calyces with pus. The infection may be tuberculous.

### Pathology
The kidney becomes converted into a pus-filled sac. Pus cells or organisms may be few or absent in the urine if the ureter is blocked, e.g. a stone. The kidney becomes fixed to nearby structures by inflammatory adhesions.

### Symptoms and signs
- Ureteric colic – precedes pyonephrosis if obstruction is the cause.
- Fever – high swinging temperature, rigors and leucocytosis.
- Pain in the loin with an enlarged, tender kidney.

- The urine may contain pus cells, red blood cells and organisms.
- Ultrasound shows the distended pus-filled kidney.

**Treatment**
- Treatment is urgent.
- Percutaneous nephrostomy under ultrasound control drains the renal pelvis.
- Intravenous antibiotics.
- A cystoscopy and retrograde ureterogram may be necessary later to locate and treat any obstruction.
- The kidney may have no remaining function and nephrectomy is needed.

## PERINEPHRIC ABSCESS

This occurs due to suppuration of diffuse cellulitis of the fibro-fatty tissue around the kidney. The infection may be blood-borne or secondary to kidney infection – infected renal calculus, hydronephrosis or tuberculosis. Symptoms are those of a loin abscess, i.e. pain and swinging fever. By the time the diagnosis is made, drainage is usually necessary through an incision in the loin.

## RENAL TUBERCULOSIS

Tuberculosis of the kidney is **always secondary to disease elsewhere,** usually from a primary lesion sited in the lung or in a lymph node from which the infection has spread via the bloodstream. It is rare in developed countries and typically occurs in young adults.

**Pathology**
In the early phase of infection tubercle follicles appear in the kidneys, usually in the region of the cortex, most of which heal. Occasionally one or more grow and becomes caseous. Spread occurs into the calyceal system leading to greater involvement and destruction of the kidney. If the pelviureteric junction becomes stenosed the kidney becomes hydronephrotic and a tuberculous pyonephrosis forms. Rarely, a tuberculous pyonephrosis calcifies, is apparently inactive, and the kidney is destroyed (so-called **auto-nephrectomy**).

The ureter is involved from infected urine and from periureteric lymphatic spread. It becomes thickened and ulcerated, with regions of stenosis that cause back pressure on the kidney. The bladder is commonly infected from the kidney; tubercles and ulcers are seen at cytoscopy on the lips of the ureteric orifices which become enlarged, stiff and gaping (**golf-hole ureter**). If healing takes place, fibrosis narrows the vesico-ureteric junction and leads to hydronephrosis. Spread via the vas deferens produces **tuberculous epididymitis**.

**Symptoms and signs**
- Low grade fever, night sweats, weight loss, anaemia
- Cystitis – painful frequency with occasional blood
- Loin pain, ureteric colic.

## Diagnosis

- Urine – pus and blood cells but sterile on ordinary culture. Staining for acid-fast bacilli on centrifuged early morning urine (EMU) specimens may prove the diagnosis. Culture takes many weeks. (**Note: sterile pyuria is most commonly seen in patients taking antibiotics for an 'ordinary' urinary tract infection.**)
- Ultrasound guided aspiration or biopsy provides an early positive diagnosis.
- Careful examination of the whole body should be made for evidence of any other foci of disease, e.g. in the lung, bones and joints, the genitalia and prostate.

## Treatment

The results of treatment of urogenital tuberculosis have been immensely improved by the use of newer antituberculous drugs. In most cases surgery can be avoided during the stage of active infection, but is indicated when healing causes fibrosis and stenosis of the renal pelvis, ureters and bladder. Combination therapy consisting typically of pyrazinamide, isoniazid and rifampicin is given for 2 months, followed by maintenance therapy of isoniazid and rifampicin for a further 4–6 months. Regular EMU samples should be cultured throughout treatment and for at least a year following cessation to ensure no recurrence.

## RENAL AND URETERIC CALCULI

Calculi ('stones') are found in the kidney, ureter, bladder and urethra. Those in the ureter come from the kidney, those in the urethra come from the bladder. In the vast majority of cases no cause for calculi can be found but it is possible to list predisposing factors under the imprecise headings **metabolic**, **stasis** and **infection**:

### Metabolic

- Inborn errors – uric acid (gout); xanthinuria; cystinuria
- Hyperparathyroidism
- Renal tubular acidosis
- Vitamin D overdosage
- Idiopathic hypercalciuria.

> **Types of calculi**
>
> - Calcium oxalate
> - Magnesium ammonium phosphate
> - Uric acid
>
> Pure stones are rare – most are mixed

### Stasis

For a stone to form there must be stasis; otherwise microcalculi would be excreted before enlarging:

- Enlarged prostate
- Bladder diverticulum
- Pelvicalyceal, pelviureteric and ureterovesical stenosis
- Anatomical anomalies
- Prolonged recumbency
- Poor urine flow – dehydration; excess sweating.

## Infection

Some bacteria (e.g. *Proteus*) split urea to form an alkaline urine in which phosphate calculi are prone to form. Foreign bodies (especially catheters) cause infection and act as a nidus for stone formation.

## Types of calculi

It is unusual to have a stone of a pure chemical substance; one component may predominate but almost always there are at least traces of others.

- Calcium oxalate stones are small, hard and dark in colour, with an irregular spiky surface ('mulberry' stones).
- Uric acid stones are hard, smooth and brownish in colour.
- Phosphate stones are grey-white in colour and often very large.

Calcium phosphate stones are white and hard, mixed phosphatic calculi are softer and paler.

Oxalate, uric acid and urate stones occur in acid urine, phosphate stones arise in alkaline urine.

## Symptoms and signs

**Stones in the kidney** Stones in the kidney can cause obstruction, resulting in hydronephrosis which can be further complicated by infection, leading to septicaemia, pyonephrosis or perinephric abscess. A stone may gradually increase in size until it fills the pelvis and the calyces, resulting in a **staghorn** calculus, which gradually destroys the kidney.

Uncomplicated stones in the kidney may be surprisingly asymptomatic but complications cause pain in the loin on the side of the problem.

**Stones in the ureter** Stones in the ureter cause ureteric colic. Nearly all stones under 5 mm in diameter will pass down the ureter and over half of all stones will eventually pass spontaneously down to the bladder.

On urinalysis there is usually a trace of blood due to the minor trauma of the stone.

**Stones in the bladder** Stones in the bladder cause pain at the tip of the penis, which is often relieved by lying down. Pain is worse at the end of micturition due to impaction of the stone and is often accompanied by a few drops of blood.

**Stones in the urethra** Stones in the urethra are very rare since most pass spontaneously. They may impact to cause sudden obstruction whilst voiding. They are relieved by catheterization to push the stone back into the bladder or by surgical excision.

## Diagnosis and investigation

- The diagnosis of stones is often made on the history alone but urinalysis invariably shows the presence of blood.
- Clinical examination is often unrewarding, although there may be renal tenderness in an obstructed kidney.
- A plain abdominal x-ray demonstrates approximately 90% of stones but the stone may be lost among other causes of abdominal calcification, e.g. pelvic phleboliths. The most common radiolucent stone is pure uric acid.

- An IVU is the best investigation for urinary stones. It can show up small stones in the ureter but also demonstrates the degree of obstruction they are causing. Delay of the contrast passing through an obstructed kidney may require a film taken many hours later to demonstrate the site of the hold-up and the stone.
- Ultrasound scan often demonstrates the stone and is especially good for showing hydronephrosis or dilated ureters. It can, however, miss small stones in the ureter.

### Treatment of stones

An obstructed infected kidney is a surgical emergency requiring the drainage of the obstructed infected urine. This can be achieved by a **percutaneous nephrostomy** – under local anaesthetic a needle is passed into the renal pelvis through the skin of the loin under x-ray or ultrasound control. A wire is passed into the dilated pelvicalyceal system over which a drainage tube is railroaded.

### Stones in the kidney

Stones in the kidney can be treated in various ways:

- **Extracorporeal shock-wave lithotripsy (ESWL)** – the stone is located with ultrasound or x-ray and a shock wave generated by an electrical spark or a piezoelectric emitter. The shock wave is focused on the stone and passes through the patient to shatter the stone. Larger stones may need more than one treatment and can be complicated by fragments of stone impacting in the ureter, causing obstruction.
- **Percutaneous nephrolithotomy (PCNL)** – a guidewire is passed through the skin of the loin into the kidney using the same technique as for a nephrostomy tube. The tract is gradually dilated over the guidewire until a nephroscope can be inserted. The calculus is located under direct vision and the stone smashed using various techniques such as ultrasonic lithotripsy (sound waves); electro-hydraulic lithotripsy (shock waves); lithoclast (pneumatic drill); and pulsed laser beam (laser energy). The fragments of stone can be washed out or grabbed via the nephroscope tube.
- **Staghorn calculi** can be removed with repeated ESWL sessions or a combination of ESWL and PCNL. If the staghorn calculus has already destroyed much of the kidney function (as measured on DMSA scan), a simple nephrectomy can be performed. A kidney with under 10% function can be removed safely as the other kidney will maintain renal function. A staghorn calculus or large renal stone can also be removed at open surgery, although advances in technology now make this treatment a rare event.

### Stones in the ureter

- **Non-obstructing stones** under 5 mm in diameter can be left in the hope they will pass spontaneously. With radio-opaque calculi, progress can be monitored with repeated plain abdominal x-rays.
- **Obstructing stones** can be treated by ureteric stenting. Using a cystoscope a ureteric cannula is inserted into the ureteric orifice on the obstructed side. Retrograde injection of x-ray contrast locates the position of the stone. Sometimes the cannula can be passed beyond the stone into the obstructed portion or the impacted stone can be flushed back into the proximal ureter. A

guidewire can then be passed up into the kidney, and a silicone stent inserted to allow the kidney to drain. Insertion of the stent relaxes the spasm in the ureter and when the oedema settles, the stone may pass spontaneously alongside the stent into the bladder.

- **ESWL** can be used, although it can be difficult to focus the beam with stones in the lower pelvis or close to the vertebral column.
- **Ureteroscope** – this can be passed via the bladder and retrogradely up the ureter. Stones can be smashed by a lithoclast or electrohydraulic lithotripsy, or a wire basket (Dormia basket) can be passed via the ureteroscope and the stone snared under direct vision.
- **Surgery** – if all else fails because of a tortuous or kinked ureter, the stone can be removed at open ureterolithotomy. This is a simple procedure through a muscle-splitting extraperitoneal incision.

### Stones in the bladder

Most stones in the bladder (Figure 32.4) can be treated with the passage of a resectoscope sheath into the bladder via the urethra. The stones can be smashed using an electrohydraulic lithotrite or lithoclast and the fragments evacuated via the resectoscope sheath. Most bladder stones are associated with prostatic obstruction and TURP may be required to gain access to the stone and will almost certainly be required to prevent further formations.

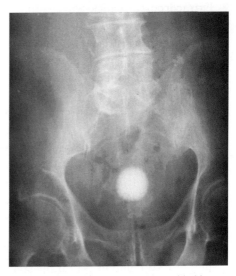

**Figure 32.4** Plain x-ray with opaque bladder stone

### Long-term treatment

Patients who develop stones are more likely to develop recurrent stones than the routine population and are very keen to avoid further problems. Stones retrieved should be sent for analysis and patients should be investigated and treated for underlying metabolic problems, e.g. hyperparathyroidism or gout.

The mainstay in the prevention of recurrent stones is maintenance of a very high fluid input to prevent stone formation and to flush through any microcalculi that are formed.

## HYDRONEPHROSIS

Intermittent or partial obstruction to the outflow of urine from the kidney leads to distension, first of the renal pelvis, then the calyces (hydronephrosis)

(Figure 32.5); later, thinning of the renal parenchyma leads to reduction of renal function. Eventually the kidney may be converted into a thin-walled functionless sac in which infection and stone formation are common sequels. Bilateral hydronephrosis may lead to renal failure and death unless the cause can be treated. Depending on the site of obstruction the ureter is also dilated – hydroureter.

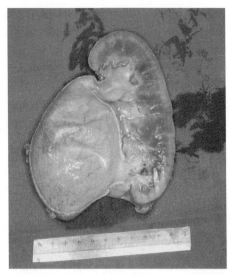

**Figure 32.5** Hydronephrotic kidney

### Pathology

- **Primary** – seen at the pelviureteric junction (PUJ obstruction). It is postulated that there is a defect of PUJ neuromuscular transmission, because no mechanical barrier exists. It can present at any age from *in utero* to adulthood.
- **Secondary** – caused by mechanical obstruction. If the block is in the bladder or urethra the hydronephrosis will be bilateral with dilated ureters. There are **myriad causes of secondary hydronephrosis** including stones, urothelial tumours, prostatic hypertophy, pelvic or colonic tumours involving the ureter, retroperitoneal fibrosis and congenital urethral valves.

### Symptoms and signs

- Renal pain fixed in the loin – often brought on by drinking large volumes of fluid (beer).
- Back pain – may be mistaken for musculoskeletal pain.
- Symptomless – during abdominal examination a painless mass is felt in the loin.
- Infection – causing pyonephrosis.
- Trauma – the distended kidney is prone to trauma and rupture.
- Renal failure and hypertension.

### Investigation

- IVU, ultrasound and radionuclide scan will demonstrate the degree of distension and the function of the kidneys.
- Cystoscopy and retrograde catheterization of the ureters, or antegrade injection of contrast into the renal pelvis may be needed to accurately define the site and nature of the obstruction.

### Treatment

The treatment of secondary hydronephrosis is treatment of the cause of the condition. Primary hydronephrosis is treated with plastic operations on the pelviureteric junction (**pyeloplasty**). It is vital to preserve renal function as much as possible, because both sides are likely to become affected. Nephrectomy is only performed for the grossly diseased kidney with absent function. In adults, primary hydronephrosis can be treated by endoureteric **pyelotomy** (using a blade and guidewire) or balloon dilatation of the narrowed segment.

## URETEROCELE AND MEGA-URETER

### URETEROCELE

Ureterocele is a congenital anomaly in which the lower ureter is dilated and projects into the bladder on the summit of an eminence of redundant mucous membrane. The ureter and renal pelvis may become dilated (hydroureter and hydronephrosis). Often there is a duplex collecting system. The condition may be recognized on IVU, since it produces a typical filling defect shaped like a **cobra's head** in the vesical shadow (Figure 32.6). Cystoscopy confirms the diagnosis. Minor degrees in adults can be treated by slitting the meatus with a diathermy knife to form a larger ureteric meatus. Large ureteroceles are excised and the ureter reimplanted into the bladder.

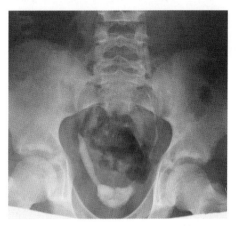

**Figure 32.6** IVU of right ureterocele – note cobra head appearance

### MEGA-URETER

Massive dilatation of the ureter is often bilateral and due to some neuromuscular defect in the lower end of the ureter or to ureteric reflux. It is often associated with stenosis of the bladder neck and occasionally urethral valves which require treatment. The ureters become very wide and tortuous, with associated hydronephrosis. Mega-ureter is usually congenital, and often gives rise to symptoms in early childhood, e.g. infection, frequency, haematuria and enuresis. Treatment is division and shortening of the ureters and reimplantation in the bladder.

## TUMOURS OF THE KIDNEY

### RENAL CELL CARCINOMA (HYPERNEPHROMA; GRAWITZ TUMOUR)

Renal cell carcinoma is the commonest malignant tumour of the kidney. The term hypernephroma was given because the cells of the tumour resemble adrenal cells but are in fact renal tubular cells. Adults aged 50 and over are most commonly affected, men more often than women.

## Pathology

The cut surface of the kidney shows a rounded and apparently encapsulated tumour, usually in the upper pole. It is typically golden yellow in colour, with areas of haemorrhage. It rarely invades the renal pelvis, but may compress it or splay out its calyces. The growth is very vascular, and processes of it may invade veins and even **project from the renal vein into the inferior vena cava,** from where tumour emboli may sometimes break off.

The tumour spreads locally to invade the perinephric fat, lymph nodes in the fat and the great vessels. Hypernephroma classically embolizes to the lungs, where it gives rise to typically rounded shadows on chest x-ray (**'cannon-ball' secondaries**). The liver and bones may be involved and metastasis may also appear in the supraclavicular lymph nodes from spread via the thoracic duct. Isolated secondary deposits in lung or bone sometimes appear years after the primary has been treated, and their removal is then well justified.

Classical presentation is:

- Frank painless haematuria
- Pain in the loin
- Mass in the loin.

Only 40% of cases have all three features but approximately 80% present with haematuria. Renal cell carcinoma is a strange tumour that can present in bizarre ways:

- **Pyrexia of unknown origin** – due to pyrogens produced by the tumour
- **Anaemia** – more from marrow toxins produced by the tumour than from the haematuria
- **Raised haemoglobin** due to erythrocytosis stimulated by tumour-produced erythropoietin
- **Hypercalcaemia** – the tumour can produce an ectopic parathormone type product but hypercalcaemia can also occur in combination with multiple bony metastases
- **Abnormal liver function** – without hepatic metastases
- **Glucagon secretion** – can lead to diarrhoea and enteropathy
- **Tumour obstruction of the left renal vein** – can put back pressure on the left testicular vein to cause a left varicocele.

## Diagnosis

Ultrasound shows a solid mass in the kidney and differentiates it from a cystic swelling. Any solid mass in the kidney must be assumed to be a potentially malignant tumour. The ultrasound demonstrates tumour progression into the renal veins or vena cava and may show enlarged para-aortic lymph nodes. An IVU is not as helpful as an ultrasound scan but confirms the normal kidney is functioning properly. CT scanning is more accurate than ultrasound and can also show up small lung metastases that can be missed on routine chest x-ray.

## Treatment

Treatment of renal cancer is **radical nephrectomy** which entails totally removing the kidney and surrounding perinephric fat. Any locally enlarged lymph nodes are also removed to allow staging. Tumour extension into the renal vein and inferior vena cava should be removed at the same time. Tumour extending above the liver and diaphragm into the right atrium needs **cardiopulmonary bypass** for total excision. In cases of renal cell carcinoma in a solitary kidney, renal arteriogram will demonstrate the vessels and help planning for a possible partial nephrectomy. Occasionally removal of the primary tumour causes regression of secondary deposits. Therapeutic embolization, leading to infarction, with autologous clot, gelatin sponge or steel coils may be an alternative to surgery in unfit patients or those with multiple metastases.

Survival rates when the tumour is isolated in the kidney are almost 100%, although prognosis deteriorates rapidly when the tumour is found to be invading the renal vein and lymph nodes.

## NEPHROBLASTOMA (EMBRYOMA; WILMS' TUMOUR)

Nephroblastoma of the kidney is **one of the few malignant tumours of children**. It very rarely occurs over the age of 7 years; usually it presents between the ages of 2 and 4. Very rarely it is bilateral.

### Pathology

The origin of an embryoma of the kidney is undecided, but it very probably arises from mesonephric tissue. The kidney is enlarged, sometimes massively, and may be completely replaced by white tumour tissue in which there is haemorrhage or cystic degeneration. It is very adherent to perinephric tissue and may cause ascites. Microscopically, an embryoma appears to be a tumour of mesenchyme, with disordered masses of spindle cells, degeneration and haemorrhage. It is unlike a teratoma in not having elements of all three embryonic layers. The tumour grows rapidly and may become very large. **Spread occurs early**, both locally and by the bloodstream.

### Symptoms and signs

- Haematuria occurs in about a third of patients or the mother may feel a mass in the child's loin when bathing.
- Enlargement of the abdomen from a rapidly growing tumour may occur. The child soon becomes wasted and anaemic, often with high fever.
- Typically there is a large swelling in the abdomen of a wasted baby.
- Diagnosis is made by feeling the mass and by intravenous urogram which shows a large filling defect or absence of function on the side of the swelling.

### Treatment

Treatment is radical nephrectomy combined with chemotherapy and radiotherapy according to staging. Nowadays, 60–80% of children survive for 4 years.

## TRANSITIONAL CELL PAPILLARY
## TUMOURS OF THE RENAL PELVIS AND URETER

Papilliferous growths are found most commonly in the bladder but these tumours also occur in the renal pelvis and ureter. Those in the renal pelvis are very prone to spread by **'seeding' in the ureter and bladder.** As in the bladder, all papilliferous tumours should be regarded as malignant.

**Haematuria is the commonest symptom.** Urography shows a filling defect in the renal pelvis or hydronephrosis; sometimes defects in the ureter may be seen. Cystoscopy may show papillomata protruding from the ureteric orifice or in the bladder near to it. Treatment is by **nephro-ureterectomy,** i.e. removal of the kidney and whole of the ureter. As the patient may later develop a bladder tumour, long-term follow-up by cystoscopy is essential.

## SQUAMOUS CELL CARCINOMA OF THE RENAL PELVIS

The presence of calculi in the renal pelvis for many years may induce metaplasia transitional to squamous epithelium and the development of squamous carcinoma. The prognosis is poor because of local and distal spread. The kidney must, if possible, be removed and radiotherapy given post-operatively.

## BENIGN TUMOURS OF THE KIDNEY

Benign tumours are rare and usually found at post-mortem examination. **Adenomas** sometimes grow to large size and show cystic formation. They may be difficult to distinguish from carcinomas. **Lipomas** and **fibromas** rarely cause symptoms. **Angiomas** are rare; they may cause haematuria and can be difficult to diagnose, for there may be no urographic signs. Angiography may be of help. Cystoscopy at the time of bleeding is important in the hope of locating the side from which bleeding is occurring. When bleeding is severe or persistent, nephrectomy may be necessary.

## POLYCYSTIC KIDNEY

- This is a developmental anomaly caused probably by a failure of fusion of the mesonephros and the duct system in the embryo.
- Both kidneys are affected, often asymmetrically.
- Massive enlargement of the kidneys at birth may cause difficulty in delivery.
- Usually the condition is not recognized until adult life, and cysts tend to grow progressively in size between areas of apparently normal-looking renal tissue.
- The cysts are lined by cuboid epithelium and contain clear or blood-stained fluid.
- The spleen, pancreas and liver may also be affected.

### Symptoms and signs
Apart from severe renal impairment in childhood, most people with polycystic kidneys are unaware of them until adult life. In some, the condition is compatible

with normal longevity and may only be found at post-mortem examination. Common presentations are the discovery of **large swellings** in the abdomen, **haematuria, hypertension** and **renal failure** with uraemia.

IVU shows elongated spidery calyces, which are splayed out and narrow; sometimes rounded indentations of the renal pelvis and calyces can be seen. Ultrasound or CT scan may be necessary for the diagnosis.

### Treatment

Nothing can be done to correct the condition. Aspiration of the cysts may relieve pain. If chronic renal failure occurs it is treated appropriately.

## SOLITARY CYSTS

Solitary cysts may reach a great size and be mistaken for tumours. The cysts are lined by flattened epithelium and are filled with clear fluid. They may cause aching pain or present without symptoms as an abdominal tumour. Urography may show a rounded filling defect in the calyceal system or only a soft tissue shadow. Scanning will establish whether the suspicious lesion is a solid tumour or a cyst and fluid can be aspirated for cytology or to relieve symptoms.

## INJURIES OF THE KIDNEY

The kidney is usually injured by a blow in the loin or by crushing. Other viscera may be damaged, especially the liver and spleen. Penetrating wounds by a knife or bullet are likely to involve other organs as well as the kidney. The kidney may be bruised, torn, or even completely avulsed from its pedicle. If a tear goes into the calyces or renal pelvis, haematuria will result. A large subcapsular perirenal haematoma may produce a mass in the loin.

### Symptoms and signs

Haematuria is the commonest symptom; it may be minimal or so severe as to require transfusion, or it may be intermittent over a period of 2 or 3 weeks. There is pain and tenderness in the loin, and if haemorrhage or extravasation of urine has occurred around the kidney (**urinoma**) a swelling may result in the loin. Evidence of other visceral injury must be sought very carefully.

### Treatment

Relatively **few renal injuries require operative treatment**. Following resuscitation an IVU reveals the state of the injured kidney and establishes that there is another functioning kidney without congenital anomalies. In minor injuries the urogram may be normal; in more severe injuries the calyceal pattern may be distorted and in very severe injuries no contrast medium may be excreted on the affected side. If there is no renal function on the injured side, an angiogram is performed.

With rest, antibiotics and analgesics most patients show decreasing haematuria and recover. An IVU is repeated 2 or 3 months after the accident to assess the state of the kidney, as occasionally hydronephrosis may result. Long-term follow-up is advisable to detect hypertension caused by residual renal ischaemia.

Operation is indicated for associated visceral injury or severe haemorrhage. In most patients requiring operation, bleeding is so severe and renal damage so great that **partial or total nephrectomy** is required.

## INJURIES OF THE URETER

- The ureter may rarely be damaged by severe crushing injury.
- **The most common injury is that caused accidentally by surgery.**

> - The ureter is particularly at risk in the operation of **hysterectomy**, because the ureter lies close to the vault of the vagina and is liable to be caught in ligature of the uterine artery. It presents early with pain in the loin due to hydronephrosis, **peritonitis** due to leaking, or late with a **ureterovaginal fistula**.

If the injury is low in the pelvis, then the ureter may be divided and reimplanted into the bladder; at a higher level the ureter is reanastomosed. **If both ureters are obstructed, anuria results,** requiring urgent laparotomy with bilateral reimplantation of the ureters or emergency bilateral nephrostomy.

---

**CRIB BOX – KIDNEY AND URETER**

Commonest symptoms are **pain, haematuria and micturition problems**

**Frank painless haematuria is assumed to be tumour** until proved otherwise

Infections are usually associated with **obstruction, stone, or stasis**

Causes of stones – **metabolic, stasis and infection**

Stones cause trouble:

- In the kidney – obstruction; infection; stag horn
- In the ureter – ureteric colic; obstruction
- In the bladder – pain; infection; obstruction; carcinoma
- In the urethra – acute retention

**Hydronephrosis** – primary (congenital); secondary (any obstruction or reflux)

**Kidney tumours:**

- Benign are rare
- Renal cell carcinoma (adults)
- Wilms' tumour (children)
- Transitional cell in the pelvis (remember seeding)

**Ureteric injuries** are usually surgical (especially hysterectomy)

# chapter 33

# BLADDER, PROSTATE AND URETHRA

## THE BLADDER

### CONGENITAL ABNORMALITIES

The bladder and urethra develop from the anterior part of the cloaca (the upper part of which becomes the urachus) with the trigone developing from the distal ends of the mesonephric ducts.

#### Ectopia vesicae

In this condition the anterior bladder wall, the anterior abdominal wall, and the pubic rami fail to fuse in the midline (Figure 33.1). The posterior wall of the bladder is clearly visible and the ureters may be seen dribbling urine. In addition, the penis is often split along its dorsal surface (epispadias) and the sphincter muscles are inevitably incomplete.

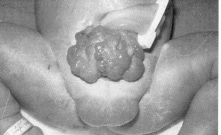

**Figure 33.1** Ectopia vesicae

Reconstructive surgery over many years is required to prevent ascending kidney infections, and to restore some bladder function.

#### Abnormalities of the urachus

The urachus extends from the vault of the bladder to the umbilicus and usually closes to become a fibrous cord – the median umbilical ligament. However, all or part may remain patent to form:

- A patent urachus – leaking urine at the umbilicus
- A urachal diverticulum – in dome of the bladder
- A urachal sinus – open at the umbilicus
- A urachal cyst – somewhere along the median umbilical ligament.

### INFLAMMATION OF THE BLADDER

- Acute cystitis – bacterial
- Recurrent cystitis – due to underlying pathology
- Chronic cystitis – tuberculous; parasitic; radiation
- Interstitial cystitis (Hunner's ulcer).

## Acute cystitis
- Common in women – short urethra, susceptible to local trauma.
- Symptoms – burning dysuria, smelly cloudy urine, frequency, some blood.
- Infecting organism usually perineal, e.g. coliforms.
- Treatment – antibiotics after MSU taken for microbiology.
- In men and children search for predisposing pathology, e.g. prostatism; ureteric reflux.

## Recurrent cystitis
- Usually results from anatomical or functional abnormality of the urinary tract.
- Investigations – IVU, cysto-urethroscopy, micturating cystography/manometry.
- Systemic factors such as diabetes must also be excluded.
- Treatment is directed at the underlying pathology.

## Chronic cystitis
- **Tuberculosis** – see page 424.
- **Schistosomiasis (bilharziasis)** – *Schistosoma haematobium*. Common in the Middle East, particularly around the Nile Delta. The cercarial stage of the parasite passes through the skin when standing or bathing in fresh water. Maturation occurs in the liver before migration into the pelvic veins. Eggs are formed in the urinary tract and it is these that cause the characteristic pathological changes. An intense local inflammatory reaction is set up around the eggs with granulation tissue and fibrosis. **Squamous cell or transitional cell carcinoma may supervene.** Bladder contraction with calcification may occur in long-standing cases, and ureteric stricture with obstructive hydronephrosis is not uncommon.
- **Radiation/chemical cystitis** – both ionizing radiation and some chemicals (e.g. cyclophosphamide) cause damage to the bladder. Radiation cystitis is characterized by new vessel formation and fibrosis. Severe haemorrhage may result from mucosal ischaemia and ulceration and the bladder wall may even break down, resulting in fistulae into adjacent organs. These changes can take several years to develop and the symptoms tend to be progressive.

## Interstitial cystitis (Hunner's ulcer)
This is almost exclusively a disease of women. The aetiology is unknown – possibly autoimmune. It is a pancystitis with inflammation throughout the bladder wall (it can be likened to Crohn's disease of bowel), resulting in fibrosis and contraction which produces symptoms of frequency, nocturia and pain. Distension of the bladder at cystoscopy causes the eponymous characteristic linear mucosal tears which ulcerate and bleed. Treatment usually comprises hydrostatic dilatation of the bladder under general anaesthetic but the symptoms recur. Bladder augmentation cystoplasty or urinary diversion is indicated for severe intractable symptoms.

## TUMOURS OF THE BLADDER

### Benign tumours
Any tissue normally found in the bladder may be the site of a benign tumour (fibroma, lipoma, leiomyoma, etc.) but all are extremely rare.

### Malignant tumours
- Transitional cell carcinoma (TCC) – most common
- Squamous cell carcinoma – rare
- Adenocarcinoma – rare.

> Almost all urothelial carcinomas are transitional cell carcinomas, but squamous cell carcinomas occur in the presence of chronic irritation, e.g. stones, schistosomiasis or chronic infection. Adenocarcinomas of the bladder are extremely rare and usually associated with congenital abnormalities, e.g. tumour arising in a urachal remnant.

## TRANSITIONAL CELL CARCINOMA (TCC)

The urothelium of transitional cell epithelium lines the urinary tract from the renal calyces to the distal urethra. TCCs can occur at any level in the urinary tract, but are **more common in the bladder as the relative stasis gives any carcinogen present in the urine time to act.** There are approximately 60 bladder carcinomas discovered for every one in the ureter.

### Aetiology
Urothelial carcinomas are strongly associated with carcinogens in the urine from industrial exposure. Initially this was **aniline dye workers and then workers in the cable and rubber industries who were exposed to naphthylamines.** Almost 100% of workers with prolonged exposure developed tumours, although some cases did not present for 30 years. It is difficult to know which of today's chemicals will be found to cause urothelial carcinoma in the years to come. Cigarette smoking and exposure to diesel fumes are probably two of the most important factors at present.

### Pathology
For practical purposes there are three types of TCC:

1 **Superficial** – limited to the epithelium or subepithelium and often papillary and well differentiated.
2 **Invasive** – tumour has spread through the lamina propria into muscle, is often solid and moderately to poorly differentiated.
3 **Carcinoma *in situ*** – these are tumour cells in the epithelial layer that have not penetrated the epithelial base membrane. Although often designated 'precancerous', this is an important lesion as it almost invariably develops into the dangerous invasive type of carcinoma.

**Spread** of tumour may be:
- **Local** – to neighbouring lymph nodes or adjacent organs (including the ureteric orifice which produces hydronephrosis and renal failure)

- **Distant** – lungs, bone and, rarely, liver. It often occurs after several years of the disease.

Death results from the effects of the local disease (i.e. renal failure) or from widespread metastases.

### Staging

The TNM system of staging has now been accepted as standard. Using this system, the local tumour (T), the lymph nodes (N), and distant metastases (M) are assessed separately (Figure 33.2).

The local tumour is assessed as follows:

- Tis – carcinoma *in situ*
- Ta – does not invade lamina propria of mucosa
- T1 – invades lamina propria
- T2 – invades superficial layers of muscle
- T3a – invades deep muscle
- T3b – invades through muscle wall

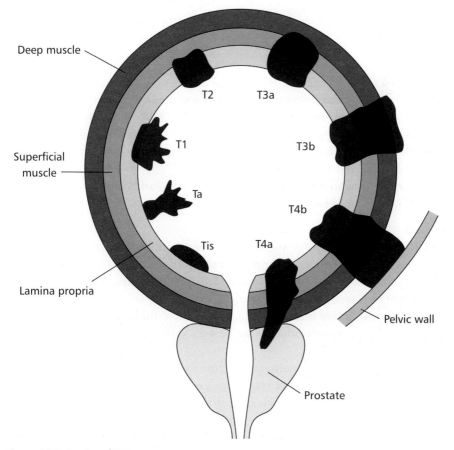

**Figure 33.2** Staging of TCC

- T4a – invades adjacent organs (prostate, uterus, vagina)
- T4b – fixed to pelvic wall.

The lymph node status is also classified: N0–N3 depending on the number of nodes, whether they are on the same side as the bladder lesion, and how far removed they are from the primary.

The presence or absence of metastases is denoted by M1 or M0.

### Clinical features

Urothelial carcinomas classically present with **FRANK PAINLESS HAEMATURIA**. Microscopic haematuria or pain in the bladder from an invading invasion lesion is less common. Clinical examination is usually negative although occasionally a suprapubic or renal mass is felt.

---

**Haematuria** is an important symptom always requiring investigation with:

- Cystoscopy – usually a flexible fibreoptic scope under local anaesthetic
- Renal tract ultrasound scan and/or intravenous urogram – to exclude other sources of bleeding in the upper urinary tract
- Urinary cytology – tumours release cells into the urine.

---

### Diagnosis

- **USS and IVU** – to exclude lesions in kidneys or ureters and to determine whether there are two functioning kidneys and if either is obstructed.
- **Urine cytology** – for malignant cells.
- **Cystoscopy** – the appearance, the number and the site of lesions should be carefully noted. A bimanual examination is performed to assess the stage, and should be repeated after endoscopic resection.
- **Ancillary investigations** – CT scanning, bone scan, and chest x-ray are helpful in staging the carcinoma.

### Treatment

1. **TURBT** (Figure 33.3) is the mainstay of treatment and may need to be repeated at regular intervals for the remainder of the patient's life. Open resection and partial cystectomy are avoided as these tumours show a remarkable propensity for seeding in open wounds.
2. **Cytotoxic instillation** into the bladder is indicated for multiple well-differentiated papillary tumours which may be very difficult to control by resection alone.
3. **BCG instillation** as immunotherapy is now frequently used instead of cytotoxics and gives similar or better results for carcinoma *in situ*.
4. **Radiotherapy** (external beam) is used to treat lesions that are poorly differentiated or have invaded too deeply into the bladder for resection.
5. **Radical surgery** (cysto-urethrectomy with urinary diversion) is reserved for invasive tumours (T2 and T3).

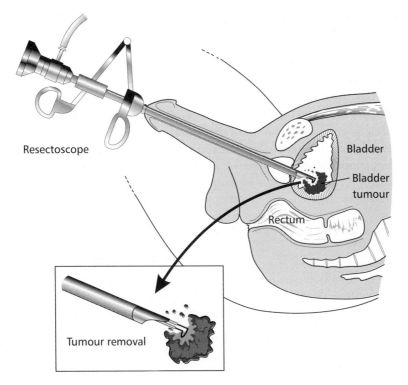

**Figure 33.3** Diagram of TURBT

## SECONDARY TUMOURS

The bladder is a not unusual site of secondary tumour involvement, commonly by local spread from adjacent organs (colon, prostate, cervix). Treatment depends on the primary site, but quite often palliation is all that is possible.

## TRAUMA TO THE BLADDER

Either closed or open (penetrating) injuries may rupture the bladder. Pelvic fractures may lacerate the bladder, causing extravasation of urine. Surgical damage may result from instrumentation or resections.

### Clinical features

- **Intraperitoneal rupture** A history of blunt or sharp trauma, in association with abdominal pain and no urine being passed, should suggest the possibility of this condition. Generalized peritonitis is a late sign unless the urine was already infected. The bladder is most susceptible to injury when full and has even been reported as rupturing spontaneously in the presence of retention.
- **Extraperitoneal rupture** Bloody urine extravasates into the extravesical tissues of the pelvis, giving rise to a painful pelvic mass. Again, usually no urine is passed or there may be some blood-stained urine appearing at the external meatus. There may be some difficulty differentiating this condition from a

ruptured membranous urethra, but the history will often give a clue to the true diagnosis. A cystogram will prove the diagnosis.

### Treatment

**Intraperitoneal ruptures** should be repaired surgically at a full laparotomy (to exclude other intra-abdominal injury) and the bladder drained, ideally by suprapubic catheter as this is more comfortable for the patient and does not traumatize the urethra. Continuous drainage of the bladder is undertaken for 7–10 days and a cystogram performed after this time confirms that the leak has sealed.

If an **extraperitoneal rupture** is small (as usually occurs when surgically induced) it is possible to treat it by simple bladder drainage for 7–10 days. Larger lacerations may require suturing although the site may be inaccessible.

## FISTULAE INVOLVING THE BLADDER

These are always secondary to another pathology, such as:
- Trauma – usually surgical
- Inflammation – diverticular disease of the colon, Crohn's disease
- Tumour – commonly colorectal carcinoma; uterus; cervix.

The fistula may be between the bladder and the body surface (external); or may be between the bladder and a neighbouring organ (internal).

### Clinical features

External fistulae are usually self-apparent. Internal fistulae may either present with the uncontrolled passage of urine by another orifice (vesicovaginal fistula) or with the passage of gas (**pnuemoturia**) and faecal debris in the urine (enterovesical fistula), commonly with symptoms of cystitis.

### Treatment

Simple external fistulae (as following suprapubic catheterization) will usually close spontaneously as long as there is no distal obstruction to urine flow. Internal fistulae usually require surgery to remove the cause (colonic carcinoma, etc.) and to close the bladder defect.

## DIVERTICULA OF THE BLADDER

Acquired diverticula are secondary to bladder outlet obstruction, causing a rise in intravesical pressure (cf. diverticular disease of the colon). They are **pulsion** diverticula or 'blow-outs' of mucosa through bands of hypertrophied detrusor muscle. Congenital diverticula contain all layers of the bladder wall and are rare. Diverticula may:
- Be the source of recurrent urinary tract infection because of stagnation
- Develop a calculus, again because of stagnation
- Produce pressure on a ureter, causing hydronephrosis
- Develop malignant change in the wall (often associated with stones in which case the tumour may be squamous cell). The prognosis of tumour in this site is usually very poor as the thin wall allows early extension into paravesical tissues.

Symptoms are usually referable to the causative pathology (usually prostatic hypertrophy) and treatment should be aimed at this with attention paid only to the diverticulum if it is large or the site of complications. Surgical excision with repair of the bladder wall is the definitive treatment.


## DISORDERS OF BLADDER FUNCTION

The bladder is made up of interwoven smooth muscle fibres of the detrusor muscle which spiral down around the bladder neck to form the internal sphincter. **The external sphincter is striated involuntary muscle (S 234) but, unlike other voluntary muscle, is in a constant tonic state and only relaxes to allow micturition.**

The detrusor muscle is controlled by parasympathetic nerves but the bladder neck area and internal sphincter is controlled by α1-adrenergic sympathetic fibres.

Urinary flow rate depends on the pressure generated by the detrusor contracting against any outflow resistance. Normal micturition is achieved by a sustained detrusor contraction and relaxation of the internal autonomic sphincter and voluntary relaxation of the external sphincter. The internal sphincter is more important in men and probably has little function in women. Failure of these mechanisms results in **urinary retention or incontinence.**

**Urinary retention** can be:

- **Acute** – complete and **painful**; caused by prostatic enlargement or urethral stricture
- **Chronic** – partial with overflow and often **painless**. Chronic urinary retention can be **primary** from a neurological problem or **secondary** to prolonged outflow obstruction.

**Urinary incontinence** is caused by:

1 **Abnormal detrusor function**
   - **Urge incontinence** – detrusor instability.
     - **Primary** due to powerful bladder contractions overcoming the external sphincter, the patient being unable to reach the lavatory in time before wetting.
     - **Secondary** to a bladder irritant, e.g. infection, tumours or stones.
   - **Overflow incontinence** – poor bladder contraction leads to incomplete emptying, residual urine and chronic retention with overflow, often the cause of bed wetting in elderly men.

2 **Poor external sphincter**
   - **Stress incontinence** – common in elderly women, following childbirth or due to uterine prolapse. Increased abdominal pressure from coughing and sneezing leads to a urinary leak.
   - **Complete loss of sphincter** action leads to a continuous dribble of urine, e.g. sphincter damage post-prostate surgery.

## Treatment

### Urinary retention

- Acute retention presents with severe pain and a hard palpable bladder. It is treated as an emergency with urethral or suprapubic catheterization followed by definitive treatment of the cause.
- Chronic retention produces a large floppy bladder with poor tone. There is no method of increasing the tone of an atonic destrusor muscle to ensure complete bladder emptying. Intermittent self-catheterization by the patient helps to keep the bladder empty and prevent complications of urinary infection and renal failure.

### Urinary incontinence

- An overactive bladder can be modified with the use of the **anticholinergic drugs** (e.g. oxybutynin), although the bladder relaxation achieved is often accompanied by the side-effects of dry mouth and nose. Bladder contractions can be further limited by a cystoplasty. The most common is the **clam cystoplasty** where the bladder is opened in the coronal plane and augmented with a length of ileum which is isolated and sewn into the defect.
- Stress incontinence can be treated by **pelvic floor exercises** to strengthen the sphincter, the **injection of silicone** into the bladder neck area to buttress the outlet and help continence or finally **surgery** to hitch up the bladder neck to prevent descent.

## THE PROSTATE

### BENIGN PROSTATIC HYPERTROPHY (BPH)

This very common condition affects men progressively from late middle age onwards; indeed, it is so common that it might almost be considered an exaggerated aspect of the normal ageing process.

### Pathology

**Hyperplasia** of the **glandular** and **muscular elements** of the prostate occurs, giving rise to adenomata which enlarge and compress the normal surrounding tissue, including the urethra. Adenomata in the lateral lobes enlarge posterolaterally and are easily palpable per rectum as a smooth, bilobed mass. Adenomata in the middle lobe encroach increasingly into the urethral lumen and may project upwards into the bladder. Middle lobe enlargement is not palpable per rectum.

As the outflow obstruction increases, the bladder detrusor muscle compensates by hypertrophy; the bladder wall thickens and at cystoscopy, instead of a smooth bladder wall, a basketwork of hypertrophied bladder muscles is seen (**trabeculation**). The high pressure required to overcome prostatic obstruction can lead to mucosal 'blow-outs' between these thickened bars, causing sacculation and eventually diverticulum formation.

### Symptoms

- The detrusor muscle usually becomes **unstable,** producing spontaneous contractions and symptoms of **urgency and frequency.**
- If the bladder remains **stable,** frequency is not a marked symptom and the raised intravesical pressure may cause **hydronephrosis and deteriorating renal function** with minimal warning symptoms.
- The bladder often empties incompletely and the resulting puddle of residual urine is an ideal site for infection and stone formation.

### Clinical features

The classical features are:

- **Frequency** – due to detrusor instability
- **Urgency** – again a symptom of bladder instability
- **Hesitancy** – a delay between attempting to micturate and actually doing so
- **Poor flow** – the stream is slow or weak
- **Terminal dribbling**
- **Nocturia** – patients need to rise several times during the night
- **Incontinence** – a rare complaint, usually due to overflow of a large capacity bladder. This symptom must be taken seriously as there may be an element of hydronephrosis and chronic renal failure.

The diagnosis is usually apparent from the history. Examination sometimes reveals a large, distended bladder (as in chronic retention with overflow) but more commonly the only physical finding is of an enlarged prostate palpable on rectal examination.

### Investigations

- **International prostatic symptom score** – a questionnaire enabling the patient's symptoms to be given a number, the total providing a rough indication of symptom severity. A score of over 20 out of a possible 35 suggests the patient has severe problems and probably needs intervention.
- **Urinary flow analysis** – a simple test where the patient urinates into a flowmeter and the maximum and average flow per second is measured. A reduction of the maximum flow rate below 10 or 12 ml/second is an indication for treatment.
- **Ultrasound** – post-micturition residual urine can be estimated in clinic with a small portable ultrasound machine. Residual volume of over 150–200 ml suggests significant bladder impairment.
- **MSU** – to exclude infection.
- **Bloods** – to check renal function.
- **Prostatic specific antigen (PSA)** – rises in prostatic carcinoma and symptoms may be identical to benign prostatic hypertrophy.
- **Cystoscopy** – usually performed at the time of surgery. Essential to exclude other pathologies, e.g. bladder stones or tumour. Bladder tumours, especially carcinoma *in situ,* may present with irritable bladder symptoms similar to prostatism.

## Treatment

Treatment is indicated when:

- Symptoms are severe
- Renal damage is being produced by obstruction
- Complications such as stone or infection supervene
- Retention occurs.

Frequency may not be alleviated by surgery, and is not therefore an indication to operate when present in isolation.

If left too long the bladder can become overstretched and the detrusor muscle loses its power to contract. This results in chronic urinary retention (even if the outflow obstruction is corrected) and can only be treated by long-term bladder catheterization or intermittent catheterization by the patient.

## Surgical treatment

- **Trans-urethral resection of the prostate** (TURP) – using a resectoscope through which a diathermy loop is passed the prostate is resected piecemeal from within the urethra. Surgery may be performed under general, spinal or epidural anaesthesia.
- **Open retropubic prostatectomy** – reserved for patients with very large glands (in whom TURP would be time-consuming) and when complications (diverticula; large stones) necessitate an open approach. The prostate is approached extraperitoneally and the adenomata enucleated from within the compressed normal gland.

## Complications of surgery

The mortality of TURP is low, and is often attributable to pre-existing medical conditions. There are, however, a number of specific complications:

- **Haemorrhage** – reactionary, and secondary at around 10 days due to infection.
- **Clot retention** – requires bladder washouts.
- **Septicaemia** – when surgery is performed in the presence of infected urine.
- **Fluid disturbance** – TURP necessitates continuous bladder irrigation and some of this fluid is absorbed into the general circulation through open prostatic veins. When this fluid was commonly water (saline cannot be used with diathermy), fluid overload, haemolysis of red cells and considerable electrolyte disturbance could occur. Nowadays, a 1.5% solution of glycine (almost isosmolar) is used, and haemolysis is no longer a problem, although fluid overload, congestive cardiac failure, cerebral oedema and renal failure is still seen (**TUR syndrome**).
- **Retrograde ejaculation** – as the internal sphincter is destroyed as part of the operation, retrograde ejaculation is common.
- **Incontinence** – if the external shincter is damaged (rare).
- **General complications** – deep vein thrombosis and pulmonary embolism, chest infection, stroke, and myocardial infarction.

## Medical treatment

Medical treatment is used mainly in primary health care. The prostate is dependent on androgens and testosterone is converted to the active androgen dihydrotestosterone by the enzyme 5α-reductase.

- **5α-reductase inhibitors** (e.g. finasteride) given over a prolonged period can eventually lead to a slight improvement in urinary flow and reduction in prostatic volume.

Up to 30% of the prostate is made up of smooth muscle rich in α1-receptors.

- **Selective α1-blockers** (e.g. indoramin) can lead to a relaxation of the prostatic muscle and some improvement in symptoms. There are side-effects such as postural hypotension and nasal stuffiness.

## CARCINOMA OF THE PROSTATE

Prostatic cancer is rapidly becoming the most common cause of malignancy in men in the United Kingdom; approximately 10 000 cases a year die from the disease. It is a disease affecting old men and probably all men in their 80s have prostatic carcinoma present if it is looked for. A large proportion of these men die with the disease but not from it. The natural history of prostatic carcinoma is not fully known but from a small malignant focus in the gland to symptomatic disease can take up to 10 years.

**In approximately two-thirds of men presenting with symptoms the tumour has already spread beyond the prostate gland, often to the bones.** About 20% of patients suffering from prostatic obstruction are found to have prostatic carcinoma.

## Pathology

The tumour arises in the posterior lobe of the prostate (below and behind the ejaculatory ducts) and spreads out through the capsule to invade neighbouring structures including the rectum. Spread via the pelvic veins to the bones of the pelvis and lumbar spine is a common feature. Local lymphadenopathy is also common. Microscopically, the tumour is an adenocarcinoma, although it may be poorly differentiated.

## Clinical presentation

- Symptoms are identical to BPH although the history is often considerably shorter.
- Pain from bony metastases.
- Blood in the urine or sperm (haemospermia).
- Ureteric obstruction due to local invasion.
- Incidental histological diagnosis following prostatic resection for presumed BPH.

## Examination and investigation

- **Rectal examination – the most important part of the examination.** The benign prostate feels rather rubbery whereas a prostatic carcinoma is felt as a harder area. As the tumour grows this harder area expands to involve the whole gland, **obliterating the medial groove** between the lateral lobes. Eventually the tumour spreads laterally towards the pelvic wall producing 'winging' of the prostate until finally there is a solid fixed hard mass anterior to the rectum.

- **Prostatic specific antigen** – PSA is an enzyme secreted by the prostate that prevents the semen gelling after ejaculation. The blood levels of PSA increase with an enlarging prostate but are markedly increased with any upset to the prostatic blood barrier, e.g. carcinoma, biopsy, surgery or prostatic inflammation. A PSA over 6 ng/ml is suspicious and over 10 ng/ml indicates probable prostatic carcinoma. A PSA over 20 ng/ml suggests spread beyond the prostate with distant metastases.
- **Transrectal ultrasound** – ultrasound screening of the prostate with a rectal probe will show quite small foci of carcinoma which can be biopsied with a fine needle under direct vision.
- **Biopsy** – with a needle during digital rectal examination or using ultrasound as above.
- **Bone scan** – and x-rays to screen for metastases. Deposits show as sclerotic dense areas on x-ray.

### Staging (Figure 33.4)

- Stage A – unsuspected and found on pathological examination of TURP specimen.
- Stage B – clinically palpable and confined within the prostatic capsule.
- Stage C – extension beyond the prostatic capsule.
- Stage D – metastatic disease.

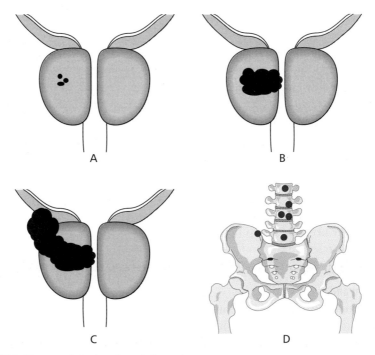

**Figure 33.4** Diagram of staging of prostatic carcinoma

## Treatment

### Stages A and B

Treatment of prostatic carcinoma confined within the capsule depends on the natural life expectancy of the patient and his general health:

- Asymptomatic elderly men with a natural life expectancy of <5 years can simply be observed.
- Men with a life expectancy of 5–10 years are probably best treated with external beam radiotherapy.
- Younger men fit for surgery can be offered **radical prostatectomy**. This is a major operation preceded by bilateral internal iliac node sampling to ensure they are clear of metastases. The prostate with its capsule and the seminal vesicles are removed *en bloc* and the urethra re-anastomosed to the defect in the bladder base. The operation is complicated by a high level of impotence and an incontinence rate of just under 10%.

### Stages C and D

Hormone ablation is the treatment of choice. The majority of prostatic cancers are dependent on testosterone. Removal or blocking the source of testosterone produces resolution of the tumour and any metastases present in approximately 60–70% of patients. The effect lasts for on average 2 years in half of these. Hormone ablation can be achieved in various ways:

- **Orchidectomy** – usually subcapsular orchidectomy, i.e. removal of the testicular contents, leaving the epididymis and tunica behind. This produces castrate levels of testosterone within 12 hours but has the complication of troublesome hot flushes.
- **LHRH agonists** (e.g. goserelin) – requires a monthly subcutaneous injection to produce castrate levels of testosterone.
- **Anti-androgens** – stilboestrol was used for many years as the drug of choice until it was found that the levels required to suppress testosterone led to a high incidence of vascular thromboembolic problems. The two main drugs today are:
  - **Cyproterone acetate** which has a local anti-androgen effect as well as a steroidal pituitary effect; it can cause quite severe liver problems and should probably not be used for more than a year.
  - **Specific androgen blockers** (e.g. flutamide) act by blocking the testosterone receptor sites on the prostate, preventing dihydrotestosterone stimulating prostatic growth.

**Radiotherapy** is used for palliation against specific bony metastases that are causing pain or problems. Hemi-body irradiation can be used in widespread metastatic tumour.

## THE URETHRA

### CONGENITAL ABNORMALITIES

#### Hypospadias

The urethra is formed by fusion of the genital folds, thus enclosing a tube of tissue. If fusion is incomplete, hypospadias results. There are varying degrees, from a minor failure of fusion at the tip of the penis to a more complete failure, leaving a bifid scrotum and a perineal opening for the urethra. The prepuce is characteristically deficient ventrally. There is very frequently a tight fibrous cord in the substance of the penis, causing a ventral curvature of the penile shaft – **chordee**. Surgery to straighten the penis and reconstruct the urethra is usually done before 2 years and gives good results.

### Epispadias

This is the reverse of hypospadias as the urethra opens on the **dorsal** surface of the penis. This is commonly associated with ectopia vesicae. Repair of minor forms is relatively straightforward using plastic surgical techniques, but more extensive malformation, as with ectopia vesicae, requires extensive, staged surgery.

### Urethral valves

This rare congenital abnormality of males can produce severe **urethral obstruction** *in utero*, resulting in a huge, thick-walled bladder, bilateral hydroureters and hydronephrosis in the newborn. Treatment must be carried out urgently, and involves bladder decompression and resection of the valves trans-urethrally. In older children, urethral valves present with infection or problems with micturition.

## URETHRAL STRICTURE

Urethral strictures can be:
- Congenital
- Iatrogenic
- Traumatic
- Inflammatory.

Urethral strictures are fibrotic narrowings composed of dense collagen with fibrosis extending from the urethra into the corpus spongiosum. The strictures restrict urine flow and cause proximal dilatation and recurrent urinary infections.

### Signs and symptoms

The presenting complaint is usually one of **slow urinary stream or recurrent infection with or without a discharge**.

A **urethrogram** (Figure 33.5) with a voiding **cysto-urethrogram** will demonstrate the location and extent of the stricture. **Urethroscopy** under local or general anaesthetic may also be required.

- **Congenital strictures** are either in the posterior urethra (posterior urethral valves) or can occur along the penile urethra.
- Most **iatrogenic strictures** are secondary to instrumentation or catheterization.
- **Traumatic injury** to the urethra, either via pelvic fracture injury or a kick to the perineum, results in fibrosis and stricture.
- The **inflammatory strictures**, which are now rare, are due to gonococcal urethritis.

## Treatment

The treatment depends on the site and type of stricture.

- Congenital urethral valves require incision.
- Congenital strictures in the bulbar or penile urethra may be dilated or incised under direct vision with a small urethrotomy knife.
- Following incision or dilatation, patients are encouraged to self-dilate using a 12 or 14F catheter to maintain urethral patency.
- Should urethrotomy fail, surgical reconstruction may be required.

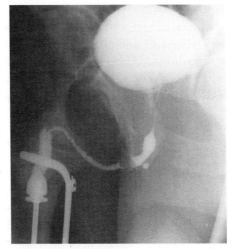

**Figure 33.5** Urethrogram

## URETHRAL TRAUMA

Damage may comprise contusion, partial rupture or complete rupture. Rupture (Figure 33.6) almost never occurs in women. Urinary extravasation follows complete and partial injuries and exacerbates the liability to stricture formation.

### Anterior bulbar urethra

- Follows a fall astride an object, a kick in the perineum or instrumentation.
- The urethra is crushed against the pubis or perforated.
- A perineal haematoma forms and blood may discharge from the external meatus.
- The patient is usually unable to pass urine and, if he tries, urine extravasates from the torn urethra into the surrounding tissues.

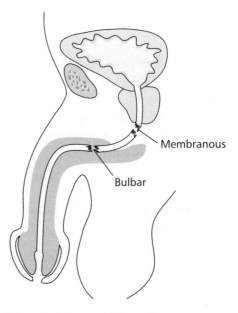

**Figure 33.6** Ruptures of the urethra

- Urine tracks into the penis and scrotum and upwards onto the abdominal wall.
- Diagnosis may be confirmed by urethrography using a water-soluble medium.

Treatment is probably best undertaken by suprapubic catheterization, without attempts at urethral instrumentation. **Vain attempts at urethral catheterization will merely convert a partial rupture into a complete rupture.** After 6 weeks, urethrography and urethroscopy will commonly reveal a short stricture which is easy to treat by standard techniques.

## Posterior membranous urethra

- Ruptures at this site usually follow pelvic fractures and other major injuries.
- The bladder and prostate are avulsed from the urethra.
- The distended bladder and prostate float cephalad on the resulting haematoma.
- There is bleeding from the external meatus.
- Rectal examination may show prostatic dislocation.

Again, urethral instrumentation should be avoided and urethrography will establish the diagnosis. Careful rectal examination will establish whether there is prostatic dislocation.

Suprapubic bladder drainage will allow the urethra to heal and subsequent urethrography and urethroscopy will delineate the limits of the stricture. This may require formal urethroplasty, but, more commonly, simple urethrotomy will be sufficient. The distal mechanism of the urethra will have been damaged by the injury, and the bladder neck mechanism is therefore of considerable importance to the patient's continence.

With wide dislocation some surgeons advocate early operation to reduce the dislocation and approximate the torn urethral ends over a catheter. Subsequent stricture formation can be treated in the standard fashion.

---

### CRIB BOX – BLADDER, PROSTATE AND URETHRA

**Tumours of the bladder**

- Benign (rare)
- TCC – *in situ*; superficial; invasive
- SCC – secondary to chronic inflammation
- Adenocarcinoma – rare; urachal remnant

Present often with **frank painless haematuria**

**Bladder rupture** – extraperitoneal or intraperitoneal

**Urinary retention**

- Acute
- Chronic – primary (neurological); secondary (obstruction)

**Incontinence** – urge; overflow; stress

**BPH**

- Symptoms due to outflow obstruction and detrusor instability
- Treat by TURP – remember the complications

**Carcinoma of the prostate is common and increasing**

- Most patients have metastases when they present
- Early tumours treated with nothing, DXT or radical prostatectomy depending on age and fitness
- Late tumours treated with hormonal manipulation

**Urethral trauma** – anterior bulbar; posterior membranous; treat with suprapubic catheter

# chapter 34

# THE MALE GENITALIA

## EMBRYOLOGY

- The male genitals ducts are derived from the Wolffian ducts at approximately 7 weeks.
- Germ cells differentiate into both **Sertoli cells** which manufacture **sperm** and **Leydig cells** which secrete **testosterone**.
- Dihydrotestosterone influences the Wolffian ducts to turn into the vas deferens, seminal vesicles and epididymis. In addition, its influence causes the phallic and genital tubercles to develop into the penis, scrotum and urethra.
- Shortly before birth the testes, which have been intra-abdominal, descend from the peritoneal cavity along the inguinal canal guided by the **gubernaculum**.

## ANATOMY

The penis contains two elements (Figure 34.1):

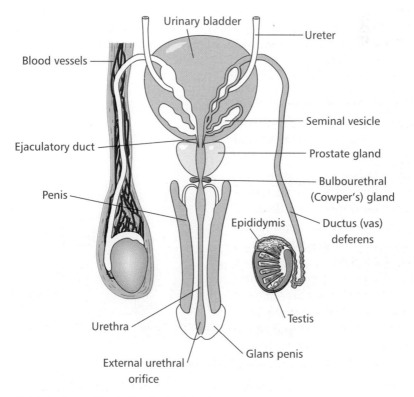

**Figure 34.1** Anatomy of the male reproductive system

- The corpora cavernosa are responsible for erectile function.
- The corpus spongiosum expands distally to form the glans penis. The urethra runs on the ventral aspect of the penis between the two corpora.
- The scrotum contains the testes, epididymis, vas deferens and the constituents of the spermatic cord made up of the **testicular artery** and **pampiniform plexus** of veins.
- The **left testicular** vein drains into the **left renal** vein.
- The **right testicular** vein drains directly into the **inferior vena cava** at the same level.
- The main nerve supply to the male genitalia is the pudendal nerve (S2–S4).
- The nerves responsible for erectile function are autonomic – parasympathetic fibres from S2–S4 and sympathetic fibres from T11–L2.

## LYMPHATIC DRAINAGE

> The **testes** drain to the para-aortic lymph nodes – **NOT TO THE GROIN**. The **penis and scrotum** drain into the inguinal lymph glands.

## AMBIGUOUS GENITALIA INTERSEX

Congenital abnormalities of the external genitalia are rare – children born with ambiguous genitalia can belong to one of two groups:
1. A genetic female who has been subject to masculinization.
2. A genetic male in whom the process of masculinization has been impaired.

- **Female** – an excessive production of adrenal androgens occurs as a result of a block in the pathway of cortisol production from the adrenal gland (**congenital adrenal hyperplasia**).
- **Male** – failure to become masculine. If there is failure of testosterone biosynthesis or a defective Y chromosome, the appearances of the external genitalia will be that of a female.
- Mild disorders of imperfect masculinization can result in **hypospadias** (failure of the male urethra to exit at the distal end of the penis – Figure 34.2). It may need surgical correction depending upon its location along the shaft of the penis.

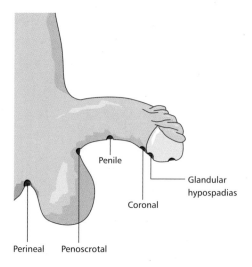

**Figure 34.2** Hypospadias

- Congenital abnormalities such as Klinefelter's syndrome (XXY), Turner's syndrome (XO) and mosaicism (XO XY) can result in ambiguous genitalia, but these are rare.

## DISORDERS OF THE TESTIS AND EPIDIDYMIS

### UNDESCENDED TESTICLE

In the fetus the gubernaculum guides the testis from its intra-abdominal position through the inguinal canal and down into the scrotum (Figure 34.3). Both testes are normally in the scrotum at birth. Absence of the testis from the scrotum occurs for one of three reasons:

1 **True maldescent** – the testis is held up somewhere along its proper course of descent. This can occur at any position – within the abdomen, in the inguinal canal or at the superficial inguinal ring. Most often it is found at the internal ring. When the testis is retained within the abdomen or in the inguinal canal it is impalpable. The testis itself is often abnormal.
2 **Ectopic** – the testis ends up in an abnormal position. This is thought to be due to an abnormal lower insertion of the gubernaculum. Thus, instead of being guided into the scrotum, it comes to rest in the subcutaneous tissue of the upper thigh, superficial inguinal pouch (most common), perineum, anterior abdominal wall or penile root, and can often be felt. The testis is usually normal.
3 **Retractile** – in most boys the testes are very mobile and easily withdrawn into the inguinal canal by the cremasteric muscle reflex. Fear or cold hands may cause retraction but by careful and gentle examination in warm surroundings the testes can be stroked into the bottom of the scrotum. Retractile testes require no treatment.

### Complications of undescended testicle

In order for spermatogenesis to occur the testis must lie within the scrotum at approximately 1–2°C cooler than body temperature.

- **Spermatogenic function** – between 12 and 18 months, undescended testes undergo a change in their histological structure; after this time they are unlikely to have normal function.
- **Trauma and torsion** – undescended testes are more liable to injury and torsion.

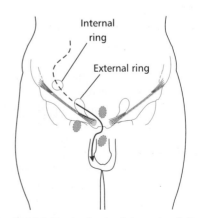

**Figure 34.3** Route of normal descent and sites of ectopic testis

- **Malignancy** – after puberty there is a significant risk of malignant change in an undescended testis. It is therefore important that the testis is in the scrotum, if only to enable regular inspection. An undescended testis diagnosed in adulthood should be removed provided there is a normal functioning testis on the other side.

### Treatment of undescended testicle

Retractile testes require no treatment. Maldescended and ectopic testes should be brought down to the scrotum as early as is practicable in the hope of preserving spermatogenesis and hormone production – usually between 1 and 2 years of age. However, many boys are referred to a surgeon later than this.

The operation is termed **orchidopexy** – via a groin incision the testis and cord are located and fully mobilized to allow placement of the testis in the scrotum without tension. There is often a hernial sac which needs excising (herniotomy). It is common practice to place the testis in a subcutaneous **dartos pouch** to keep it in position in the scrotum.

Abdominal testes can be located with MRI scans or laparoscopy and transferred to the scrotum using microvascular surgery. Alternatively, if the other testis is normal, an abdominal testis can be excised to avoid risk of future malignancy.

## INFECTION

Infections of the testicle and epididymis can be **acute or chronic**. It is also important to differentiate between infections of the testis (orchitis) and infections of the epididymis (epididymitis).

- **Acute orchitis** – rare and associated with a viral infection such as mumps, or coxsackie. Mumps orchitis in adults, which occurs in approximately 15% of cases, may cause testicular atrophy and **sterility**.
- **Acute epididymitis** – usually caused by *Escherichia coli* or *Klebsiella*, particularly following **instrumentation or catheterization** of the urinary tract. In younger men, *Chlamydia* is often responsible. **An acutely painful swollen hot scrotum** is the normal presentation. It was previously described as 'epididymoorchitis' but is usually predominantly an epididymitis. A **secondary hydrocele** can occur. Clinically, the patient is pyrexial and toxic.

  **Investigations** – culture of urine and any urethral discharge. **Ultrasound** scan shows a normal testis and acutely swollen epididymis.

  **Treatment** – bed rest, analgesia, scrotal support and intravenous antibiotics. If *Chlamydia* is the organism, the treatment of choice is oral tetracycline for 4 weeks.

**IMPORTANT LESSON**

It is essential to distinguish an acute swollen **infected scrotum** from torsion of the testis. Torsion is usually in a **different age group** (approximately 11–25 years) and the **onset of symptoms and pain** are more acute. However, if any doubt exists in a younger man, surgical exploration as an emergency is mandatory.

### Chronic infection of the testis and epididymis

Chronic infection of the testes is rare in the Western world, and is due to **syphilis** or **tuberculosis**. A primary source of tuberculosis should be sought, in both the genitourinary tract and the chest. Diagnosis is often based on a urine specimen or pus specimen with acid-fast bacilli. Treatment requires a prolonged course of antituberculous medication but also may require an orchidectomy.

## TORSION OF THE TESTIS

- Torsion (twisting) of the testis and spermatic cord is a **urological emergency** and requires immediate exploration once diagnosed (Figure 34.4).

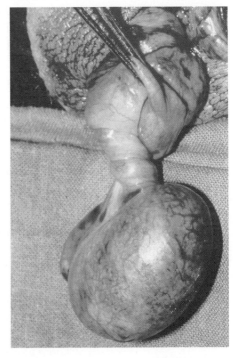

- It can occur in an undescended testis or present in infancy.
- Commonly torsion presents in early teenage years.
- The history is of an **acute painful testicle of sudden onset** which usually brings the young adult to hospital immediately.
- Torsion impedes blood flow through the spermatic vessels in the cord to produce testicular ischaemia and ultimately infarction and atrophy.

### Signs and symptoms

- The testicle is **acutely tender** and swollen, and lies **horizontally** and **higher** than normal.
- **Elevation of the testis increases the pain**, in contrast to **epididymitis** where **elevation eases the discomfort.**
- In the classical presentation no investigations are required and the patient is taken to theatre immedi-

**Figure 34.4** Torted testis (Courtesy of The Wellcome Trust)

ately. It is imperative to untwist the torsion within 4–6 hours of the onset of the pain if spermatogenic function is to return.
- If there is doubt about the diagnosis, urine **microscopy** to identify pus cells in the urine to rule out acute epididymitis may be helpful. The use of **colour flow Doppler** ultrasound imaging may confirm the presence or absence of blood flow.

### Treatment

- The patient is taken to theatre for immediate scrotal exploration if there is any doubt. If the testis is not untwisted **within 6–12 hours it will infarct.**

- At surgery the scrotum is explored and the twisted testicle untwisted. If its colour returns it is anchored to the scrotum with three non-absorbable sutures to prevent recurrence. **In addition, the testis on the opposite side is also fixed** with three non-absorbable sutures. If the testis is black and infarcted it is removed.

## TORSION OF THE APPENDIX TESTIS

A vestigial remnant, called the **appendix testis or hydatid of Morgagni,** exists at the upper pole of the testis. This can twist (torsion) and cause similar symptoms to torsion of the testis.

### Signs and symptoms

- **Acute pain** in the testis is experienced in **early teenage** patients without signs of classical torsion. A 'blue' spot of approximately $0.5 \times 0.5$ cm can often be identified through the scrotal skin at the upper pole of the testis – this is the infarcted appendix testis.
- **Treatment** – testicular exploration is performed and the appendix testis excised.

## CANCER OF THE TESTICLE

- Cancer of the testes is the commonest cancer in men under the age of 35. It is rare before puberty.

- The majority of testicular tumours arise from the **germinal cells** which line the seminiferous tubules. Rare benign tumours can arise from the Sertoli cells or the Leydig cells. The germinal cells produce more than 96% of the testicular tumours.
- The germinal epithelium cell is **totipotent** and, when it becomes malignant, can result in a **seminoma** or an **embryonal carcinoma (teratoma and choriocarcinoma).** The seminoma and teratoma are the two most common.

### Tumour markers

- Germ cell tumours produce abnormal amounts of protein which can be detected by radioimmuno assay – beta human chorionic gonadotrophin (**beta-hCG**) and alpha-fetoprotein (**AFP**).
- Beta-hCG is produced by approximately 60% of non-seminomatous germinal cell tumours and 7% of seminomas.
- AFP is elevated in patients with embryonal carcinoma and teratoma. Elevated levels are not present in patients with seminoma.
- These tumour markers are useful in the diagnosis and management of patients with testicular tumours and, if present prior to surgery, should fall to zero after orchidectomy. Persistently raised tumour markers following orchidectomy generally indicates metastatic spread.

### Metastases

- Testicular germ cell tumours almost always spread via **lymphatics first** and **haematogenously later**.

> - Lymphatic metastases follow a predictable path from **the testis to the para-aortic lymph nodes – NOT TO THE GROIN NODES**.

### Examination and investigation

- The most common presentation is **painless enlargement,** often described as a 'heaviness'.
- The testis is enlarged, heavy, hard and insensitive, with loss of anatomical detail.
- **Metastatic deposits** may be felt in the **epigastrium,** or **supraclavicular nodes**.
- Around **20%** of patients present with **metastatic disease**.
- Ultrasound scanning of the testis usually confirms the suspected diagnosis.
- CT or MRI scanning of the chest and abdomen shows metastases.
- Chest x-ray will show pulmonary metastases.
- Blood is taken for **tumour markers prior to surgery**.

> **IMPORTANT LESSON**
> Any painless testicular swelling must be considered malignant until proved otherwise.

### Surgery

- Via a groin incision the spermatic cord is divided at the internal ring and the testis removed.
- Following surgery tumour markers are again taken on day 3 and day 5.

### Pathology

- Seminomas show a white cut surface without haemorrhage or necrosis. It is clearly defined and separate from the normal testicular tissue.
- Non-seminomatous tumours contain complex elements of more than one germ cell and the cut surface reveals a cystic lesion with gelatinous or mucoid material. Various amounts of solid tissue are also identified.

> - It is important to distinguish between **seminomatous** and **non-seminomatous** tumours pathologically as the treatment and prognosis of each is different.

### Tumour staging

- Stage 1 – tumour confined to the testis
- Stage 2 – tumour in the regional lymph nodes with retroperitoneal nodal masses <10 cm
- Stage 2b – tumour in the regional lymph nodes with retroperitoneal nodal masses >10 cm
- Stage 3 – tumour beyond the diaphragm.

## Treatment and prognosis

Following orchidectomy and clinicopathological staging further treatment is instituted.

### Seminoma

- Standard therapy for a stage 1 seminoma is radiotherapy to the lymphatic drainage area as these tumours are radio-sensitive, lymphatic spread is orderly and early haematogenous spread is rare.
- Treatment for stage 2b and stage 3 seminomas is chemotherapy.
- Patients with stage 1 tumours have a 95% normal life expectancy.

### Non-seminomatous germ cell tumours

These tumours are classically understaged in 15–20% of cases.

- Stage 1 are treated with combination chemotherapy. In the USA prophylactic retroperitoneal lymph node dissection is performed for stage 1 disease instead of chemotherapy.
- Stage 2 and 3 disease requires chemotherapy and may require surgery to remove bulky residual disease in the retroperitoneum following the chemotherapy.
- The **prognosis** for patients with non-seminomatous germ cell tumours is poorer than that for seminoma but with early stage disease should be approximately 75%. However, the prognosis for stage 2b and above is much poorer.

## DISORDERS OF THE TUNICA AND CORD

During its descent from the abdominal cavity, the testis pushes forward a pocket or diverticulum of peritoneum which it pulls down into the scrotum. This peritoneal process or **processus vaginalis** normally seals off at birth to form the investing **tunica vaginalis** around the testis.

Appreciation of this embryology gives a better understanding of hydroceles and hernias. For example, the indirect inguinal hernia sac in a neonate is, in effect, a processus vaginalis which has failed to seal off and is sufficiently widely patent to admit bowel. If the processus remains patent but very narrow, only peritoneal fluid can pass through and a communicating or congenital hydrocele exists.

## HYDROCELE

A hydrocele is a collection of fluid within the tunica vaginalis (Figure 34.5). A hydrocele may be primary or secondary.

### Primary hydrocele

This is associated with a normal underlying testis and can be:

- Congenital
- Infantile
- Idiopathic vaginal
- Encysted hydrocele of the cord.

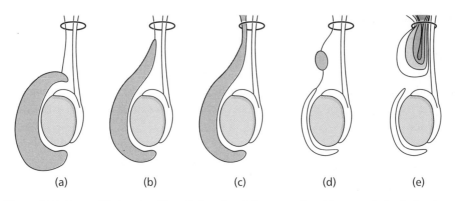

**Figure 34.5** Types of hydrocele with an indirect hernia for comparison. The upper limit of a hernia cannot be defined. (a) Vaginal, (b) infantile; (c) congenital (communicating); (d) encysted hydrocele of cord; (e) indirect hernia

Congenital, infantile and encysted hydroceles are the product of the processus vaginalis which has either failed to occlude completely, has occluded high in the inguinal canal, or has occluded in part to leave a cyst in the cord – **they are all common in infancy.**

Congenital (communicating) hydroceles vary in size during the day as peritoneal fluid drains in and out of the tunica through the **patent processus vaginalis.**

In the idiopathic vaginal type the tunica vaginalis is distended with a straw coloured fluid – they are common in **elderly** men.

### Secondary hydrocele

This is due to underlying disease of the testis – either **inflammation** of the **testis or epididymis** or a **testicular tumour.**

### Signs and symptoms

* Hydroceles present with a smooth, globular swelling in the scrotum which slowly enlarges without pain (Figure 34.6a).

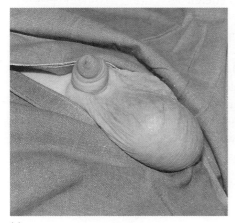

(a)

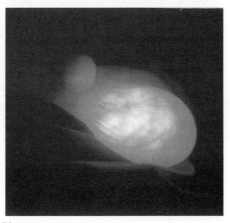

(b)

**Figure 34.6** (a) Infantile right hydrocele with (b) transillumination

- On examination it is possible to get above the swelling and feel the contents of the cord.
- A hydrocele usually **transilluminates** well (Figure 34.6b).
- It is usually not possible to palpate the testis as it is surrounded by fluid.
- **Underlying testicular pathology must be excluded** – ultrasound scanning will rule out any abnormality of the testis and diagnose the hydrocele with confidence.

> **IMPORTANT LESSON**
> Large hydroceles and hernias are common in clinical examinations. You can 'get above' a hydrocele and it transilluminates.

### Treatment

Treatment is usually sought by adult men when the hydrocele is large enough to cause discomfort or embarrassment. Most hydroceles in neonates resolve spontaneously but, if still present after 1 year, need treatment.

- In infantile (communicating) hydroceles the patent processus vaginalis is ligated.
- An encysted hydrocele of the cord is easily excised.
- Aspiration of a hydrocele is a temporary measure as the fluid will re-accumulate.
- Vaginal idiopathic hydroceles require excision of the tunica vaginalis surrounding the testis to prevent re-accumulation of fluid.

## EPIDIDYMAL CYSTS

- Small cysts can develop between the epididymis and the testis (Figure 34.7). These are diverticula of the collecting tubules of the vasa efferentia testis.
- Unlike hydroceles, the testis can be palpated separately from the cyst.
- Unlike hydroceles, they are multiloculated and rarely require surgical treatment unless they become large and are causing problems for the patient.
- They do transilluminate but not as well as a hydrocele and once again diagnosis is usually confirmed by ultrasound.

## VARICOCELE

- Varices of the pampiniform plexus of veins surrounding the testis are **common**.

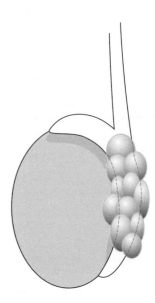

**Figure 34.7** Epididymal cysts

- They are more common on the **left side,** due to the anatomical drainage of the left testicular veins into the left renal vein. They are thought to be due to retrograde flow via the renal vein or increased blood flow via the adrenal vein to the testicular vein.
- Left varicocele is said to be rarely associated with left hypernephroma – tumour invading the left renal vein supposedly obstructs the testicular venous return.

### Signs and symptoms

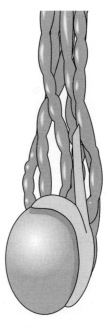

- Varicoceles are generally **not noticed** in the majority of patients until they become large and cause a dragging sensation in the groin (Figure 34.8).
- More commonly they present at the time of investigations for **male infertility** as it is proposed that the presence of the increased blood circulation around the testis increases its temperature and therefore affects spermatogenesis.
- In teenage males large varicoceles can result in a smaller testis on that side.

### Treatment

- **Conservative** management is recommended in most cases.
- In young men who have been noted to have a small testis and who are symptomatic, surgical **ligation** is recommended.
- Whether a **varicocelectomy** should be performed for infertility is still unclear although the majority of patients will request surgery to try to improve their sperm count. Surgery can be undertaken by **ligating the two to three testicular veins** in the inguinal canal or, alternatively, via a retroperitoneal approach to ligate the single testicular vein at the level of the internal inguinal ring.

**Figure 34.8** Varicocele

- **Laparoscopic clipping** of these vessels can be performed intra-abdominally, which allows excellent exposure to draining vessels with good results.

## TRAUMA TO THE TESTIS

- Occurs usually in association with contact sports.
- The history of trauma is usually followed by a period of swelling and pain in the scrotum.
- The entire scrotum can become large, distended and bruised.
- The treatment depends on the extent of the injury.
- Testicular ultrasound will confirm the presence or absence of a tear in the tunica albuginea.
- If there is significant testicular disruption, exploration with removal of the blood and devitalized tissue and closure of the tunica is required.
- Conservative management can be undertaken if only a small tunica tear is identified with no extrusion of tissue seen on ultrasound.

## VASECTOMY

- Scrotal vasectomy under local or general anaesthetic is one of the commonest forms of male contraception.
- The vas is identified, delivered through the scrotal skin, a segment removed and the ends ligated. The vas should be separated into two facial planes to prevent spontaneous recanalization.

### Complications

- Immediate – haematoma and swelling with or without infection.
- Late – epididymal discomfort and pain and often a palpable sperm granuloma.
- Testicular discomfort following vasectomy is a common cause of scrotal pain.

## MALE INFERTILITY

- **Investigations** include identification of **normal testicular anatomy, normal hormone profile** and an **analysis of semen**. The hormone profile is checked for serum testosterone, follicular stimulating hormone (FSH) and luteinizing hormone (LH). FSH is elevated in patients with atrophy of the seminiferous tubules.
- **Examination** – size, shape and consistency of the testis, and the presence of an epididymis and whether it is enlarged (obstructed). The vas is palpated along its length in the scrotum to ensure its presence.
- **Semen analysis** (Figure 34.9) is performed on a fresh specimen, looking at **sperm density**, which should be greater than 20 million/ml. **Sperm motility** should be greater than 60% and sperm morphology should have greater than 60% of normal forms. Semen analysis will reveal **oligospermia (reduced sperm count)** or **azoospermia (absent sperm)**.

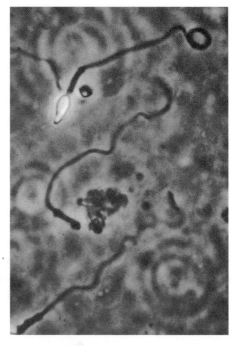

**Figure 34.9** Sperm analysis (Courtesy of The Wellcome Trust)

### Treatment

Provided the testicular anatomy is normal and the hormone profile is normal, patients with oligospermia or azoospermia have a defect in the delivery system either between the testis and the epididymis, in the epididymis itself or a problem along the vas deferens. Testicular exploration, biopsy and vasograms will aid diagnosis.

New treatments where sperm can be aspirated from either the testis or the epididymis itself and the sperm then injected into a single egg retrieved from the female (**intracytoplasmic sperm injection – ICSI**) has transformed the treatment and management of male factor infertility. The pregnancy rate is approximately 20% following implantation of the fertilized embryo.

## THE PENIS

### The foreskin
The foreskin is attached by adhesions to the glans penis up to approximately 3 years of age but thereafter is usually retractible.

### PHIMOSIS

Phimosis can occur both in early infancy or in adult life and results in a tight foreskin which cannot be retracted. Ballooning of the foreskin or inflammation of the glans with irritation of the foreskin (balanitis) can occur.

### Treatment
- Circumcision is only required for **recurrent balanitis, severe ballooning of the foreskin** and **narrowing of the preputial skin**. Adult circumcision is required for patients who cannot retract the foreskin and for discomfort during intercourse.
- A rare form of balanitis in adults is known as **balanitis xerotica obliterans (BXO)**. The foreskin becomes partly ischaemic and sclerotic, white and shrunken with a resultant pinhole meatal orifice. Circumcision is often required to allow normal voiding.

### PARAPHIMOSIS

This occurs when the retracted foreskin gets trapped at the base of the glans penis and cannot be reduced back over the glans. It is a very painful condition resulting in severe oedema of the penis with necrosis of penile skin and infection.
- It is a **common complication of catheterization** following which the **foreskin is not replaced** in its normal position.
- Treatment of paraphimosis is to replace the foreskin in its normal position by compressing the glans penis and pulling the foreskin over it.
- If the paraphimosis has been present for many days a small incision may be required over the tight ring of tissue (**dorsal slit**) to allow reduction. Once it has been reduced, a circumcision may be required at a later date.

### CARCINOMA OF THE PENIS

Penile carcinoma occurs on the glans or foreskin and spreads locally initially. It is almost **never seen in circumcised men**. It disseminates to the **inguinal lymph glands** and later to those in the pelvis. When the tumour extends to the corpora cavernosum, haematogenous spread occurs.
- Stage 1 – tumours are confined to the foreskin or glans penis.
- Stage 2 – the cancer invades the shaft to the penis.

- Stage 3 – the tumour has invaded around the glans and to the scrotum.
- Stage 4 – the inguinal lymph nodes are involved.

All these tumours are **squamous cell carcinomas** and a diagnosis is made initially by excision biopsy. Circumcision may be required to achieve full visualization of the lesion.

### Treatment
- Stage 1 penile cancers are usually **excised locally** or can be treated with **radiotherapy**.
- Failure of radiotherapy or lack of local control requires **partial or complete penile amputation** with or without an *en bloc* **dissection of the inguinal lymph glands**.

## PENILE WARTS

Penile warts (Figure 34.10) and condylomata acuminata can occur in the urethra but are generally seen around the meatus, on the glans or extending on to the shaft of the penis. They are caused by papilloma virus and are **sexually transmitted**. The lesions can be treated with topical **fluorouracil** to the penile and glandular regions but those in the meatus and distal urethra require excision and diathermy.

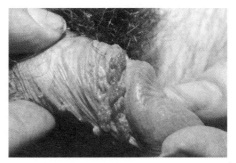

**Figure 34.10** Penile warts

## PEYRONIE'S DISEASE

A plaque-like lesion occurring on one side of the corpora cavernosum can occur in middle-aged men. The presenting complaint is one of **penile pain with erections and curvature of the penis**. Penile deformity may prevent adequate penetration for intercourse. There is no pain or deviation of the penis in its flaccid state.

### Signs and symptoms
On examining the penis, a palpable dense plaque of tissue can be felt along a portion of the shaft. The condition is sometimes associated with Dupuytren's contracture.

### Treatment
Symptomatic treatment of pain and vitamin E may be beneficial in the initial stages of this disease. Surgical correction of the deformity should be avoided until the pain subsides (usually approximately after 1 year). Surgical correction to straighten the penis requires plication or excision of a wedge of tunica from the corpora on the opposite side, which corrects the bend.

## ERECTILE DYSFUNCTION

- Penile erection requires an intact neurovascular supply.

- The nerve supply from the autonomic erection centre consists of both parasympathetic and sympathetic branches via the pelvic plexus which is located between the prostate and the rectum in the perineum.
- The cavernous nerves travel along the posterolateral aspect of the seminal vesicles and prostate and then to the hilum of the penis at the level of the distal urethral bulb. Terminal branches of the cavernous nerves innervate the helicine arteries and the trabecular smooth muscle and are responsible for the vascular events during tumescence and detumescence.
- The vascular supply for erectile function comes from the internal pudendal artery which branches into the urethral, dorsal and cavernosal arteries. The cavernosal artery supplies the corpus cavernosum and the dorsal artery of the glans penis.

### Mechanism of erection

- Increased arterial inflow fills the the corpora cavernosa. As the corpora cavernosa expand with blood they compress the venous drainage channels with resultant turgidity and erection.
- The increased arterial flow into the corpora appears to be initiated by smooth muscle relaxation. It is thought that this process is aided by nitric oxide at a local level.

Erectile dysfunction is classified as:

1 Psychogenic (majority)
2 Neurogenic
3 Hormonal
4 Arterial.

- Direct injury to the cavernous or pudendal nerves from **trauma, radical prostatectomy or rectal surgery** can interrupt neural pathways and result in impotence.
- **Diabetes mellitus** (i.e. diabetic autonomic neuropathy) is the most common hormonal disease associated with erectile failure, and disorders of **thyroid function** or the pituitary will also affect erectile dysfunction.
- Adequate arterial pressure is essential (**Leriche syndrome**).
- **Drugs** causing impotence are **antihypertensives, antidepressants, oestrogen, cimetidine or cyproterone acetate.**
- **Systemic diseases** that contribute to impotence are **diabetes, renal impairment,** particularly patients on dialysis, and patients recovering from myocardial infarction.
- Investigation requires a detailed medical history and physical examination with associated hormonal profile investigations of FSH, LH, testosterone and prolactin.

### Management

- Intracavernosal injection of prostaglandin E2 causes local vasodilatation and tumescence lasting approximately 20 minutes and is now the most popular form of treatment for erectile failure.
- Vacuum erection devices are also used.
- As a last resort, the insertion of a penile prosthesis in each corpus creates an artificial erect penis.

# THE SCROTUM

The main scrotal pathologies consist of sebaceous cysts and infection.

- Sebaceous cysts of the scrotum are treated in the same way as sebaceous cysts on the rest of the body. They may be multiple and require numerous surgical procedures but are not associated with any intrascrotal pathology.
- Inflammatory conditions of the scrotum consist of **contact dermatitis, atopic dermatitis, psoriasis** and, more rarely, **infestations** with **pediculosis pubis** (pubic lice) or **scabies**.
- Fungal infections with *Candida* are often common in this area.
- Bacterial infections are usually staphylococcal in nature and many inflammatory dermatoses may be secondarily infected by *Staphylococcus aureus*.

## FOURNIER'S GANGRENE

- An **idiopathic synergistic gangrene** of the scrotum and penile skin. It may follow minor trauma and is more common in **diabetic** patients.
- Aerobic and anaerobic organisms cause gangrene and sloughing of the scrotal and surrounding skin. This condition can be fatal.
- Rapid debridement of the entire area back to fresh tissue is mandatory, and combination triple antibiotic therapy with penicillin, gentamicin and metronidazole. Plastic surgical repair of the resulting defect is often necessary.

---

**CRIB BOX – MALE GENITALIA**

**Lymphatic drainage**
- Of the **testis** is to **para-aortic nodes** – NOT THE GROIN
- Of the penis and scrotum is to the groin

**Undescended testicle**
- True maldescent – testis may be abnormal
- Ectopic – testis usually normal
- Retractile – normal and needs no treatment

**Torsion** of the testis is an emergency which needs surgery – differentiate from infection

**Testicular cancer**
- Most common cancer in men <35 years
- Seminoma
- Non-seminomatous (embryonal – teratoma and choriocarcinoma)
- Tumour markers – AFP and $\beta$-hCG

Understand the patent processus vaginalis and its relation to hernias and hydroceles

Understand the difference between phimosis and paraphimosis

**Carcinoma of the penis is squamous** – almost exclusive to **uncircumcised** men

**Erectile dysfunction** – psychogenic; neurogenic; hormonal; arterial

# chapter 35

# TRANSPLANTATION

Transplantation of a healthy organ to replace a diseased or failing one has been a long-standing aim in surgery. The technique of vascular anastomosis is fundamental to organ transplantation and was first described by Alexis Carrel in 1902.

**Rejection** of the engrafted organ by the host was for many years a hurdle to progress. In 1954 the first successful kidney transplant was performed between identical twins and this paved the way forward for cadaveric transplantation.

The development of powerful **immunosuppressive drugs**, originally steroids, then azathioprine and cyclosporin, has transformed organ transplantation.

- Treatment using organ transplantation depends on the availability of donors.
- Currently there is a world wide shortage of donors.
- Medical staff should recognize potential donors and manage them appropriately.

**Table 35.1** Types of transplantation

| Solid organ | Tissue | Cell |
| --- | --- | --- |
| Kidney | Bone | Bone marrow |
| Heart | Skin | Hepatocytes |
| Lung(s) | Cornea | Islet cells |
| Liver | Heart valve | Endothelial cell |
| Pancreas | | Neural transplantation |
| Small bowel | | Myoblast |

## ORGAN DONATION

There are three types of organ donation:

1 Living donation
2 Non-heart-beating cadaveric donation
3 Heart-beating cadaveric donation.

- **Living donation** from a relative or spouse is important in countries that do not have brain stem death legislation and therefore lack cadaveric transplant programmes. Living donation is a relatively common source of bone marrow and kidneys.

- **Non-heart-beating donation** is not new – before the introduction of brain stem death legislation it was the only available method of cadaveric organ collection.
- **Heart-beating donation** resulted in a loss of interest in the former source, but this has changed and kidney retrieval from non-heart-beating donors is becoming more common.

> The majority of organs come from cadaveric heart-beating donors previously diagnosed as brain stem dead. The concept of brain stem death is essential to the process of cadaveric heart-beating organ donation.

Shortage of donors (due primarily to increased road safety) has led to attempts to increase the pool of donor organs in several different ways:

- Public and medical staff awareness initiatives
- Donor card schemes
- National and international organ exchange networks, e.g. UK Transplant Support Service.

**Potential donors** include any patient deeply unconscious on a ventilator as a result of severe irreversible brain injury of known aetiology:

- Spontaneous intracranial haemorrhage
- Cerebral trauma
- Cerebral anoxia from diverse causes.

Following identification of a potential organ donor, a clinical assessment of the patient is performed to confirm the presence of **brain death**.

### Brain death

> **Two sets of brain stem function tests** are performed by **two independent physicians**. The criteria for the diagnosis of brain stem death in a deeply comatose person maintained on a ventilator are:
> - Fixed and dilated pupils not responding to light
> - Absent corneal reflexes
> - No motor response to painful stimuli
> - No reflex activity except at spinal cord level
> - No oculocephalic reflex (doll's eyes)
> - Absent vestibulo-ocular reflexes (tested by flushing ice cold water into the ear and observing eye movement)
> - No gag or cough reflex in response to bronchial stimulation
> - No respiratory movement if mechanical ventilation is stopped for long enough to ensure the arterial $P\text{co}_2$ rises above the threshold for stimulation of ventilation.

Brain stem tests must not be performed if there is a history of ingestion of alcohol or neurodepressant drugs such as barbiturates, or if metabolic abnormalities such as hypernatraemia are present.

Permanent functional death of the brain stem equates to brain death. Following diagnosis, further artificial support is of no benefit and should be withdrawn unless organ donation is contemplated.

Doctors involved with diagnosing brain stem death should not be involved in organ retrieval or the subsequent transplantation of any organ from that donor.

## DONOR MEDICAL MANAGEMENT

Correct management of the potential donor is important to maintain and improve his/her overall condition.

Medical management includes:
- Early treatment of haemodynamic instability
- Treatment of diabetes insipidus
- Maintaining a good blood pressure
- Avoiding complications related to brain death
- Continued supportive care.

Supportive care includes:
- Frequent turning of the patient to prevent pressure sores
- Lubrication and protective closure of the eyes
- Suctioning of airways and physiotherapy to prevent atelectasis and pneumonia
- Nasogastric aspiration and free drainage to prevent aspiration of gastric contents
- Central venous pressure monitoring to maintain optimum hydration
- Urinary catheter to monitor hourly urine output
- Warming blankets to maintain a temperature above 35°C and optimize cardiac, renal and hepatic function.

Exclusion criteria for organ donation are:
- Severe untreated systemic sepsis
- AIDS
- Active viral hepatitis B or C
- Viral encephalitis
- Malignancy excluding primary brain tumours
- Creutzfeldt–Jakob disease and recipients of human pituitary growth hormone.

Relative contraindications to organ donation are:
- Prolonged cardiac or respiratory arrest
- Diabetes mellitus
- Severe alcohol abuse
- Chronic disease affecting the organ to be donated.

Investigations to assess potential donors include:
- ABO and rhesus blood grouping

- Haemoglobin, platelet and white blood count
- U&Es
- LFTs
- Arterial blood gases
- Blood for subsequent tissue typing
- Chest x-ray
- Electrocardiogram
- Blood and sputum cultures
- Viral studies – HIV; hepatitis B surface antigen (if available core antibody also); hepatitis C antibody; cytomegalovirus; Epstein–Barr virus (consider in young children).

## MULTI-ORGAN RETRIEVAL

The donor retrieval team take the donor to theatre with full anaesthetic support. The chest and abdomen are opened through a midline incision. Following inspection of the organs, cannulas are placed in the aorta for perfusion of the abdominal organs, and into the portal vein for perfusion of the liver. The chest team prepares the heart and lungs for perfusion and ventilation of the donor is stopped. The various organs are then perfused with a cold preservative solution. The heart and lungs are removed first, followed by the liver, pancreas and kidneys. Part of the spleen and some lymph nodes are also removed for **tissue typing**. The individual organs are then stored in preservation fluid within sterile containers at 4°C and transported on ice.

The length of time that organs can be preserved (the cold ischaemic time) varies significantly:

- The heart and lungs must be transplanted within 6–8 hours
- Liver and pancreas within 20 hours
- The kidneys within 30 hours.

Delay in implantation will result in **graft dysfunction or non-function** and will jeopardize the recipient's chances of survival.

## INDICATIONS FOR TRANSPLANTATION

Organ transplantation is indicated in the presence of end stage failure, either acute or chronic, that no longer responds to medical treatment and is unsuitable for other forms of surgical management. Exceptions to this are patients with systemic infection, AIDS, malignancy, other life-threatening disease and those who are unable to comply with post-transplant treatment.

## COMMON INDICATIONS FOR TRANSPLANTATION

### Cardiac
- Cardiomyopathies
- Ischaemic heart disease

### Renal
- Glomerulonephritis
- Diabetic nephropathy
- Reflux and analgesic nephropathy

### Liver
- Chronic liver failure – primary biliary cirrhosis; primary sclerosing cholangitis; hepatitis B, C; autoimmune hepatitis
- Acute liver failure – drug-induced (paracetamol toxicity); unknown
- Inborn errors of metabolism
- Unresectable hepatic malignancies, e.g. neuroendocrine tumours
- Miscellaneous, e.g. Budd–Chiari, polycystic disease

## ORGAN RECIPIENT

The immunology of organ transplantation is complex. Potential recipients are:
- Blood group compatible
- Tissue type matched (human leucocyte antigen – HLA) to a varying degree
- Lymphocyte cross-match negative (donor lymphocytes not lysed in recipient serum).

In practice 'histocompatibility' is not as crucial to organ survival or rejection as might be assumed, as long as donor and recipient are of the same ABO blood type. Heart and liver transplants appear to be less immunogenic than kidney. Furthermore, immune tolerance of the recipient to the donated organ is modified by immunosuppression.

## POST-TRANSPLANT COMPLICATIONS

As in all forms of surgery, complications can be:

1 Local and general
2 Early, intermediate and late.

Specific surgical complications relate to the wound and anastomoses:
- Post-operative haemorrhage
- Wound infections/haematoma/seromas
- Vascular complications – anastomotic haemorrhage; thrombosis; stenosis; pseudo-aneurysm formation
- Biliary, ureteric, bronchial anastomotic leaks or strictures due to ischaemia
- Lymphoceles.

Any complication, but particularly those related to anastomoses, is likely to compromise graft function. **Rejection and infection**, however, remain the major factors to be controlled in order to achieve good long-term results.

## REJECTION

**Acute rejection** occurs most commonly in the first month after organ transplantation. Late episodes are usually associated with inadequate levels of immunosuppression.

**Chronic rejection** occurs insidiously after many months and its pathophysiology is not fully understood. It is characterized by a steady decline in graft function and must be differentiated by biopsy and/or radiological imaging from other causes of dysfunction such as ischaemia due to anastomotic stricture formation.

Even with perfect tissue typing, rejection can still occur so the alternative approach is to suppress the immune system.

## IMMUNOSUPPRESSION

Reduction of the immune response aims to prevent and treat rejection and prolong graft survival. Unfortunately, immunosuppression therapy at present is non-specific and thus **renders the patient more susceptible to infection and malignancy**.

- **Infection** with common bacteria may be severe. Immunosuppressed patients are also vulnerable to uncommon pathogens, some of which may be transmitted with the donor organ (e.g. viruses) (see Table 35.2).
- **Malignancy** of all types is increased, but particularly those thought to be associated with viruses:
  - Lymphoma
  - Squamous cell skin cancer
  - Cervical cancer
  - Kaposi's sarcoma.

**Table 35.2** Pathogens that can cause infection after organ transplantation

| Bacterial | Viral | Fungal and parasitic |
| --- | --- | --- |
| Tuberculosis | Cytomegalovirus | Candida |
| Legionella | Epstein–Barr | Aspergillus |
| Nocardia | Herpes simplex | Pneumocystis |
| Listeria | Herpes zoster | Toxoplasma |

## IMMUNOSUPPRESSIVE DRUGS

- **Cyclosporin** interferes with cytokine production and blocks activation as well as proliferation of lymphocytes. Side-effects of cyclosporin include:
  - Renal impairment (partially reversible)
  - Hypertension
  - Neurotoxicity (tremor, headaches, confusion, convulsions)
  - Gingival hyperplasia
  - Hirsutism
  - Gastrointestinal toxicity (nausea and vomiting)
  - Lymphoproliferative disorders.
- **Tacrolimus** is a newer immunosuppressant that acts in a way similar to cyclosporin, but is 100 times more potent. Its side-effects are similar, although it does not produce hirsutism and is rarely a cause of gingival hyperplasia. However, it can produce hyperglycaemia, causing diabetes mellitus.
- **Steroids** such as prednisolone have cushingoid side-effects.
- **Azathioprine** inhibits nucleic acid synthesis and causes bone marrow suppression.
- **Anti-lymphocyte antibodies** are capable of producing profound immunosuppression, which in turn causes an increased number of infective complications.

**Immunosuppressive regimens** use various **combinations** (often triple therapy) of drugs as treatment for rejection and as prophylaxis.

## THE FUTURE

The surgical techniques of transplantation are well established and improving. Further advances rely on improved donor organ preservation, and increased knowledge and modification of the immune system.

---

**CRIB BOX – TRANSPLANTATION**

Transplantation of **kidney, liver and heart** – well established

Good prospects – **small bowel and pancreas**

Donor shortage – can use non-heart-beating donors for kidneys

Commonest **indication** – acute or chronic end stage failure

Post-transplant **complications** – surgical, rejection and infection

**Immunosuppresssion** is presently non-specific and causes **infection and malignancy**

# INDEX

Note: page numbers in *italics* refer to figures and tables

nose 216–17
nutrition 32–5
  burns 88
  *see also* diet
nutritional assessment 33

obesity prevention 108
occupational health 108
occupations associated with cancer *94*, 438
octreotide 391
oculomotor nerve pressure 119
odontogenic keratocysts 215
oesophageal atresia 293, 302, 337
oesophageal diverticula 345–6
oesophageal sphincter 338, 339–40
oesophageal tumours *93*, 323, 342–4, 346
oesophagitis 66, 339–40, 341, 342, 346
oesophagus 337, 338
  achalasia 338–9
  barium swallow 338, 343
  bird's beak 338, *339*
  bleeding 346
  dysphagia 337–8
  epithelium 337, 346
  motility 339
  mucosa 337, 340
  perforation 344–5, 346
  strictures 341
oestrogen, gynaecomastia 230, 231
oligodendroglioma 116
oligospermia 464
oncogenes 91
onychogryphosis 177
operating staff HIV precautions 69
operation 6–7
opioids 38, *39*, 40, 41, 42
orchidopexy 456
orchiectomy 449
orchitis 456
organ donation 469–71
  assessment of potential 471–2
  brain stem function tests 470–1
  cold ischaemic time 472
  heart-beating 470
  living 469–70
  non-heart-beating 470
  recipient 473
organ donor 471–2, 475
oropharynx infection 58
orthopaedic surgery, infection 56
osteitis fibrosa cystica 204
osteomyelitis, acute/chronic 215
ostium secundum defect 267
ovarian ablation, breast cancer 237, *239*
ovarian cyst 324, 326
oxygen 15, 73

paediatric fluid regimens 30, *31*

paediatric pain 38, 42
paediatric surgery 293, 305
  abdominal pain 303–4
  appendicitis 334
  congenital diaphragmatic hernia 303
  congenital hypertrophic pyloric stenosis 294–5
  congenital intestinal atresia 301
  hernias 293–4
  Hirschsprung's disease 299–300
  imperforate anus 301–2
  intestinal obstruction 298–302
  intussusception 295–7
  Meckel's diverticulum 297–8
  meconium ileus 300–1
  mesenteric adenitis 304
  oesophageal atresia 302
Paget's disease of nipple 231, 233
pain
  abdominal 303–4, 305, 314–15, 326–7
  anorectal disease 405
  assessment 39, 44
  chronic 45
  colonic 393
  continuation 37
  definition 36–7
  gynaecological causes 325–6
  intestinal obstruction 319
  ladder 44, 45
  leg 131
  measurement 37–8
  neurophysiological basis 37
  paediatric 32, 48
  pathways 45
  penile 466
  perception 36–7
  peritonitis 323
  rest 129, 130
  scales 38
  shoulder tip 315, 324, 363, 379
  treatment 38–9
  urinary tract 420
pain management 36, 45
  acute 39–43
  Acute Pain Service 39
  cancer 44–5
  ladder 38–9
  non-malignant chronic 43
painful short procedures 43
palatal repair 221
palliation, surgical for cancer 102
palliative care 44
Palliative Medicine Service 44
pampiniform plexus 454
  varicocele 462–3
pancreas 206, 208, 374–9
  carcinoma 377–8, 381

pancreas – *contd*
  ectopic tissue 297
  trauma 379
pancreatic cysts 378–9
pancreatic enzymes 301, 374
pancreatic pseudo-cyst 376, 378, 379
pancreatic tumour 99
pancreatico-duodenectomy 378
pancreatitis 66, 381
  acute 87, 374–6
  chronic relapsing 376–7
panproctocolectomy with permanent
    ileostomy 399–400
papillary muscle dysfunction/rupture 261
para-aortic lymph nodes 459, 468
para-scapular pulsation 270
paraganglioma 255
paralytic ileus 319, 332, 386
paraneoplastic syndromes 100–1
paraphimosis 465
parathyroid glands 203–5
parathyroid hormone 203, 204
parathyroid mass, mediastinal 255–6
parathyroid related protein 101
parenteral nutrition 34–5
  short gut syndrome 389
  small bowel resection 325
Parkland formula 84
paronychia 176–7
parotid gland 212
  tumours 95, 212
parotidectomy, superficial 212
parotitis 212
patella tendon weight bearing prosthesis
    138
patent ductus arteriosus 268–9
pathogenicity of bacteria 48
patient
  ASA classification of condition 7
  identification 17
  mix in wards 50
patient-controlled analgesia 40
pediculosis pubis infestation 468
pelvic abscess 332
pelvic floor exercises 444
pelvis 77
  collateral circulation 131
pelviureteric junction surgery 429–30
Pendred's syndrome 190
penetrating injury 75, 76
penicillin 54
penile warts 466
penis 453–4, 465–7, 468
peptic ulcer 66, 349–57, 360
  acid status 349
  *H. pylori* 348
  haemorrhage 355–6
  malignancy 351

Meckel's diverticulum 297, 298
  operations 351–2, *353*
  perforation 353–5
  pyloric stenosis 356
percutaneous nephrolithotomy (PCNL)
    427
percutaneous transhepatic
    cholangiography (PTC) 365
percutaneous transluminal coronary
    angioplasty (PTCA) 258
perforation, peptic ulcer 353–5
perianal abscess 409, 418
perianal haematoma 408
perianal sepsis 68
perianal tags 408
perianal warts 411–12
pericardectomy 266
pericardial disease 266–7
pericardial tamponade 14
pericardiocentesis 267
pericarditis 266–7
pericardium 273
perineal trauma 78
perinephric abscess 424
peripheral nerve injuries 125
peripheral neuropathy 145, 157–8
peripheral vascular disease 43
peristalsis, absence 338
peritoneal defences 323
peritoneal lavage 376
peritoneum, metastases 100
peritonitis 316, 322–4
  appendicitis 329
  bowel paralysis 323
  infarction 325
  peptic ulcer perforation 353
  small bowel obstruction 384
  strangulated hernia 308
  ureter injury 435
peritonsillar abscess 218
Peutz–Jeghers syndrome 385
Peyer's patches, hyperplasia 295, 296
Peyronie's disease 466
phaeochromocytoma 202–3
pharmacopoeia, limited 39
pharyngeal pouch 211, 345–6
pharyngoplasty 221
phenol lumbar sympathectomy 138
phimosis 465
phleboliths 159, 426
phosphate calculi 426
pilar cyst 178, 179
pilonidal sinus 416–17
pith balls 386
pituitary tumours 117, 206, 208
platelet count, shock 15
pleura 241–6
  empyema thoracis 245–6